Pharmaceutical Reform

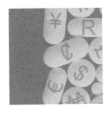

Pharmaceutical Reform is available as an interactive textbook at **http://www .worldbank.org/pdt.** The electronic version allows communities of practice and colleagues working in sectors and regions, as well as students and teachers, to share notes and related materials for an enhanced, multimedia learning and knowledge-exchange experience.

Pharmaceutical Reform

A Guide to Improving Performance and Equity

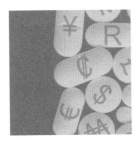

Marc J. Roberts and Michael R. Reich

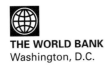

THE WORLD BANK
Washington, D.C.

ISBN 978-0-8213-8760-3
eISBN 978-0-8213-8771-9
DOI 10.1596/978-0-8213-8760-3

Library of Congress Cataloging-in-Publication Data
Roberts, Marc J.
  Pharmaceutical reform : a guide to improving performance and equity / by Marc J.
    Roberts and Michael R. Reich.
      p. ; cm.
  Includes bibliographical references and index.
    ISBN 978-0-8213-8760-3 — ISBN 978-0-8213-8771-9 (eISBN)
  1. Pharmaceutical policy. 2. Pharmaceutical industry. 3. Health care reform.
    I. Reich, Michael, 1950- II. World Bank. III. Title.
  [DNLM: 1. Drug Industry—organization & administration. 2. Health Care Reform—
    organization & administration. 3. Pharmaceutical Preparations. QV 736]
    RA401.A1R63 2011
  615.1—dc22
    2011012020

CONTENTS

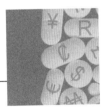

Figures

Tables

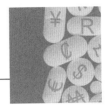

FOREWORD

Ensuring reliable access to, and appropriate use of, safe, effective, and affordable medicines is one of the core functions of an effective health system. Medicines are important beyond their therapeutic utility: they are often seen by the public as the most tangible representation of health care, and their availability is taken (sometimes problematically) as an indicator of the quality and accessibility of services.

Yet despite the integral role of medicines in health system performance, the availability and appropriate use of essential medicines in developing countries continues to be a challenge. Each year, more than 10 million children in the developing world die of conditions that could be prevented or cured with existing vaccines or medicines. Similarly, an estimated 1,000 women die every day from complications during pregnancy or childbirth, many of whom could be saved with access to appropriate care—including medicines. Poor-performing pharmaceutical systems and policies that fail to ensure the equitable distribution and timely provision of essential medicines to populations that need them cost lives every day.

The critical importance of medicines to health care outcomes, combined with the challenges of information asymmetries in the pharmaceutical sector, make policy reform imperative. This requires a clear understanding of the functions, norms, and policies that shape pharmaceutical demand and provision. However, it is also necessary to understand the institutional, cultural, political, and economic contexts within which pharmaceutical and health systems operate. Indeed, the pharmaceutical sector is a microcosm of the challenges that health sectors face overall—financing, defining appropriate services, training and deploying human resources, generating and using information, demand management, and effective governance. There is more to medicines than just their therapeutic or prophylactic qualities and logistics.

This publication, which is based on the unique methodology and tools developed for the World Bank Institute/Harvard School of Public Health Flagship Course on Health System Reform and Sustainable Financing, provides a powerful set of resources to help policy makers better navigate the complicated process of reforming pharmaceutical systems. Its problem-solving approach complements technical resources and training curricula available on the discrete elements of a pharmaceutical sector.

The application of the Flagship approach to the pharmaceutical sector is both useful and timely. Ensuring the availability of medicines and the effective management of their procurement and distribution is central to the drive to achieve coverage and access to basic health care that is both universal and financially sustainable. Together, the methodology and case materials contained in this publication provide a rich resource from which policy makers in developing countries may draw to guide their efforts to meet these challenges.

Maria-Luisa Escobar
Manager, Health Systems Practice
World Bank Institute

Saul Walker
Senior Health Advisor
Department for International
Development (U.K.)

The views expressed by Mr. Walker are his own and do not necessarily reflect the policy of the U.K. Department for International Development.

PREFACE

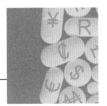

The origins of this project go back to a meeting in London, in fall 2007, between Michael R. Reich and Michael Borowitz, then at the U.K. Department for International Development (DFID). At that meeting they agreed to pursue the idea of offering a short executive course on health system reform, in London in March 2008, for DFID officials from around the world. That was the first step toward developing a larger course focused on pharmaceutical policy reform, in connection with DFID's new pharmaceutical initiative, known as the Medicines Transparency Alliance (MeTA). The plan was to draw on the analytical methods and substantive arguments in the intensive three-week Flagship Course on Health Sector Reform and Sustainable Financing, presented by the World Bank Institute, the training arm of the World Bank.

That program had been jointly developed over the previous decade by a team at the World Bank Institute and the Harvard School of Public Health (in which both of the authors of this book played a major role), along with other partners. During that period, the Flagship Course had been successfully offered numerous times and in various forms to senior health sector planners and managers around the world, as well as to participants from many international agencies. It was offered as a global course in Washington, D.C., as a regional course at various partner institutes, and as national courses in more than 40 countries (Shaw and Samaha 2009). It had also been extended and adapted to provide the basis for courses focused on more specific topics. The Flagship approach to health system reform had also been discussed in the book *Getting Health Reform Right*, written by the two of us and our two colleagues William Hsiao and Peter Berman (Roberts et al. 2004).

In spring 2008, the "mini Flagship" was offered in London, with the support of Rifat Atun of Imperial College. During that time an agreement was reached with Saul Walker of DFID, who had assumed responsibility for the MeTA initiative, to proceed with the larger course. This book originally was developed as a background note to support that course, which was offered in Jordan in January 2010, with delegations representing multiple stakeholders from all six countries that belong to MeTA.

Since then, we have continued to work on pharmaceutical policy issues, including offering a specialized two-day module using this material in the global Flagship Courses at the World Bank in 2009 and 2010. We have also supported the development of additional teaching cases and used some of this material in our courses at the Harvard School of Public Health. Recently, we also used parts of the text and some of the case studies as the basis for a one-week pharmaceutical policy course in Cape Town, South Africa, for multi-stakeholder delegations from 14 countries organized by the Southern Africa Development Council (SADC). In the midst of these developments, the leader of the Health Flagship Team at the World Bank Institute, Maria-Luisa Escobar, suggested that we turn the background note and associated teaching cases into a book for publication by the World Bank. This book is the result of her suggestion and subsequent support.

The Flagship Framework

How should a country approach the task of improving its pharmaceutical sector? After all, the sector is both extremely important and extremely complicated. Pharmaceutical expenditures as a percentage of total health spending in 2000 reached as high as 53 percent in Armenia, 44 percent in Burkina Faso, and 40 percent in the Arab Republic of Egypt. In 2006, medicines accounted for about 30 percent of total health spending in low-income countries (see table 1.2, chapter 1). Most important, access to medicines has a major impact on health status. But access to medicines is often very uneven. Financial and other access barriers are substantial for many products around the world (Frost and Reich 2008).

The performance of the pharmaceutical sector is shaped by many actors, public and private, individual, corporate, and bureaucratic. They interact in a complex set of processes, from manufacturing and importation, to purchasing and distribution, to final sales and use. Those processes are shaped by problematic government actions—from the highest levels of budget allocation and legislative policy making to the more mundane details of law enforcement and direct service provision—and by the complex and imperfect ways that markets work in the pharmaceutical sector (Reich 1994). Moreover, pharmaceutical policies respond to multiple stakeholders whose goals can conflict. The ministry of health might focus on improving population health and responding to patient expectations, the ministry of finance on minimizing financial burdens on the government and fostering economic development, and industry and professional groups on promoting their own economic interests.

This book is designed to help participants gain a better understanding of all that goes on in the pharmaceutical sector. As noted above, it uses the Flagship Framework that we helped develop over the past decade. The essence of that approach is *not* to try to tell policy makers in detail what they should do. Rather it comprises a set of analytical tools that are combined into an overall, structured methodology for developing, adopting, and implementing reform proposals. The Flagship Framework also includes a comprehensive review of reform alternatives and a systematic review of their strengths and weaknesses in various situations.

Our approach is based on the principle that any reform initiative must be developed with deep knowledge of a particular country's social, economic, political, and administrative circumstances. In general, only local reformers have that kind of knowledge, and only they can judge whether the proposals of international experts make sense in their situation. Moreover, as the book emphasizes, in the course of any reform process, important philosophical and political choices are made about priorities and purposes. And as anyone who believes in democratic government has to recognize, only the citizens of a country and their leaders can legitimately make those decisions.

Our experience with the Flagship Framework shows that it can be a helpful tool for developing reform proposals. In the courses mentioned above and in other settings, it has been used by dozens of country teams to analyze their situations and develop reform plans. It has also been successfully applied by senior leaders in several countries to develop their own health sector reform efforts (Shaw and Samaha 2009).

Throughout this book we have used the Flagship Framework to structure our analysis of pharmaceutical reform, continuously and explicitly applying its methods and concepts to the pharmaceutical sector. With a few minor exceptions, all the examples and all of the reform options come directly from pharmaceutical reform efforts around the world. We have also given specific attention to issues in pharmaceutical policy related to reproductive health. Two teaching cases are particularly relevant here: those concerning efforts to register misoprostol in Sri Lanka and preparation for the introduction of microbicides in South Africa.

The Role of the Cases

We believe that effective reform of a nation's pharmaceutical sector can be best understood—to borrow a phrase used to describe clinical medicine—as "a craft informed by science." By "craft" we mean an area of human activity that is characterized by a dedication to practical improvement in the context of imperfect knowledge. One could offer many examples of this kind of activity—from playing an instrument, to preparing a soufflé, to tackling an opponent in football, to making a campaign speech, to sailing a small boat in a high wind, to writing software for a video game. Science is relevant in all of those activities. We know a lot about acoustics, food chemistry, crowd psychology, and fluid dynamics. But the science alone does not tell us what we need to know. In such arenas it is not possible for those who want to act effectively to be guided by simple rules and precise "how-to" instructions. The underlying systems are just not sufficiently understood. They may be too poorly studied, or too varied and unpredictable, or too complex, or too reactive and interactive. In these situations, results depend not only on what is done, but on how it is done.

At the same time, the skills to deal successfully with such tasks can be systematically developed. For all of human history especially adept basket weavers, buffalo hunters, and commanders of sailing ships have passed on their skills, through apprenticeships and opportunities for supervised practice, to those they were mentoring.

In more recent times, professional schools (notably, to begin with, Harvard Business School) have developed instructional methods that adhere to those same principles. Students are given actual case examples to study and analyze. Usually these examples are descriptions of management problems that stop at a key decision point. Students have to decide, and come to class prepared to argue about, what to do next—while the teacher guides and comments on the analysis they offer. This experience is probably less fun than having the tribe's master hunter watch you as you try to stalk and kill an antelope, but it serves much the same purpose.

Both of us have used these case-based methods for many years to teach economic and political analysis and to stimulate student thinking about heath sector reform. Case discussions play a major role in the Flagship course, and they also play a major role in the pharmaceutical Flagship activities that we have organized. Indeed, the cases in this book were developed explicitly for those activities.

Unfortunately, we cannot be in the room with everyone who will read this book, and we cannot personally guide the discussion of the cases that are presented. We wish we could, for we often learn a great deal from such discussions. Instead, readers will have to provide some of that experience on their own. We urge readers, as they finish a chapter, to turn to the suggested cases. Begin with the study questions that come before each case. Then read the case, keeping those questions in mind. To get the most from the experience, make some notes to yourself as you go along and try to formulate an explicit answer to the study questions when you finish. Only then turn to the brief discussion note at the end of the case to check your thinking against the ideas that previous students have offered when they encountered the same material. We know this may seem like a laborious way to deal with the cases—and it is. But there are no shortcuts when it comes to genuine skill development.

This reminds us of an old New York City joke that is relevant here. A young woman in her twenties is walking down a midtown street, seeming a bit lost in the big city. She approaches an older man who is walking energetically down the street. She asks, "How do I get to Carnegie Hall?"—the city's premier concert hall. He stops, looks at her quizzically for a moment, and in an emphatic voice answers, "Practice!" before striding off.

References

Frost, L. J., and M. R. Reich. 2008. *Access: How Do Good Health Technologies Get to Poor People in Poor Countries?* Cambridge, MA: Harvard University Press.

Reich, M. 1994. "The Political Economy of Health Transitions in Developing Countries." In *Health and Social Change in International Perspective*, ed. L. Chen, A. Kleinman, and N. C. Ware, 413–51. Boston: Harvard School of Public Health.

Roberts, M. J., W. Hsiao, P. Berman, and M. R. Reich. 2004. *Getting Health Reform Right: A Guide to Improving Performance and Equity.* New York: Oxford University Press.

Shaw, R. P., and H. Samaha. 2009. *Building Capacity for Health System Strengthening: A Strategy that Works.* Washington, DC: World Bank Institute.

ACKNOWLEDGMENTS

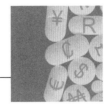

This book on pharmaceutical reform would not have been written without the initiative and support of Michael Borowitz and Saul Walker of the U.K. Department for International Development (DFID). We are especially appreciative to DFID for financial support to write the first version of this book and the associated teaching cases, which we used as a textbook for the Medicines Transparency Alliance (MeTA) course in Jordan in January 2010, and for funding to develop and offer that course on pharmaceutical reform. We are equally appreciative of our more recent financial, intellectual, and administrative support from Maria-Luisa Escobar of the World Bank Institute and her team (especially Marilou Bradley). We would like to also acknowledge the financial support of the government of the Netherlands, provided through the Bank-Netherlands Partnership Program, to publish this book. We thank Rifat Atun of Imperial College London and the Global Fund for his help in organizing the initial course, his support of the curriculum development effort, and his continuing advice. We never would have gotten to this point without the aid of all of these individuals and their belief in our work.

We deeply appreciate the willingness of our co-authors of *Getting Health Reform Right*, William Hsiao (at Harvard) and Peter Berman (recently returned to Harvard from the World Bank), who have played major roles in developing the Flagship Framework over the years, to let us draw so heavily on the product of our joint intellectual effort. We have also drawn on the work of other colleagues at Harvard, especially Tom Bossert (on decentralization) and Norman Daniels (on ethics). In addition, over the years our understanding of the Flagship Framework has benefited greatly from our collaboration with Paul Shaw and Anne Johansen at the World Bank.

We are also deeply grateful to some of the world's experts on pharmaceutical policy, including Andreas Seiter, of the World Bank, and Loraine Hawkins, an independent consultant, who have been extraordinarily helpful to our process. In addition, we appreciate the many comments on various drafts of this manuscript from Saul Walker, Veronika Wirtz, Wilbert Bannenberg, Marianne Schurmann, Anita Wagner, Corrina Moucheraud, Paul Shaw, Peter Berman, and Alex Preker.

We thank the authors and co-authors who helped write the teaching cases. Their work illuminated the details of what happened in pharmaceutical reform around the world and contributed a great deal to our thinking. Those individuals are acknowledged for each case, but we would like to thank them here, as well: Anya Levy Guyer, Tory Ervin, Nathan J. Blanchet, Eric O. Moore, Laura Rock Kopczak, Prashant Yadav, Wilbert Bannenberg, Ramya Kumar, Pamela Norick, and the authors of the original report on microbicides in South Africa. We also thank the research assistants who contributed to the initial version of the book, including Nathan Blanchet, Anya Levy Guyer, Jean Leu, Hope O'Brien, Kate Powis, and Meghan Reidy, as well as Seemoon Choi and Juhwan Oh for their comments on case study C.

We also express our appreciation to those who helped make possible the various versions of the course that played such a large role in the development of our ideas. They include Anne Mathiot and Tatiana Schofield at Imperial College London; Susan Gilbert and Anya Levy Guyer of the Harvard School of Public Health; and Wilbert Bannenberg, Elodie Brandamir, and Marieke Devillé of the MeTA Secretariat. Wilbert in particular has been our consultant, adviser, commentator, and, in Jordan, a co-teacher, in ways that have contributed much to our thinking and understanding.

We thank Susan Gilbert for preparing a first draft of the glossary and Corrina Moucheraud for helping us organize the permissions for tables and figures. When it came time to put the manuscript into production, we received much help from the team at the World Bank's Office of the Publisher, including our production editor, Mark Ingebretsen, our copy editor, Nancy Geltman, and others.

Lastly, we express our deep appreciation to the more than one hundred individuals from more than a dozen countries who participated in the mini-Flagship in London, the MeTA Pharmaceutical Flagship in Jordan, and the two pharmaceutical modules we offered at the Flagship Course in Washington, D.C. Their energy, interest, suggestions, examples, and advice have made the book more detailed and realistic than it would have been otherwise. Of course, neither they, nor any of our other partners and friends, are responsible for the views we take or for the errors that remain despite their efforts to prevent us from making them.

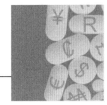

CHAPTER 1

Introduction

Why Care about Pharmaceutical Policy?

Pharmaceutical policy has a significant impact on health system performance in low- and middle-income countries. It influences the health of the population, public satisfaction (and dissatisfaction) with the health sector, and the cost-effectiveness of the care provided. Pharmaceuticals also are major area of expenditure in these systems, including out-of-pocket payments by poor people. Thus it plays a big role in determining the economic burden that the health system puts on all payers, from the ministry of finance to struggling farmers.

Public policy greatly influences how this important sector functions. In most low- and middle-income countries, the public sector provides a significant share of the overall pharmaceutical supply, which is directly subject to government decision making. Equally important, from product registration through quality monitoring to professional and facility licensing and price setting, much of the private pharmaceutical sector is heavily regulated and thus also is subject to public policy choices.

It may seem obvious enough, but it is worth noting at the start of this analysis that medicines, when properly used, can produce great health benefits. This book agrees with scholars who have argued that public health measures and improved living standards account for much of the past decrease in infectious disease mortality in upper-income countries (better housing, improved diet, better sanitation and clean drinking water, and changed relationships between infectious agents and human hosts) (McKeown and Record 1962). At the same time, however, modern medicines today can have a major impact on population health in low- and middle-income countries. Unlike the 19th century, many effective medicines are now available not only for malaria, tuberculosis (TB), and human immunodeficiency virus (HIV), but also for everyday respiratory, intestinal, and urological infections. And in low-income countries, such infections are major sources of mortality (table 1.1).

As the "epidemiological transition" advances and chronic diseases become ever more important in these countries, the role of medicines in improving health status will increase. Examples include the use of insulin for diabetes, antidepressants for mental health, statins for high cholesterol, and antihypertensives for high blood pressure. Projections for 2030 indicate that the leading causes of death in low- and middle-income countries will increasingly resemble those in high-income countries (Mathers and Loncar 2006). Add in the tropical diseases (such as schistosomiasis, filariasis, and soil-transmitted helminths) that are major sources of morbidity, and the

Table 1.1 Top 10 Causes of Death by Income Group, 2004

High-income countries			Low-income countries		
Rank	Cause of death	% total deaths	Rank	Cause of death	% total deaths
1	Coronary heart disease	16.3	1	Lower respiratory infections	11.2
2	Stroke and other cerebrovascular diseases	9.3	2	Coronary heart disease	9.4
3	Trachea, bronchus, lung cancers	5.9	3	Diarrhoeal diseases	6.9
4	Lower respiratory infections	3.8	4	HIV/AIDS	5.7
5	Chronic obstructive pulmonary disease	3.5	5	Stroke and other cerebrovascular diseases	5.6
6	Alzheimer and other dementias	3.4	6	Chronic obstructive pulmonary disease	3.6
7	Colon and rectum cancers	3.3	7	Tuberculosis	3.5
8	Diabetes mellitus	2.8	8	Neonatal infections	3.4
9	Breast cancer	2.0	9	Malaria	3.3
10	Stomach cancer	1.8	10	Prematurity and low birth weight	3.2

Source: WHO 2008.

role for compounds ranging from simple pain control medications and contraceptives to cancer chemotherapy agents, and the potential benefits of better pharmaceutical supply and use become quite evident.

Although medicines have the potential to improve health status significantly, policy makers are often concerned about the pharmaceutical sector because these products may not be used in the most cost-effective fashion. As a result, the money spent on them by patients and families (and by governments and donors) may produce less good than it could. Indeed, inappropriate spending on, and use of, drugs can cause significant harm. Patients who take a needlessly expensive or inappropriate drug will be sicker or poorer than they need be. Adverse effects can spread beyond the individual, for example, when misuse produces antimicrobial resistance. Misuse has promoted the emergence of multidrug-resistant TB (Ormerod 2005) and the loss of efficacy of such antimalarial drugs as chloroquine and sulfadoxine-pyrimethamine (White et al. 1999).

The causes of misuse are complex. On the demand side, consumers often behave in ways inconsistent with expert advice. Concerned about quality, they may choose expensive brand-name products over less-expensive generic equivalents. Eager for the health gains, they may use antibiotics when they are not needed and then may not take the full course, to save medication for later illnesses. In response to cultural norms and practices, people may spend money on tonics and elixirs of dubious value (though they may experience gains via the placebo effect) and ask for injections when they are not indicated. Many patients inappropriately discontinue taking their chronic disease medications because of costs, side effects, or lack of evident benefits.

On the supply side, providers and sellers of medicine all too often promote inappropriate medicine use in response to their financial interests. Those interests typically include higher profit margins on brand-name drugs, incentives from distributors and manufacturers, and the profits to be made from dealing in counterfeit compounds. Even when physician prescribing occurs, doctors eager to reduce their workload in public clinics, or to respond to patient desires in their private practices, may give patients inappropriate or multiple prescriptions to get them through quickly or encourage them to return. Both buyers and sellers can also be the targets of marketing efforts that use emotional appeals or incomplete or inaccurate information to try to influence them. All of these factors can contribute to misuse and overuse and can reinforce patients' preferences for brand-name products, promoting cost escalation.

Another important reason to care about the pharmaceutical sector is that it constitutes a significant portion of all health expenditures, especially in low- and middle-income countries. As table 1.2 shows, pharmaceutical spending was around 30 percent of total health spending in low-income countries in 2006, and low-income countries spent more of their health budgets on medicines than middle- or high-income countries. With many claimants competing for limited "fiscal space" (including education, economic development, and security), governments in low-income countries face great challenges in financing medicine expenditures. As a result, many rely heavily on external financing from donors to cover these costs and also leave much of the burden to be paid for in the private sector (over 75 percent by the estimates in table 1.2), largely by consumers out-of-pocket. That can place an enormous burden on low-income individuals, who may face a choice between doing without medicines and incurring serious financial hardship. (The book will term this a lack of "financial protection," as explained below.) In middle-income countries, where per capita spending on pharmaceuticals is higher than in low-income countries, the questions of what to cover and how to finance the growing costs are major sources of public controversy. (The same is true in many high-income countries as well.) Table 1.2 also shows how little low-income countries spend on medicines per capita (less than US$8), compared to others; the average is over US$400 in high-income countries.

Because of both the potential health benefits and the fiscal burden, access to medicines and the pharmaceutical policies that influence it are a significant source of concern to citizens in all countries, regardless of income level. But especially in low- and middle-income countries, these issues are so salient that they are a major determinant of public attitudes about the adequacy of the nation's health system and even of attitudes toward government in general. Because drugs provide tangible benefits, citizens become

Table 1.2 Pharmaceutical Expenditures by Country Income Level, 2006

Income level of country	Medicine spending as % of total health spending (mean)	Medicine spending in the private sector (%)	Per capita total medicines spending (US$ at exchange rate)
High	19.7 [46 countries]	38.7 [42 countries]	431.60
Upper-middle	23.1 [37 countries]	61.2 [31 countries]	84.10
Lower-middle	27.6 [44 countries]	66.5 [34 countries]	31.30
Low	30.4 [34 countries]	76.9 [27 countries]	7.61

Source: Lu et al. 2011.

Note: Countries are classified into income level according to World Bank methods (for 2009). Low = gross national product per capita under US$995; lower-middle = US$996–US$3,945; upper-middle = US$3,946–US$12,195; high = US$12,196 or more.

unhappy when medicines are unavailable in the public sector and difficult to afford in the private sector. Many countries have experienced persistent calls for improved access to medicines from political parties, nongovernmental organizations (NGOs), and the mass media, as well as from international organizations (Frost and Reich 2008).

What Is Pharmaceutical Policy?

To understand what is meant by "pharmaceutical policy" and why it matters, we need to understand the pharmaceutical system and the way it operates. The system involves eight complex subsystems that influence the impact of medicines on citizens' health and satisfaction (figure 1.1).

The set of medicines available in a country begins with (1) research and development and proceeds through (2) clinical trials to (3) registration. Registration occurs at the national level, but the first two processes may occur in other countries. After registration, the next question is (4) where and how the product is manufactured (including its formulation and packaging). Then, for each country, (5) procurement and importation, both public and private, determine which medicines are available nationally. Those medicines flow through (6) multiple supply chains to various outlets (including vendors, shops, stalls, clinics, and health centers), where (7) dispensing and sales occur. The final process is (8) how patients use the medicines once they have acquired them.

By "pharmaceutical policy" we mean the conscious efforts of national governments to influence the functioning of these subsystems. Many other actors play a role in what occurs—from multinational pharmaceutical companies and the World Trade Organization to the World Health Organization (WHO) and the Global Fund to Fight AIDS, Tuberculosis and Malaria, to faith-based delivery systems and local medicine sellers. But although this book offers suggestions for these other stakeholders at various points, its focus is on what national governments can and should do to influence both public sector and private sector performance, as well as the actions of citizens in using medicines, because they play a vital role in overall outcomes.

Figure 1.1   The Pharmaceutical System

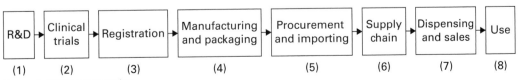

Source: Authors' representation.

Note: R&D = research and development.

Considering these subsystems reveals the many points of contact between the actions of national government, on the one hand, and the behavior of the pharmaceutical system and the ultimate outcomes that we seek to achieve, on the other. Governments in industrialized countries, where the major pharmaceutical companies are based, play the largest roles in pharmaceutical research and development and clinical trials, and hence those receive less attention in this book. In every low- and middle-income country, however, governments have a major part in the rest of the pharmaceutical system. They register medicines, license manufacturers, compile essential medicines lists, procure supplies for the public sector, operate public sector supply chains, and dispense a substantial share of medicines through public facilities. They also regulate (to varying degrees in different countries) the prices, products, and staff qualifications of private wholesalers and retailers, inspect medicines for quality, collect taxes and tariffs, train pharmaceutical personnel, and conduct campaigns to influence patient behavior. The resulting complex collection of laws, rules, expenditure patterns, financing choices, regulatory decisions, and managerial initiatives constitutes a nation's pharmaceutical policy.

Because these decisions may be taken by different government entities at different times, a nation's policy may not be fully coherent or consciously designed. Even specialists may not be aware of how some government decisions influence the performance of the pharmaceutical system. The central purpose of this book is to explore these connections and help governments manage their choices and actions more effectively.

The authors believe that governments can perform better in the pharmaceutical sector. If governments spend more on medicines, and spend those funds wisely, availability in the public sector can improve. If quality control and product registration are carried out effectively, the presence of counterfeit drugs can be reduced. Subsidies and price controls, educational campaigns, and supply chain improvements—government action on all of these components of the pharmaceutical system can produce important gains if properly implemented. That is a significant if, of course, and one that we pay attention to throughout the book.

The approach of this book to pharmaceutical policy differs slightly from that of the World Health Organization. WHO officially recognized the importance of a national policy for medicines in 1975, when the World Health Assembly passed a resolution (WHA28.66) calling for countries to formulate this kind of policy. In 1988, WHO published guidelines for developing a national drug policy, and it updated them in 2001 (WHO 1988; 2001). These WHO publications emphasize a single government document that provides "a commitment to a goal and a guide for action . . . [and] provides a framework within which the activities of the pharmaceutical sector can be coordinated" (WHO 2001, 4). The WHO approach also uses a list of policy components different from the one in this book, starting, for example, with the selection of essential drugs, reflecting WHO's own substantive and strategic views on pharmaceutical policy. The approach of the book is both more inclusive (in not focusing only on a national policy document) and less normative (in not prescribing particular values or substantive approaches). Seiter (2010) uses an approach similar to ours in a recent book on pharmaceutical policy. The two approaches are broadly compatible, however.

What the Book Seeks to Accomplish

The purpose of this book is to help policy analysts, program managers, and decision makers in low- and middle-income countries develop reforms that will improve the performance of their pharmaceutical sectors. To do that, we draw on a large body of research and analysis that has been developed over the last eleven years for the Flagship Program on Health Sector Reform. The program has been offered by the World Bank in regional and national courses in more than 40 countries around the world (Shaw and Samaha 2009).

The Flagship Framework provides a systematic and disciplined approach to pharmaceutical policy making. It begins with tools and concepts for identifying performance problems in the sector and setting priorities among them. Then it moves to methods for identifying the causes of poor performance, devising effective responses to the problems, and bringing countries to adopt them. Readers should know that what follows does not offer detailed, technical solutions to specific problems. Instead, the book's approach is to provide readers with methods for developing policy responses that are appropriate in each country's specific national circumstances.

In addition to numerous examples that are discussed in the text, the book relies heavily on case studies of the processes of formulating, adopting, and implementing a variety of pharmaceutical policy initiatives in countries around the world. Some of the cases are retrospective and describe in detail how events unfolded. Others are prospective. They are designed to pose analytical and conceptual problems to readers, so that they can practice the skills that the book seeks to communicate. Engaging with the cases along with the text, in a back-and-forth manner, takes maximum advantage of what the book has to offer.

The book is divided into three parts. The first part, chapters 2 through 6, is devoted to general concepts and methods. It discusses how to identify the most important performance problems in the pharmaceutical sector and diagnose their causes, and it explores the role of political and ethical analysis in those processes.

The second part, chapters 7 through 11, explores the roles of what we call the "control knobs" for improving pharmaceutical sector performance. The five control knobs—financing, payment, organization, regulation, and persuasion—reflect specific arenas in which governments can intervene to improve the functioning of their health systems in general and their pharmaceutical sectors in particular.

The third part comprises the cases, together with brief notes after each that highlight the main points that we hope readers will take away from considering them. As suggested above, the authors hope that readers will interrupt their progress through the text to take time to consider each case as it becomes relevant (indicated by notes in the text).

Because the book is directed at policy makers in low- and middle-income countries, it does not spend much time on industrial policy for the pharmaceutical sector in high-income nations. Governments in those countries have to decide whether to support or oppose various pharmaceutical industry mergers, whether to allow private firms to make use of science developed with public dollars, how to spend public research funds, and how to support the export activities of their local manufacturers. All are important questions, and some are becoming critical issues in middle-income countries with strong pharmaceutical industries (such as India and China). But they are largely beyond the scope here.

To use a chess metaphor, this book is focused from the "side of the board" of low- and middle-income country governments. It does not explore the perspective of international or donor organizations that are trying to decide which countries to engage, which priorities to foster, and which policy developments to support. Although the analytical frame employed here can be helpful in reaching those decisions, they do not receive much space in the book. Nor is much attention devoted to recent international initiatives, including public-private partnerships to promote product development for neglected tropical diseases, or research alliances. Instead, these issues enter into the discussion as forces that national decision makers need to consider in seeking their policy objectives.

Finally, vaccines and immunization policy are also generally outside the book's scope. Those are issues of great importance, inasmuch as immunization is often the most cost-effective health intervention a nation can support. But many of the relevant actors, delivery systems, and policy choices in such activities are specialized, and space and time constraints prevent their consideration here.

It is also important to recognize that the performance of the pharmaceutical sector depends on many external factors. What is happening in the health system generally? How well does the government operate, and what is the country's broader socioeconomic context? In discussing aspects of pharmaceutical policy reform, we will identify these broader connections to help readers understand both the constraints and the opportunities for change that they provide.

References

Frost, L. J., and M. R. Reich. 2008. *Access: How Do Good Health Technologies Get to Poor People in Poor Countries?* Cambridge, MA: Harvard University Press.

Lu, Y., P. Hernandez, D. Abegunde, and T. Edejer. 2011. "Medicine Expenditures." In *The World Medicines Situation 2011.* Geneva: WHO. Available at http://www. who.int/medicines/areas/policy/world_medicines_situation/en/index.html.

Mathers, C. D., and D. Loncar. 2006. "Projections of Global Mortality and Burden of Disease from 2002 to 2030." *PLoS Medicine* 3 (11): e442.

McKeown, T., and R. G. Record. 1962. "Reasons for the Decline of Mortality in England and Wales during the Nineteenth Century." *Population Studies* 16: 94–122.

Ormerod, L. P. 2005. "Multidrug-Resistant Tuberculosis (MDR-TB): Epidemiology, Prevention, and Treatment." *British Medical Bulletin* 73–74: 17–24.

Seiter, A. 2010. *A Practical Approach to Pharmaceutical Policy.* Washington, DC: World Bank.

Shaw, R. P., and H. Samaha. 2009. *Building Capacity for Health System Strengthening: A Strategy that Works.* Washington, DC: World Bank Institute.

White, N. J., F. Nosten, S. Looareesuwan, W. M. Watkins, K. Marsh, R. W. Snow, G. Kokwaro, J. Ouma, T. T. Hien, M. E. Molyneux, T. E. Taylor, C. I. Newbold, T. K. Ruebush II, M. Danis, B. M. Greenwood, R. M. Anderson, and P. Olliaro. 1999. "Averting a Malaria Disaster." *Lancet* 353: 1965–67.

WHO (World Health Organization). 1988. *Guidelines for Developing National Drug Policies.* Geneva: WHO.

———. 2001. *How to Develop and Implement a National Drug Policy.* Geneva: WHO.

———. 2008. "The Top Ten Causes of Death." Fact Sheet 310, WHO, Geneva.

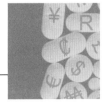

CHAPTER 2

Using the Flagship Framework to Reform Pharmaceutical Policy

How to Begin the Process of Reform

The Flagship Framework is designed to help analysts and policy makers develop reform initiatives that improve their health care systems in general and, as used in this book, improve pharmaceutical sector performance in particular. The framework is based on the argument that effective policy development has to start by identifying the *performance deficiencies*—that is, the outcomes—that reformers want to improve. We call this step "identifying the problem." The logic here is simple: you are unlikely to reach a goal unless and until you identify the goal that you are trying to reach.

Proceeding in this way is not always easy or obvious. Pharmaceutical reformers often do not begin their efforts by identifying the outcome deficiencies that they are unhappy with. Rather, they immediately focus on perceived *process failures* that they want to correct or on particular *solutions* that they favor. They might say, "Our problem is that we need to decrease leakage of medicines from the public sector supply chain," or "We need to regulate the high profit margins on brand-name drugs in private sector pharmacies."

A key feature of the method that we propose is that such statements are premature at the beginning of the pharmaceutical reform process. It might turn out that supply chain leakage or high private sector margins are critical causes of the poor performance that a reformer wants to correct. And it might turn out that a particular policy would be a plausible response. But given their complexity, most pharmaceutical systems suffer from multiple failures. How is a reformer to know which process failures to address or which initiatives to try? The answer is that reformers need to begin by identifying which aspects of the performance of the system they want to improve (Berwick, Godfrey, and Roessner 1990). To someone who leaps directly to improving the supply chain or regulating certain prices, our response is, Why do that? What improvements in system performance will such changes bring about? The answers to such questions will begin to reveal the implicit *problem definition* behind the proposals in question, the *performance deficiencies* whose improvement can and should be understood as the actual policy objective.

Disciplined thinking about identifying problems is especially important because the world is awash in consultants and donors eager to convince countries to adopt particular solutions. How are a nation's policy makers to know whether improving the nation's clinical laboratory, or imposing "regressive margin" price regulation, or contracting out logistic functions, is a sensible strategy? Reform advocates are often enthusiastic about their particular solution precisely because they are advocates. An old saying in the international-advice-giving world is, "To someone with a hammer, every problem looks like a nail."

Although such experts may have much to offer, our experience teaches us that local knowledge and local inputs are critical to developing effective pharmaceutical system reforms. Only local governments can legitimately decide on priorities or resolve the value conflicts that inevitably arise in reforming the pharmaceutical sector. Moreover, local experts often know best how their own systems actually function. They are often those best able to judge which ideas will, or will not, work in their particular cultural and political context and with the available financial and administrative resources.

As discussed further below, serious value conflicts are all too common in pharmaceutical reform. To strike a balance among competing goals, responsible and effective reform efforts have to combine technical analysis with both ethical and political considerations. For example, should countries spend limited funds on improving access to basic drugs for the rural poor or on helping those with life-threatening illnesses to secure expensive cancer chemotherapy agents? The pervasiveness of such value conflicts provides yet another reason for reformers, as they begin the process, to stop and reflect on exactly which aspects of pharmaceutical sector performance they most want to improve.

Those decisions require reformers to think deeply about such issues as the meaning of fairness in setting policy objectives and the extent to which governments should respond to what people want as opposed to what they need. By involving various stakeholders and interest groups (from civil society organizations to local importers) in a discussion of these questions, a nation's planners and policy makers will be able to identify conflicts among objectives and resolve them in an open and accountable way. One example of an international effort to promote this process is the Medicines Transparency Alliance, which was launched in 2008 by the U.K. Department for International Development (DFID), in collaboration with the World Health Organization (WHO) and the World Bank (*Lancet* 2008). Proceeding in that way has both philosophical and practical virtues. A well designed, participatory process meets the test of legitimacy set by democratic political theory. And in the realm of practical politics, it can be an important step in marshaling support for reform (even as a badly designed process can open up decision making to undue influence from well-funded and organized interests).

Ultimate Performance Goals

How should policy makers decide which performance problems in the pharmaceutical sector they most want to fix? The Flagship Framework suggests that health system performance problems in general, and pharmaceutical sector performance problems in particular, can be usefully sorted into three categories referred to as "ultimate goals." These are *health status, citizen satisfaction*, and *financial protection*. Moreover, reformers may care about more than a nation's *average level* of performance in these areas. *Variations* in performance across population groups (that is, the equity aspects of that performance) often are, or should be, of concern.

Health Status

Improving the health status of the population is a central goal of much pharmaceutical policy making (and of health sector reform generally). If citizens do not get artemisinin-based combination therapy (ACT) for malaria or antiretroviral therapy (ART) for HIV, not to mention oral rehydration salts for diarrheal disease or appropriate antibiotics for various infections, their health status will suffer. However, deciding on health status in general as a major performance goal is only the beginning of the process of problem identification. The questions then are, Which aspects of health status most need attention? Is it the prevalence of conditions that create an especially high burden of disease in a particular country (for example, malaria in parts of East Africa)? Is it poor performance versus comparable countries on a basic health status index, such as under-five mortality rate? The discussion below of the ethics and politics of priority setting will have more to say about these questions.

Some studies of pharmaceutical policy use formal analytical methods to try to measure the potential health status impact of alternative interventions (for example, by calculating their comparative cost-effectiveness in terms of gains in Quality Adjusted Life Years), and a growing number of countries consider these studies as part of their licensing requirements for new medicines (Taylor et al. 2004). As discussed further below, these methods make a series of assumptions about how to value various kinds of outcomes (for example, the value of saving the young versus the old, or the productive versus the disabled) (Musgrove 2000). Thus using such tools does not, in itself, solve the priority-setting problem in an accountable way. Instead, reformers have to be aware of, publicly acknowledge, and accept as valid for their situation, the assumptions that particular methods employ.

Citizen Satisfaction

In considering pharmaceutical policy, public health professionals tend to focus on objective measurements such as health status. In contrast, both politicians and economists pay great attention to how citizens feel about their situation, that is, to their levels of satisfaction. Economists do so because, within their analytical framework, a good system of pharmaceutical supply is one that responds to market demands—to what people *want* (rather than to what people may *need* to improve their health status). Politicians may or may not share economists' goals, but they do have to be concerned about satisfaction (and respond to dissatisfaction) to recruit support for themselves and their policies.

That is so regardless of the political system in which they operate. Even in countries without meaningful elections, most national leaders are at least somewhat concerned about responding to popular demands. As with health status, the distribution of satisfaction (or dissatisfaction) may influence the importance that reformers attach to it. For example, how politically powerful are the dissatisfied, and are they allies or opponents of the governing coalition?

Financial Protection

Most people most of the time are not sick. Evolution has seen to that. Thus some of the burden of illness takes the form of the relatively infrequent large costs of serious illness. Such catastrophic costs, when they occur, can devastate a family economically (Blumenthal and Hsiao 2005) or can constitute a major barrier to care so that patients do not receive adequate treatment.

The cost of medicines, however, often follows a somewhat different pattern. That pattern involves the costs of treating an occasional childhood (or adult) case of infectious disease, the kind of pharmaceutical expenses that are associated with ordinary primary care. Unlike the costs of infrequent major illnesses, they are relatively predictable (on average) on an annual basis. Every family expects that some fevers or diarrheal diseases will occur among the household each year.

Purchasing medicines to treat those illnesses can be financially burdensome—especially when epidemiological and economic bad luck coincide. But they may well be manageable much of the time for much of the population (provided the drugs in question are not too expensive). Because much drug purchasing takes this relatively modest, almost routine (rather than catastrophic) form, a great deal of out-of-pocket purchase of medicines in the private sector occurs, even in low-income countries. Again, the impact on a family's welfare of even routine illnesses—for example, through the short-term adjustment of food purchases—can be substantial. But the high value that citizens place on medicines leads them to make those adjustments, despite the hardships involved.

In addition, in many low- and middle-income countries, as noted above, chronic diseases are increasingly important. They may not generate sudden, short-term, catastrophic medicines costs. Indeed, the costs of routine treatment for conditions such as diabetes and cardiovascular disease (as well as HIV), once diagnosed, may be quite predictable. However, the ongoing pharmaceutical costs may also be unaffordable for many, especially when reliable supplies of low-cost medicines are not available in the public sector (Mendis et al. 2007).

In response to this complex reality, an important performance goal for many governments has been to provide citizens with *financial protection* in the face of (1) low-probability, expensive short-term risks; (2) the ongoing costs of medicines for routine infectious diseases; and increasingly, (3) the long-term costs of chronic disease treatment. It is worth noting that protecting citizens against infrequent large costs is an insurance or risk-pooling problem. However, helping lower-income individuals carry the burdens of routine medicine expenses for chronic and infectious disease is a redistributive problem. It is a matter of finding a funding mechanism to cross-subsidize certain expenses for people who would otherwise have difficulty affording them.

A source of information on the last point is the surveys conducted by WHO and HAI (a Dutch nongovernmental organization, Health Action International). These surveys, in various countries, compare the costs of common medicines to the pay of low-wage public sector workers and document the nontrivial burden that such expenses often impose on large parts of the population (WHO and HAI 2008).

These three goals appear as the ultimate performance objectives in our Flagship Framework for a health system, as shown in figure 2.1. The other elements of the framework—the control knobs and the intermediate performance measures—will be discussed in detail farther on in the book.

Figure 2.1   The Flagship Framework for Health System Performance

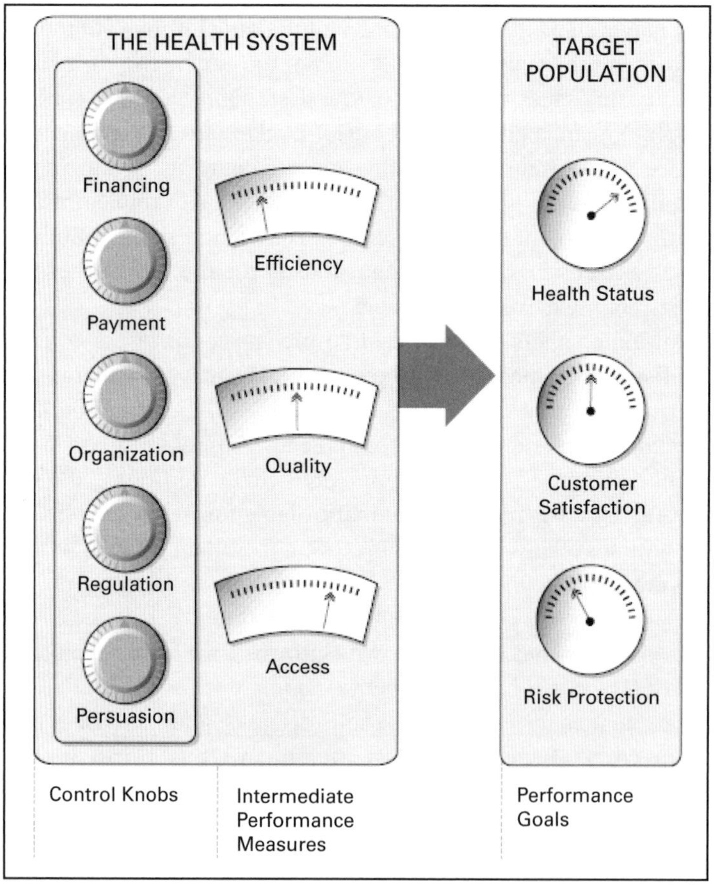

Source: Roberts et al. 2004, 27. By permission of Oxford University Press, Inc.

Before proceeding, it is important to note that the pharmaceutical sector poses difficult problems for policy makers when it comes to potential conflicts and tensions among these goals. Suppose that low-priced generics are available, but poor citizens choose to buy expensive branded products instead (increasing their satisfaction but undermining their financial situation). To what extent should policy makers see those choices as a priority problem? Similarly, the tension between improving health status and increasing citizen satisfaction can be significant. Citizens might believe that they have not received care if they do not receive an injection; or they might favor inexpensive elixirs and unproven traditional remedies; or they might want antibiotics when they are not indicated (see case study H, "Changing the Use of Antibiotics in Peru"). In these instances, policy makers have to decide how much importance they should attach to responding to citizen preferences. These issues will be discussed extensively in the following chapters.

The Role of Cost in Setting Reform Goals

The costs of a nation's health care system in general, and its pharmaceutical sector in particular, are critical in setting reform goals. In the short run, budget limitations constrain public sector choices. In the long run, economic growth may increase "fiscal space"—making more funds available (Heller 2006). In addition, taxes can be raised or budgets reallocated to improve pharmaceutical sector funding. And the expansion of external support (for

Figure 2.2 Cost-Performance Trade-Offs

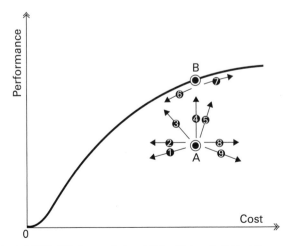

Source: Roberts et al. 2004, 100. By permission of Oxford University Press, Inc.

example, from the Global Fund) may also be possible. Moreover, the question is always present whether to shift medicines expenditures from the private to the public sector—or vice versa—which can significantly affect the financing burden in the public sector. In Ghana, for example, public pressure to end its cash-and-carry policy pushed the government to provide medicines with public sector funds (see case study J, "Drug Coverage in Ghana's National Health Insurance Scheme").

Figure 2.2 provides a simplified illustration of these choices. The vertical axis is a measure of the performance of the pharmaceutical sector that combines the three performance goals into a single index to make the diagram possible. The curve in the diagram relates spending to the maximum possible performance that is theoretically obtainable for that cost. The shape of the curve reflects our belief that maximum possible performance begins to level out at some point. (It probably even turns down eventually, to reflect the effects of inappropriate overuse, but that is not the part of the curve that is relevant in low- and middle-income countries.)

Before exploring this diagram, however, a word of warning is in order. The figure is meant as a conceptual exercise. Few countries actually know where they are in such a diagram. They are not able to measure their performance, nor do they know what the maximum level of performance could be for any given spending level. Indeed, given the large role of private, out-of-pocket spending on medicines, many countries do not even know with much precision where they are on the horizontal axis, that is, how much they and their citizens are spending on pharmaceuticals. Indeed, since "cost" in the diagram includes both public and private sector expenditures, as well as foreign aid and donations, the ability of governments to "move" the nation in this cost-performance space may be somewhat limited.

Leaving all that aside for the moment, we believe that in general, a nation's pharmaceutical sector performance will put it at a point such as point A in figure 2.2. Because the sector is not perfectly efficient, better performance with the existing resources would be possible. As a result, performance is below the curve that reflects the maximum possible outcomes. In such a situation, the cost-performance problem that a national government confronts can be formulated in five ways, as indicated by arrows 1 to 5 in figure 2.2:

(1) Reduce costs, even if performance declines.

(2) Reduce costs—but maintain current levels of performance.

(3) Reduce costs and improve performance.

(4) Maximize performance for current costs.

(5) Improve performance even if costs increase.

Arrows 1 and 2 reflect the kind of overwhelming commitment to decreasing costs that typically occurs only when an economy has collapsed (for example, in a post conflict situation). In many cases, high-spending nations formulate their problem as arrow 3, obtaining better performance and lower costs (such as Japan's efforts to decrease drug spending in recent decades) (Ikegami, Ikeda, and Kawai 1998). Alternatively, a nation may view its goal as represented by arrow 4, maximizing performance for a given budget—as reflected, for example, in Germany's regional pharmaceutical spending caps (Delnoij and Brenner 2000) and in efforts to increase the "rational use" of medicines. Poorer countries often view the situation as 5. That reflects the belief that they need to increase total drug spending, while also spending those funds more effectively to improve overall performance. In the poorest countries, national policy makers often seek to raise much of the increased expenditure from international sources, as discussed below in the chapter on financing.

What about the other arrows in figure 2.2? Ministries of health—especially when negotiating for budgets with ministries of finance—sometimes claim that they are starting not at point A but at point B, already achieving maximum performance for current costs. Thus, they claim, the choices before the government are to spend more to get more, or to cut the budget and get less (arrows 7 and 6). Although rhetorically popular, that argument is not empirically persuasive. It is doubtful that many low- and middle-income nations have public and private pharmaceutical sectors that together are already maximally efficient.

Similarly, a country that engages in poor policy making could produce a move as shown by arrow 8, resulting in higher costs without improved performance, or even 9, higher costs and lower performance. That is not a move that policy makers are likely to make intentionally, unless they value some goal other than health—such as supporting a domestic pharmaceutical industry—so highly that they are willing to spend money and decrease health gains to achieve it. Nevertheless, some policy changes can have that effect as an unintended consequence. For example, political decisions to decentralize procurement to less-than-competent provincial bodies have resulted in reduced performance and increased costs in some nations' pharmaceutical sectors.

The Role of Politics and Ethics in Identifying Problems and Choosing Reform Priorities

As argued above, reformers need to decide on their goal—how they want to improve the performance of the system—before they can develop a reasonable plan for reaching it. That requires them to identify where and how each of the performance goals is not being met, and once they have identified the problems, to make choices about how to set reform priorities. In considering the roles of politics and ethics in that process, readers should keep in mind some of the complexities involved:

- Each of the broad performance goals mentioned above has to be made specific. That is, a decision has to be made on how to measure outcomes (for example, which health status measures to use or how to gather data on citizen satisfaction).

- The relative priority of different objectives, both within and across the performance goals (for example, which diseases or what aspects of popular discontent), has to be addressed and resolved.

- Equity considerations (which groups are of special concern) have to be clarified for each of the objectives and for the reform process as a whole.

- The role of cost considerations has to be clarified.

To understand why these decisions are so difficult, we now turn to the interlinked questions of how these questions *will* be decided (politics) and how they *should* be decided (ethics) in the formulation of a pharmaceutical reform initiative.

The process of setting reform priorities is inevitably political in several senses. First, in countries with elections, many participants in the policy process will take positions about pharmaceutical policy with an eye to their political careers. Even in systems with low levels of political competition, such calculations will influence not only current and would-be officeholders but also lobbyists, industry executives, citizens groups, and even bureaucrats.

Second, the goals of a reform effort will be political in the sense that they almost always emerge from a political process—a set of decision-making arrangements, both legislative and bureaucratic, involving players both inside and outside the government. Committees will be formed, reports written, memoranda drafted, and votes taken. Coalitions will be formed, arguments made, obligations invoked, and bargains struck. The outcomes of all these processes will reflect the political resources, positions, strategies, and commitments of the various players. This topic, including how to analyze and influence such political processes, is discussed in more detail in chapter 6.

Finally, the decision will be political in the sense that it will not (indeed cannot) be entirely technical. The role that an expert can and should legitimately play in telling a national government which problems it should focus on or which priorities it should adopt has significant limits. The expertise of experts consists in their ability to help governments predict the likely consequences of alternative actions and to explain to governments how to achieve their goals. In this sense they are like travel agents. They can tell you which place is likely to have good snow, if you want to go skiing, and how to get a cheap flight and a clean hotel. But they cannot tell you how much you should spend (whether to choose a 3 star or a 4 star hotel). And they cannot tell you if you *should* go skiing or scuba diving. Similarly, experts cannot legitimately tell a nation how much emphasis it should give to improving access to medicines for the rural poor, versus the urban middle class, or what weight to give to responding to patient wants versus patient needs.

We recognize that particular ethical points of view are implicitly embedded in many forms of expertise, in their basic concepts and analytical methods. Contemporary economic theory, for example, defines good outcomes in terms of responding to market demand (Van de Graaf 1957). In contrast, public health professionals often believe that governments can appropriately be somewhat coercive to achieve improvements in health status (for example, supporting smoking bans). But that does not mean that one or another of these perspectives should be uncritically accepted by a country as it embarks on its own reform efforts.

Indeed, because reform priorities always reflect *someone's* values, we believe that such decisions should depend critically on democratic political processes. By responding to citizens' views, democratic processes accomplish two important goals. First, popular input and accountability give citizens some control over important aspects of their own lives. Second, such processes help legitimate the resulting policy decisions in the minds of citizens. That in turn fosters what some political scientists call "the mobilization of consent," which is crucial to the survival of any effective government.

But politics is about more than the pursuit of private gain. In addition, competing views about what a good society should be also come into play. Philosophers and writers on ethics have been grappling with that question for thousands of years. Not only are their proposals relevant to pharmaceutical policy choices on their merits, but in fact they are also often influential in the thinking of many of those involved in pharmaceutical policy making. For example, debates about pharmaceutical policy in recent years have been filled with claims about rights to access to medicines, about the property rights of patent holders, and about the obligations of the rich North of the world toward the poorer South. How is one to assess these claims without first understanding where they come from, how they are justified, and what they imply? For that reason, we believe that just as politics is, and should be, a part of the policy process, the same is true for ethical arguments.

In chapter 4 we discuss various ethical and philosophical arguments that have been made about public policy and see how they apply to the choice of reform priorities in the pharmaceutical sector. We do so to help participants in the debate understand more clearly both their own views and the views of others. In a sense, the question asked is, Which arguments can someone coherently make (to themselves and others) about how to set reform goals and priorities from various points of view?

The Reform Cycle

Identifying the *performance problems* that a pharmaceutical reformer wants to fix is the first stage of what we call "the reform cycle." This cycle is not meant to represent what always happens. Rather it is an ideal type, a simplified description of what would and should happen if the process were to proceed in a logical and disciplined way (depicted in figure 2.3). The cycle idea is not unique to us. Various forms of it have been offered by writers on quality management and process improvement (Juran and Godfrey 1999), as well as by writers on policy reform in the political science literature. What is distinctive is how we apply this approach to health sector reform in general and pharmaceutical sector reform in particular.

Once the problem has been identified, the second stage of the cycle is *diagnosis*. The task is to go on what some have called a "diagnostic journey." As the Japanese quality management expert Ishikawa (1988) put it, diagnosis requires asking the question, Why? five times. For example, suppose the

Figure 2.3 The Reform Cycle

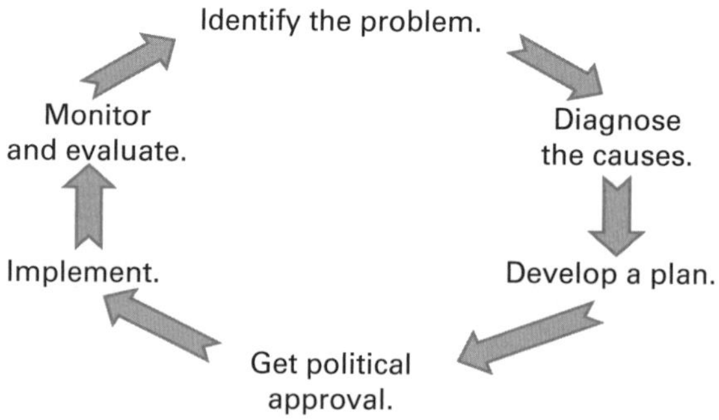

Source: Authors' representation.

problem identified is a high burden of morbidity and mortality from malaria among the rural population. If we ask, Why? we might discover a number of causes: stock-outs in the public sector, high prices for treatment in the private sector, and problems in malaria diagnosis. For each of these we need to ask, Why? and Why? again, until we have thoroughly understood the causes, the causes of the causes, and so on. A systematic way of conducting such a diagnosis is discussed in chapter 5.

After diagnosis comes *policy development*. Again, this topic is discussed in more detail below. Here we want to make two preliminary points. First, how the process of policy development is done matters. The way the process is conducted affects both the substance of what is produced and its political and social legitimacy. This point is illustrated by the Medicines Transparency Alliance (MeTA) initiative, which DFID supported in a variety of countries and which used a multistakeholder process (involving government, civil society, and the private sector) to promote pharmaceutical policy reform.

Second, smart policy developers try to foresee both political acceptability and any potential implementation difficulties in formulating their ideas. The objective of the policy development stage should be the production not just of a nice-sounding plan, but of a plan that can be adopted politically and then implemented successfully. Reformers have many places to look for innovative policy ideas. But the test should always be, Will it work here? International experts may have much to say about experience around the world, but they will not always be the best ones to answer that question—especially if they are not deeply familiar with the country under discussion.

The fourth step in the reform cycle is *political approval*. Chapter 6 discusses both how to map the key stakeholders in a political process and the strategies that are available to reformers to obtain that approval. It has been the authors' experience that technical experts often do not know how to manage local political processes and sometimes even resist examining the political aspects of a reform effort. But as we have stressed, given the value-laden nature of pharmaceutical policy choices, politics is both inevitable and appropriate. Technical experts who want to be effective in pharmaceutical reform efforts, therefore, need to learn how to operate effectively in the political arena.

Next comes *implementation*, a stage that has contributed much to pharmaceutical policy failure around the world. Some of the failure has been due to the inherent difficulties of the problem, and some has occurred because not enough attention was paid to what is and is not feasible in a specific national context. Some of the failure also reflects a tendency of economists and public health experts to downplay the role of management expertise and organizational leadership in improving service quality. For example, many countries experience serious difficulties in providing high-quality services, free of corruption, in the public sector, difficulties that greatly transcend matters of medicines supply.

At the same time, it is now widely recognized in the pharmaceutical arena how hard it can be to make systems that look good on paper actually function effectively in the field. As a result, implementation issues are now more salient in conversations on pharmaceutical reform than they are in many other areas of health system concern. (For example, efforts are now under way in many countries to improve the operational details of pharmaceutical purchasing or supply chain management.)

The final stage is *monitoring and evaluation*. We argue below that the time to plan for such activities is at the policy design stage. A good evaluation requires that data be collected before a new policy is initiated. In that context, serious consideration also needs to be given to pilot project approaches and phased implementation, to allow for learning by doing, before a reform is rolled out nationwide. Unfortunately, all too often too few resources are spent on monitoring and evaluation, or the process is merely designed to justify (or in some cases to undermine) some government policy. Those failures can seriously limit a nation's ability to learn from its own experience and improve its reform activities.

Notice that in figure 2.3 an arrow leads from "monitor and evaluate" back to "identify the problem." Experience teaches that many reforms do not work out exactly as intended. Instead, they often create their own, unanticipated problems. An example is what has happened in some countries that have made efforts to control market prices for generic drugs to enhance their affordability. In a number of cases, the controls have led private sector pharmacies not to carry those drugs because of the small profit they provide, or else to push consumers to purchase higher-cost branded products (see case study J, "Drug Coverage in Ghana's National Health Insurance Scheme"). When such outcomes are revealed in the monitoring and evaluation stage, a wise policy maker starts again with the process of problem identification, diagnosis, and policy development. Indeed, experienced reformers know that reform is not a one-time affair. Instead, it is an ongoing process of adjustment and readjustment as economic developments, new technology, and the responses of various players create new dilemmas and new needs.

The Control Knobs

As a guide for the process of policy development, the Flagship Framework organizes possible policy interventions under five headings, which we call the "control knobs." If the ultimate performance goals represent the dependent variables in our framework, then the control knobs are the independent variables—the things that pharmaceutical policy makers can change to produce the outcomes they desire. We call them "control knobs" because we have in mind the metaphor of a large factory, such as an oil refinery or steel mill, where managers must cope with the complexity of designing and adjusting many different, interrelated processes at once. We imagine that reformers are like the engineers who are sitting in the control room above the shop floor, adjusting dials to change the temperature of, or the mix of inputs going into, a blast furnace (or adjusting the design of the furnace itself) to alter what kind of steel is made and to improve the performance of the production process.

The second part of this book reviews each of the control knobs, discussing what is known from international experience about how adjusting each of them can influence performance in the pharmaceutical sector. The five knobs considered are the following (see also figure 2.1):

- **Financing** focuses on how the money for pharmaceuticals is raised and how those choices affect the distribution of use and costs across the population. We also explore how financing options affect financial protection.

- **Payment** decisions alter what and how various organizations and individuals in the pharmaceutical system are paid and the incentives that those payments in turn create. The relevant receivers of payment include everyone from manufacturers responding to national procurement efforts, to local wholesalers and retailers, to private physicians and public sector health centers.

- **Organization** deals with how activities in the pharmaceutical sector are divided among public and private entities and across centralized and decentralized agencies. We describe how these divisions, and the managerial patterns that they create, influence the incentives and motivation of frontline workers, their job performance, and the performance of the system as a whole.

- **Regulation** allows governments to alter behavior in the private (and to a lesser extent the public) sector by imposing rules that are backed by sanctions. Varying the rules can have a major impact on the quality and cost of medicines and in turn on the health status, satisfaction, and levels of risk protection of the population.

- **Persuasion** efforts involve governments' attempts to persuade key actors (doctors, patients, dispensers, and so on) to change their behavior through various kinds of educational and marketing initiatives.

These control knobs do not function in isolation. Instead, reformers often discover that they have to "turn" more than one knob to be effective. For example, educating dispensers about the importance of providing a full course of treatment (persuasion) may not be enough to change their behavior, unless the policy reform package also includes positive incentives (payment) or potential negative consequences (regulation).

It is also important for the process of policy development to be evidence based. Too often, in our experience, reformers are swept up by an idea—be it decentralization, or private health insurance, or making hospitals autonomous—without thinking through how it would actually produce the improvements in system performance that they seek and without examining prior experiences with the same reforms in other relevant settings. Although definitive statistical studies (with before-and-after observations and well-designed control groups) are often lacking, experience in other, comparable countries are a good place to begin. Reformers need to ask, How are we the same or different from the country whose experience we are considering? Can we match their resources and expertise? and, Are there cultural or political differences we need to consider?

Government Failures and Market Failures

Before concluding this chapter, we want to briefly discuss some of the causes of poor performance that are common to the pharmaceutical sectors in many low- and middle-income countries. To go back to figure 2.2, why is it that most systems do not produce higher levels of performance for the resources being used? That is, why are countries closer to point A in that diagram than to point B?

Market Failures

Economists define market failures by asking how real markets differ from ideal markets—the ideal being defined by a highly simplified set of concepts that are grouped together as the model of "perfect competition." In that model, all buyers and sellers make perfect decisions in pursuit of their own interests. The whole world is, in a sense, frictionless. It is not meant as a description of the real world but rather as an ideal against which imperfect reality can be judged. By exploring that ideal, one can develop a set of categories to describe different kinds of problems that exist in the real world.

Let us start with consumers. In a perfect market, all buyers are presumed to have total external and internal knowledge. They know in detail about the quality and prices of all available products. They also have perfect knowledge about their own tastes and preferences and how they will react to all possible outcomes. Thus consumers can perfectly predict how various alternative purchasing decisions will affect their well-being (Samuelson and Nordhaus 2009). Never ambivalent or conflicted or unable to make up their mind, consumers in a perfect market always act to maximize what economists call their "utility," that is, how well-off they are.

In the pharmaceutical context, this means that medicines buyers would know all about the quality and efficacy of all alternative products, whether generics or brand names. Such ideal buyers would know what was and was not effective, and what was and was not a counterfeit. Thus they would have no need of advice from doctors or medicines sellers. Even this brief description suggests just how far pharmaceutical markets are from the ideal.

On the producer's side, in the model of perfect competition, all the manufacturers of any given product use the same production technology, and what they produce is assumed to be exactly the same. For any one product there are numerous producers, so all sellers have to "take" (sell at) the price they find in the marketplace. Moreover, they are all motivated by, and only by, maximizing their profits. That means that they expand production until the costs of added output (their "marginal costs") are equal to the price in the market. Again, pharmaceutical markets rarely resemble this ideal, as is illustrated by the examples of patent protection, brand names, and limited numbers of sellers at many points along the supply chain.

Economists have constructed elaborate mathematical arguments to show that if the entire economy of a country were made up of such ideal markets, then the economy as a whole would be "efficient." By that, economists mean there is no way to improve the well-being (or utility) of some individuals without making others worse off. In other words, no slack or underused resources would exist anywhere in the system.

Economists use that model of perfect markets to identify and characterize various kinds of "market failure." But as we use that framework to analyze pharmaceutical markets, readers need to be reminded that the "failures" are defined relative to a specific goal, namely, the goal of giving buyers exactly what they would want if they had perfect knowledge. In other words, it is very much *not* a need-based model; rather it is a demand-based analysis.

Market Failures on the Buyer Side (Demand)

- *Buyers have limited knowledge and information.* The most serious buyer-side market failure in pharmaceutical markets is that most buyers have limited information about the characteristics and quality of the available products and limited knowledge of their likely benefits. Consequently, they often purchase more or less of a good, or a different good, than they would if they were better informed. As a result, they may well pay more, get fewer health benefits, and end up less satisfied because of poor results and the stress of the decision. To compensate for their ignorance, buyers rely on a variety of strategies, which may make sense from their point of view, but which do not necessarily improve their decision making:

- ○ Rely on brand names. Buyers who cannot judge quality often rely on brand names as a tool for avoiding mistakes. This is an approach that even sophisticated consumers (such as the readers of this book) follow in many markets. Such patterns undermine price competition by allowing originator brands, and so-called branded generics, to be sold at higher prices than unbranded products of equal quality.

- ○ Judge quality by observable characteristics. Consumers who cannot know the actual potency of various alternative medicines often rely on product characteristics that they can observe, such as taste, smell, or packaging—or even price—to guide their choices. But because such characteristics are not always closely related to pharmacological quality, again consumers can be led astray.

- ○ Rely on sellers. In the pharmaceutical arena, buyers often rely on sellers to advise them about what to buy. Economists call this an *agency relationship*. The problem is that the prescribers or dispensers who fulfill this function often respond—at least in part—to their own incentives and not to the buyer's interests. Thus they may encourage buyers to choose more expensive (and profitable) products even when they offer no additional value.

- *Buyers confront subsidized prices.* The model of perfect competition assumes that buyers face prices that reflect the actual costs of products. Yet in the pharmaceutical sector, to decrease financial burdens and lower price-based access barriers, countries often provide free or subsidized medicines in the public sector or through insurance schemes. That can lead patients to acquire more medicines than is economically optimal. When drugs are available in the local clinic, citizens may come in and ask for medicines that they do not need or visit multiple clinics to stockpile supplies for future use. Similarly, they may inappropriately overuse antibiotics by taking them for viral infections.

The issue of subsidized prices in the pharmaceutical area is complicated because the prices that various players in the supply chain—including governments—actually pay are often far above marginal production costs. The reason is that intellectual property rules and other market failures (discussed below) function to limit price competition. As a result, a significant number of pharmaceutical policy initiatives (such as the Affordable Medicine Facility for Malaria, which provides subsidized ACTs for sale in private sector pharmacies, and global pressures for concessionary prices from manufacturers of antiretrovirals [ARVs]) are designed to lower costs to consumers, despite the risk of overuse that lower costs might conceivably create.

- *Buyers fail to consider external effects.* Sometimes buyers' decisions influence other people ("external" to the buyer) in either positive or negative ways. But because those effects happen to someone else, the buyers have no incentive to take them into account. In pharmaceutical policy, a relevant example is the effect of medicine use (and misuse) in creating antimicrobial resistance. A mother pressing a local clinic to treat her child's fever with ACTs, without going through the cost and delay of a rapid diagnostic test for malaria, is in exactly that position.

Market Failures on the Seller Side (Supply)

- *Limited price competition.* Pharmaceutical markets are full of situations in which limited competition allows sellers to be *price makers*, instead of *price takers*, and thus to set prices far enough above their costs to create substantial profits. Such high prices lead to several adverse effects, particularly to inappropriately low use. Buyers who could benefit from taking the medications in question (or their governments) are discouraged from purchasing them by the high prices. There is also an equity effect because high prices, and the resulting high profits, redistribute wealth from (often poor) buyers to (often better-off) sellers—including the owners and managers of international pharmaceutical companies. Such limited price competition arises in several ways:

  o Patent-based monopoly. The most extreme form of imperfect competition is a monopoly (a single seller). Monopolies are widespread in some pharmaceutical arenas because of the exclusive (albeit time-limited) intellectual property claims created by the patent system. Whether the shorter-term use-discouraging effect of patents is a worthwhile price to pay for patents' role in encouraging the development of new medicines is an issue well beyond the scope here.

  o Oligopoly. When a market is dominated by a small number of sellers, economists call it an "oligopoly." In such cases, firms may collude implicitly or explicitly (for example, by forming a cartel or engaging in bid rigging) to keep prices up. Such limited price competition can arise at many stages along the pharmaceutical supply chain, especially in small countries when there is not enough room in the marketplace for many competitors to undertake activities such as importation or distribution. And in many rural areas that have relatively few retail medicines sellers, limited competition often leads to high prices.

- ○ Regulatory barriers to entry. Would-be sellers must have regulatory permission to conduct many activities in the pharmaceutical sector. Many countries license pharmacists and retail outlets at various levels. They also may regulate importers, brokers, testing laboratories, and wholesalers (not to mention doctors, hospitals, and clinics). All these rules create what economists call "barriers to entry" and have the effect of limiting the number of competitors in various markets.

- *Product differentiation.* Another kind of market failure arises when sellers convince buyers that their product is different and special and thus deserves to be purchased despite its higher price, leading customers to spend more than it is in their interest to spend. Advertising and other marketing efforts—intended to develop brand loyalty and brand identification—are designed to produce these effects. A combination of consumer anxiety ("I don't want to risk buying something bad") and limited knowledge about product quality creates fertile ground for such efforts. Lower-level vendors also may have limited knowledge, and thus they may be as much influenced by branding and product differentiation as are their ultimate consumers.

- *Unfair trade practices.* Sellers can use a variety of practices to distort or undermine effective market competition. Examples include bribes, kickbacks, fraud, demands for exclusive access, and knowingly supplying substandard products. Such practices also include "predatory pricing," or temporarily setting low prices to drive out a competitor and then raising them once that competitor has been eliminated. These unfair practices can occur at many market stages in the medicines supply chain. They all have the ultimate effect of limiting competition, raising prices and profits, and discouraging customer use.

Government Failures

Just as defining market failure requires the concept of an ideal market to use as a reference point, defining government failure requires us to have as a baseline a notion of how governments ought to function. But students of government do not have the same degree of agreement about that ideal as economists do about the model of perfect competition. Absent such an agreement, we propose to divide the actions of government into three stages and ask about appropriate actions at each stage: (1) Does it pursue the "right" goals? (2) Does it enact the best possible policies to achieve those goals? (3) Does it implement those policies effectively?

However, because not everyone agrees on which goals governments should pursue, serious differences of opinion are likely to arise with regard to the first kind of failure. For example, from the point of view of someone concerned with pharmaceutical access, a decision to continue the sales tax on medicines to raise more revenue could look like a failure to pursue the right goals. To someone focused on promoting government fiscal responsibility, the same decision could look like a success. With that caveat, however, we suggest that readers distinguish among three types of government failures within the pharmaceutical arena.

- *Goals/priorities failure*. The failure of a government to choose the "right" goals and priorities for pharmaceutical reform is almost always a function of a country's political system, broadly defined. By that we mean the way elections are structured, the way executive and legislative institutions are designed, the pattern of political parties, and the power of interest groups. (Such political processes are discussed in more detail in chapter 6.) Together these can produce policy goals and priorities that a particular outside observer regards as mistaken.

- *Policy design failure*. A failure of this kind occurs when a government tries to reach the right goals but fails to do so because the policies it chooses are poorly designed. Sometimes this occurs because powerful stakeholders have shaped reforms to protect their own interests. In other instances, those who developed the policy have not done a good job. Perhaps they have been limited by their own ideological or professional beliefs, or by limited data, poor analysis, or lack of knowledge, or they have given in to emotion or prejudice.

- *Implementation failure*. When a policy has the potential to be effective but is not, the reason is typically poor implementation. Such failures have many possible roots, including inadequate worker effort, badly designed production systems, and lack of needed resources. These causes, in turn, are likely to be rooted in other, more fundamental issues such as inadequate management, a lack of commitment to improved service delivery on the part of political leaders, restrictive incentive and personnel systems, and patterns of patronage and corruption. When these failures are limited to pharmaceutical sector agencies and institutions, they may be corrected more easily than when they reflect general, governmentwide difficulties and patterns.

In practice, these failures can overlap. A flawed policy design can reflect deep political forces, and those design flaws in turn can lead to implementation difficulties. Suppose, for example, that a nation adopts a health insurance scheme that is decentralized to the regional level to respond to ethnic tensions and separatist pressures. And suppose further that the scheme is badly implemented and troubled by corruption, at least in some provinces. Is that a goals and priorities failure because of its responsiveness to concerns other than creating a good insurance scheme? Or is it a policy design failure because it was a mistake to assume that the provinces had enough administrative capacity to run their own insurance plans? Or is it an implementation failure because of the corruption? In truth, it is an example of all three. In another country, however, such decentralization might lead to quite different results, and that is exactly why a context-specific analysis is always so important.

Of course there are also simpler cases. A policy intended to allow a few well-positioned citizens to be funded for expensive cancer chemotherapy abroad might represent a failure in problem identification in the eyes of many, but it could still be well designed and implemented. Similarly, a push distribution system intended to serve the reasonable goal of getting drugs to rural health centers could produce a great deal of waste—exactly because its flawed design was conscientiously carried out.

Government failures and market failures can be interdependent. Pressures from various players—such as manufacturers, pharmacists, or doctors—can push governments into policy failures that create or reinforce market failures. Stakeholders often pursue such efforts precisely to undermine competition and increase their profits. Similarly, private sector actors can exploit government failures—such as poor performance by regulatory agencies—in ways that make existing market failures even worse, for example, by illegally importing and selling unregistered or counterfeit medicines.

Summary on the Flagship Framework

Systematic analysis can significantly improve the chances of success for pharmaceutical reform. That is why we urge reformers to take seriously the concepts and analytical tools in the Flagship Framework. Think carefully about the entire reform cycle. Pay attention to the process of defining problems in terms of ultimate performance goals as the place to begin. Take the politics and the ethics of your decisions seriously. Worry about implementation issues from the beginning. Do a diagnosis, and base your consideration of how to use the control knobs on the evidence. Have a monitoring and evaluation plan in place, and be prepared to learn from your mistakes. And think systematically about the kinds of market failures and government failures that affect the pharmaceutical sector in your country.

The rest of this book examines these topics in more detail, in a way that is intended to be of practical value to readers engaged in the work of improving the performance of their national pharmaceutical systems.

References

Berwick, D. M., A. B. Godfrey, and J. Roessner. 1990. *Curing Health Care: New Strategies for Quality Improvement*. San Francisco: Jossey-Bass.

Blumenthal, D., and W. Hsiao. 2005. "Privatization and Its Discontents—The Evolving Chinese Health Care System." *New England Journal of Medicine* 353: 1165–70.

Delnoij, D., and G. Brenner. 2000. "Importing Budget Systems from Other Countries: What Can We Learn from the German Drug Budget and the British GP Fundholding?" *Health Policy* 52 (3): 157–69.

Heller, P. S. 2006. "The Prospects of Creating 'Fiscal Space' for the Health Sector." *Health Policy and Planning* 21: 75–79.

Ikegami, N., S. Ikeda, and H. Kawai. 1998. "Why Medical Care Costs in Japan Have Increased Despite Declining Prices for Pharmaceuticals." *Pharmacoeconomics* 14 (S1): 97–105.

Ishikawa, K. 1988. *What Is Total Quality Control? The Japanese Way*. Translated by David J. Lu. Englewood Cliffs, NJ: Prentice Hall.

Juran, J. M., and A. B. Godfrey, eds. 1999. *Juran's Quality Handbook*. 5th ed. New York: McGraw-Hill.

Lancet. 2008. "MeTA: A Welcome Force for Access to Medicines." *Lancet* 371: 1724.

Mendis, S., K. Fukino, A. Cameron, R. Laing, A. Filipe, Jr., O. Khatib, J. Leowski, and M. Ewen. 2007. "The Availability and Affordability of Selected Essential Medicines for Chronic Diseases in Six Low- and Middle-Income Countries." *Bulletin of the World Health Organization* 84 (4): 279–88.

Musgrove, P. 2000. "A Critical Review of 'A Critical Review': The Methodology of the 1993 World Development Report, 'Investing in Health,'" *Health Policy and Planning* 15 (1): 110–15.

Roberts, M. J., W. C. Hsiao, P. Berman, and M. R. Reich. 2004. *Getting Health Reform Right: A Guide to Improving Performance and Equity*. New York: Oxford University Press.

Samuelson, P. A., and W. D. Nordhaus. 2009. *Microeconomics*. 19th ed. Boston, MA: Irwin/McGraw-Hill.

Taylor, R. S., M. F. Drummond, G. Salkeld, and S. D. Sullivan. 2004. "Inclusion of Cost Effectiveness in Licensing Requirements of New Drugs: The Fourth Hurdle." *British Medical Journal* 329: 972–75.

Van de Graaf, J. 1957. *Theoretical Welfare Economics*. Cambridge, U.K.: Cambridge University Press.

WHO (World Health Organization) and HAI (Health Action International). 2008. *Measuring Medicine Prices, Availability, Affordability and Price Components*. 2nd ed. Geneva: WHO and HAI.

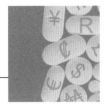

CHAPTER 3

Introduction to the Pharmaceutical Sector

Any effort to reform pharmaceutical policy must take into account several broad trends affecting the sector, especially patterns in the world pharmaceutical market, the emergence of new producers in middle-income countries, the drive toward consolidation in the research and development–oriented industry, and conflicts over product pricing. These trends shape the pharmaceutical problems that arise in low- and middle-income countries—the problems that policy reformers seek to resolve—and are related to both the market failures and the government failures described in chapter 2. We briefly review these four trends in the pharmaceutical sector to provide the broader context for our explanation of how to undertake pharmaceutical policy reform.

The World Pharmaceutical Market

The worldwide pharmaceutical industry is characterized by the concentration of consumption, production, and innovation in a relatively small number of high-income countries. In 2008, countries in North America and Europe, plus Japan, accounted for 82 percent of global pharmaceutical sales (by value) (IMS Health 2009a), and their share of production was even higher. During the 1980s and 1990s, the share of global production accounted for by high-income countries increased gradually, from 89.1 percent in 1985 to 92.9 percent in 1999 (WHO 2004, 5). Low-income countries accounted for less than 3 percent of the world's total pharmaceutical production (by value) in 1999. At the same time, pharmaceutical production in middle-income countries has been growing significantly, especially in India and China.

On the consumption side as well, middle-income countries are playing a larger role in the world pharmaceutical market. High-income markets showed slow growth (1 percent to 4 percent) in the early 21st century, and the U.S. pharmaceutical market actually declined by 1 percent to 2 percent in 2009, reflecting the effects of the economic crisis on demand and sales (IMS Health 2009b). Meanwhile, seventeen countries known as the "pharmerging" markets have been growing at rapid rates (13 percent to 16 percent) (including China, Brazil, India, the Russian Federation, Mexico, Turkey, Poland, República Bolivariana de Venezuela, Argentina, Indonesia, South Africa, Thailand, Romania, the Arab Republic of Egypt, Ukraine, Pakistan, and Vietnam, in descending order of market size) (IMSIHI 2011). China was the world's fifth-largest pharmaceutical market in 2009 and became the third-largest in 2011 (after the United States and Japan), with an annual growth rate estimated at 26 percent in 2008 (Campbell and Chui

Figure 3.1 Growth Forecasts for Global Pharmaceutical Sales by Region

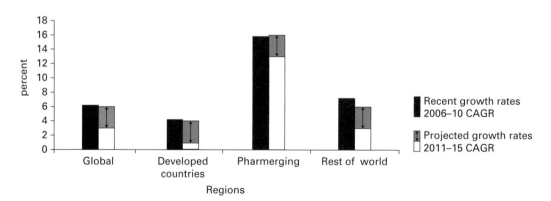

Note: CAGR is the compound annual growth rate expressed in U.S. dollars at constant exchange rates. Developed countries includes United States, Japan, Europe 5 (Germany, France, Italy, Spain, and the United Kingdom) plus Canada and the Republic of Korea. "Pharmerging" countries include China, Brazil, India, and Russia, plus 13 additional countries (Mexico, Turkey, Poland, República Bolivariana de Venezuela, Argentina, Indonesia, South Africa, Thailand, Romania, the Arab Republic of Egypt, Ukraine, Pakistan, and Vietnam, in descending order of market size). "Rest of world" is all other countries.
Source: IMSIHI 2011.

2010). Figure 3.1 shows recent growth rates and growth forecasts for global pharmaceutical sales by region. The double-digit-growth countries are now the strategic focus points for many multinational pharmaceutical companies. Global consumption of medicines by value is very unevenly distributed. As shown in figure 3.2, from the World Health Organization (WHO), high-income countries account for 16 percent of the world's population and 78.5 percent of total pharmaceutical expenditures. At the other end of the income scale, low-income countries account for 17.6 percent of the world's population and only 1 percent of total pharmaceutical expenditures. The differences reflect the huge disparities in per capita income and per capita spending on medicines, as well as huge differences in access to medicines and in the nature of the pharmaceutical markets (and health care) in those countries.

The growing importance of India, in particular, as a producer and exporter of medicines can be seen in figure 3.3, on the balance of trade in medicines by country. India has become a net exporter of medicines, while several high-income countries are net importers (such as the United States and Japan). China is also a major exporter, but it has remained a net importer, probably reflecting large volumes of imports of branded medicines. As India and China have become major exporters of medicines, especially off-patent medicines and bulk active ingredients, their internal policies have become

Figure 3.2 Distribution of Population and Total Pharmaceutical Expenditure by Country Income Level, 2005–06

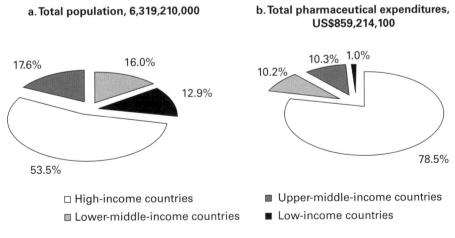

a. Total population, 6,319,210,000

17.6%   16.0%   12.9%   53.5%

b. Total pharmaceutical expenditures, US$859,214,100

10.2%   10.3%   1.0%   78.5%

□ High-income countries   ■ Upper-middle-income countries
▨ Lower-middle-income countries   ■ Low-income countries

Source: Lu et al. 2011.

Figure 3.3   Medicines in Countries' International Trade, Exports minus Imports, 2009

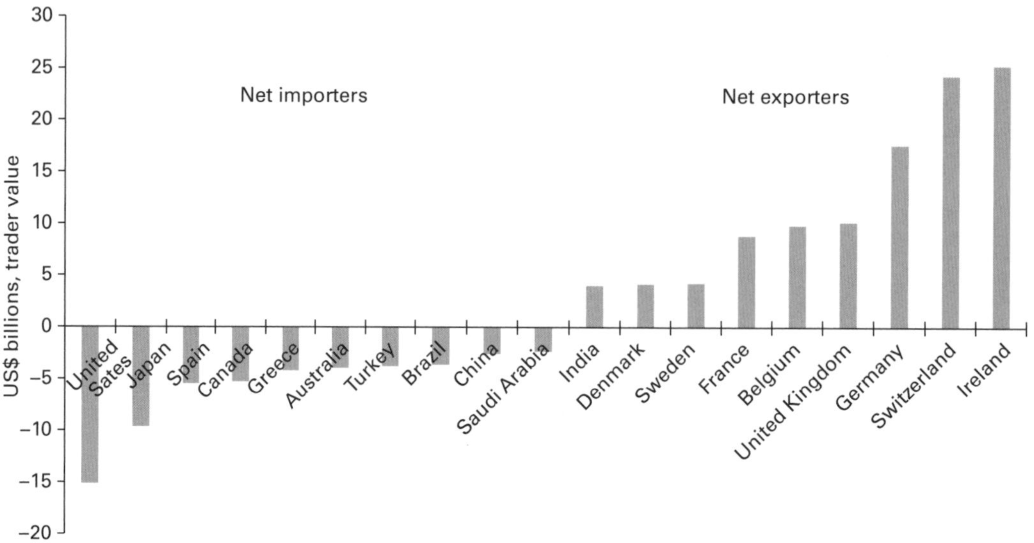

Source: UN Comtrade database, DESA/UNSD.

increasingly important to pharmaceutical policy in all countries around the world. In the United States, for example, the federal Food and Drug Administration (FDA) views the growing globalization of pharmaceutical manufacturing as a major risk for product safety, inasmuch as "the vast majority of medicines [in the United States] contain imported ingredients, increasingly obtained from suppliers in India and China" (Okie 2009). Ensuring quality in low- and middle-income countries is a major challenge because of their limited regulatory capacity, as discussed below.

For pharmaceutical research and development (R&D), high-income countries dominate expenditure in both the public and private sectors. In 2005, for example, 97 percent of health R&D occurred in high-income countries; pharmaceutical companies spent around US$80 billion on R&D in high-income countries and only about US$1.6 billion in low- and middle-income countries (Burke and Matlin 2008, 27–28). According to statistics from the Organization for Economic Cooperation and Development (OECD), shown in table 3.1, the U.S. government spent an amount equal to 0.22 percent of gross domestic product (GDP) on health-related R&D, while the U.S. pharmaceutical industry reportedly spent an amount equal to 0.3 percent of GDP on R&D. In several other high-income countries (Japan, France, and Germany), the pharmaceutical industry spent significantly more than the government on health-related research activities (OECD 2009). As a result of the dominance of both private and public

Pharmaceutical Reform

Table 3.1 R&D Expenditures by Government and the Pharmaceutical Industry in Selected High-Income Countries, 2008

Country	Government health R&D spending		Pharmaceutical industry R&D spending	
	% of GDP, 2008	US$ billions	% of GDP, 2006	US$ billions
Canada	0.095[a]	1.1	0.09	1.1
France	0.053	1.1	0.18	3.6
Germany	0.036	1.1	0.16	4.3
Japan	0.028	1.2	0.23	9.4
United States	0.220	31.8	0.30	39.6

Source: OECD 2009.

a. 2006 figure.

investment in pharmaceutical R&D in rich countries, five countries (the United States, United Kingdom, Japan, Germany, and France) account for a substantial portion of new pharmaceutical patents filed around the world. For example, these five countries accounted for 70 percent of pharmaceutical patents filed in 2004–06 under the Patent Co-operation Treaty, with the so-called BRIICS (Brazil, Russia, India, Indonesia, China, and South Africa) together accounting for about 5.5 percent, according to OECD data on health-related patents (OECD 2009).

The dominance of high-income countries in pharmaceutical R&D also affects the allocation of research funds toward conditions found in those markets. A substantial portion of pharmaceutical R&D is conducted by a relatively small number of multinational companies. Those companies have typically focused on the discovery and development of new chemical entities that can become "blockbuster" drugs. Blockbuster products are those that, while on patent, can achieve global sales over US$1 billion per year (almost entirely in rich-country markets) and produce significant profits for the originator company. This blockbuster business model has driven the economics and business strategies of the research-based pharmaceutical companies. These market dynamics help explain why the research-based companies have focused their research efforts and marketing forces on disease conditions in rich-country markets—where their products could be sold at high prices, with patent protection, for large numbers of patients, and often with health insurance coverage. The business model does not encourage spending limited R&D dollars on developing a new medicine that could be sold only to poor patients in poor countries at low prices, where most patients lack health insurance and must purchase medicines with their own money.

In recent years, however, the viability of the blockbuster business model has come into a growing question in the pharmaceutical industry, as the pipeline for new drugs has decreased and countries around the world have sought to control national health care costs, especially by limiting pharmaceutical expenditures and promoting generic substitution (*Economist* 2007). In 2011, the pharmaceutical industry confronted patent expirations on 10 blockbuster medicines that previously had global sales of around US$50 billion a year (Wilson 2011). All of the major companies are struggling to come up with new strategies to address the huge declines in sales revenue. Many pharmaceutical companies are turning to emerging markets: countries with large populations and market growth potential, especially those with expanding social health insurance and rising individual purchasing power (SustainAbility 2009, 2). This change creates both challenges and opportunities, especially for middle-income countries.

Figure 3.4 Evolution of the Pharmaceutical Sector in Countries of Different Income Levels

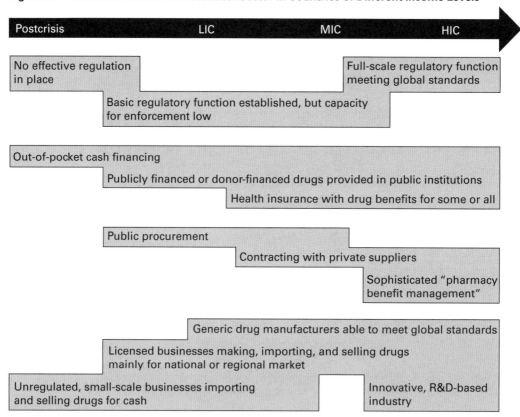

Source: Seiter 2010, 13.

Note: LIC = low-income country; MIC = middle-income country; HIC = high-income country; R&D = research and development.

In thinking about the world pharmaceutical market, one must recognize that production takes different forms in different countries. Manufacturers in the most sophisticated nations perform the full cycle of production activities: (1) manufacturing the active ingredients of medicines, (2) formulating the active ingredients into deliverable dosage forms, and (3) packaging the pills, capsules, or liquids into containers and boxes, labeled and ready for consumer sale. Production in low-income and many middle-income countries usually involves only the last two stages, as active ingredients are imported, along with other materials required for formulation. Even middle-income countries that produce some active ingredients focus mostly on small molecules—that is, on relatively simple medicines. These countries tend to avoid the large molecules characteristic of biotechnology products that are difficult to manufacture, although they are becoming more involved in this area and in vaccine production. This evolution of production capacity parallels other changes in the development of the pharmaceutical sector, shown in figure 3.4: growing capacity for effective regulation, shifts from out-of-pocket to public financing and health insurance, transitions in the organization of procurement, and transformation of the businesses involved in the sales and production of medicines. These dimensions of the evolution of the pharmaceutical sector are addressed in specific chapters in this book.

With the R&D-oriented companies focused on high-income markets, developing countries often have relied on other companies as their sources of medicines. Many imports into low- and middle-income markets come from other developing countries, as shown by the example of Uganda (63 percent from developing countries) in table 3.2. (It is worth noting,

Table 3.2   Top 10 Pharmaceutical Importing Countries in Africa, 1998

Importer	Industrialized country sources (US$ millions)	Developing country sources (US$ millions)	Imports from developing countries as % of total
South Africa	565	36	6.0
Tunisia	164	8	4.7
Nigeria	79	39	33.1
Kenya	78	27	25.7
Uganda	20	34	63.0
Senegal	49	2	3.9
Tanzania	19	22	53.7
Mauritius	32	6	15.8
Madagascar	13	3	18.8
Togo	13	1	7.1

Source: Bale 2001, 17.

however, that a few African countries nonetheless imported substantial portions of their pharmaceutical supplies from industrialized countries, for example, Senegal at 96 percent and Togo at 93 percent, as shown in table 3.2.) Until 2005, the developing country sources of supply benefited from the lack of product patents in national laws; that allowed products to be copied, manufactured, and exported with impunity. Similarly, the importing countries did not require product patents for medicines, so the products could be legally imported.

In recent years, China and India have moved steadily up the value chain through massive investments in the pharmaceutical industry and research capacity. These two countries have become increasingly important producers not only of generic products (for domestic markets and exports) but also of biopharmaceuticals (large-molecule products), and they export active ingredients for all sorts of medicines for formulation by companies around the world (Attridge and Preker 2005). The changing structure of the global pharmaceutical market has important implications for all aspects of pharmaceutical policy in low- and middle-income countries.

Consolidation of Research and Development Companies

Recent years have witnessed a steady consolidation among the world's leading R&D-based pharmaceutical firms, and larger and larger agglomerations have been formed. Much of the merger activity has combined individually significant firms. As one of many examples, SmithKlineFrench and Beecham merged into SmithKline Beecham; Glaxo Holdings and Burroughs Wellcome merged to form Glaxo Wellcome; and then those two new companies merged to form GlaxoSmithKline, now known as GSK. Consolidation has also taken the form of large companies' buying up smaller ones that had developed expertise in a specific therapeutic area or a promising product that seemed ready for the marketplace. In some cases, larger companies have purchased a small company to block a competitive product from reaching the market; in others, a large company has purchased a small company to bring a promising medicine to a global market. In recent years, consolidation has reduced the number of major companies in the global pharmaceutical industry from 22 in 1993 to 8 in 2009 (Singer 2009).

Three major reasons explain the trend toward consolidation. First, research-based companies perceive advantages in risk-spreading and portfolio diversification. As in the stock market, a diversified portfolio of investments produces less-variable returns over the long run because some stocks will do better even when others are faring worse. For research-based companies, that principle translates to a similar incentive: to assemble a large portfolio of research and development projects to ensure that it will have enough successes to support long-run corporate growth. As the cost of developing successful new products increases, the size of R&D investments needed to reach that goal increases steadily. Indeed, diversification requires spreading investments over relatively distinct realms of activity. So, to use a hypothetical example, a company with a strong portfolio of cardiac products might seek a merger with one competent in psychopharmacology to gain the advantages of diversification.

Second, consolidation allows companies to take advantage of economies of scale in marketing. A given sales representative can, in theory, effectively pitch a range of products in a single sales call. Similarly, a company's national sales office can often negotiate with the government and wholesalers for a broader range of products without much added cost. A manufacturer with a broader product range is also better positioned to negotiate favorable treatment from wholesalers and others in the distribution chain.

A third explanation lies in the economics of innovation over time. For at least a century, economists have known that the opportunities for innovation in a given industrial area vary over time in what have been called "long waves" (Atkinson 2004). The late 19th century, for example, was dominated by opportunities connected to railroads, steamships, and steel. The early 20th century was the time of automobiles, steel, and oil. The middle of the 20th century revolved around automobiles, home appliances, telephones, and aircraft. The late 20th century marked the beginning of the era of consumer electronics (and the rise of cell phones and the Internet), as well as aircraft and pharmaceuticals.

The current question is, Which industries will drive innovation and growth in the first half of the 21st century? Some observers of the international pharmaceutical industry believe that its best days are behind it and question whether the blockbuster model will be able to sustain the research-oriented companies in the near future. Many chronic conditions (cardiac diseases, diabetes, and depression) already can be treated by relatively effective medicines—many of which have recently come off patent. Although tuberculosis, HIV, and malaria cannot yet be treated by inexpensive magic bullet medicines, some effective therapeutic options exist for all these diseases.

Cancer treatment is a promising area given the increasing number of patients and the absence of effective treatments. But the genetic variation among different strains of cancer suggests that the future of that industry may lie in small markets for very expensive, personalized medicines that respond to a particular patient's cancer cells.

In recent years, as the research-oriented companies have searched for new markets, they have also pushed toward expanding the sale of patent-protected, originator-branded products in low- and middle-income countries, especially in the "pharmerging" markets, where double-digit growth is occurring. It is true that in many low-income countries, the highest-priced brand-name products are consumed mainly by the urban middle class. However, as these sales expand, purchases of such higher-priced medicines can create significant financial burdens for buyers, especially those at lower income levels. The trend also raises serious ethical and business strategy questions for the companies with respect to how to set prices across countries with dramatically different levels of per capita GNP.

The continuing consolidation of the research-oriented companies has complex implications for low- and middle-income countries. In the face of rising competition from firms based in India and China, the major Western companies are seeking to remain a dominant force in the global industry. Whether they can increase their sales of medicines in low- and middle-income countries depends at least in part on their pricing strategies, to which we turn next.

Pharmaceutical Pricing

Manufacturers of on-patent compounds face a pricing problem that is much discussed in introductory economics textbooks, that of a *discriminating monopolist*. Such a manufacturer can set the price it charges for that product and thus is a *price maker* (subject, of course to government policies such as price controls). A producer in a competitive market, however, has to sell at the existing market price to compete with other, identical products and thus is a *price taker*.

Monopolists maximize profits by taking into account how much buyers are influenced by price, known as the "price elasticity of demand," in each market. The less sensitive demand is to price, the higher is the optimum price in that market. A discriminating monopolist will keep increasing the price in each market until the revenue that would be lost from discouraged sales (if prices were increased a bit more) begins to exceed the revenue that would be gained from charging a higher price on the items that are still sold. This logic (also known as "differential pricing") shows that it can be in a manufacturer's interest to offer lower prices in poorer countries where demand is more price sensitive. Selling a product at a lower price in such markets generates more total profits because the higher volume that it creates outweighs the smaller profit per unit sold. (Note that this is true as long as the price charged by the monopolist is above the marginal cost of producing added units of the product, which is generally the case since that cost is typically quite low for medicines based on simple molecules.)

A number of problems affect how that general theory of differential pricing works in practice in the pharmaceutical sector. First, prices paid by end-user purchasers are typically much higher than the manufacturer's selling price because middlemen and distributors add their own margins to the selling price to secure their own profits. Monopolists have to take these effects into account when they set wholesale prices. Second, companies have to guard against the possibility that medicines sold in low-price markets will be resold into higher-price markets (a process termed "parallel imports"). That would threaten to reduce the monopolist's higher-profit sales in the higher-price markets. Third, companies also fear that richer countries will use the prices in poor countries as a basis for reducing prices in their own markets. That can occur either through the regulatory mechanism known as "reference pricing" (discussed below) or if the countries use information about how much less others pay as a bargaining device in their own price negotiations with the manufacturers. A major challenge then becomes the extent to which the companies follow the logic of differential pricing; that is, how do companies decide to price their products in different markets? Do they lower their prices in poorer countries to achieve a larger market share?

Even producers of on-patent products, however, do not always choose to act as classic monopolists. When the first of a new class of medicines proves promising in introductory clinical trials, other manufacturers often try to develop similar medicines that are just different enough to produce a patentable product. That is the reason popular drug categories such as statins for cholesterol control, SSRIs for depression, and ACE inhibitors for hypertension have so many pharmacologically similar products.

These "me-too" drugs, as they are often called, are typically released a few years after the "first-in-class" medicine along the path of development and adoption. The leading drug has great "first-mover advantages," as it develops publicity for its breakthrough status, and physicians and patients become familiar with its use before it has any imitators. The imitators, in contrast, face the difficult marketing challenge of winning doctors and patients away from using a medicine with which they are already familiar. In addition, head-to-head clinical trials that compare competing medicines are rare, so that only limited evidence is available to show the incremental benefits of newer products. To develop a competitive advantage, new entrants are sometimes designed to be simpler to take and manage. The followers also typically set their prices somewhat below the price of the first product. As those medicines develop their own reputations, their presence in the marketplace can force the market leader into price reductions. In effect, the demand for the original product becomes more price sensitive as other, similar products create competition.

When a patent expires, it then becomes legal for other companies to produce the same molecule as a *generic*, and the price of the originator medicine is forced down even more. However, the price premium that the name-brand medicine commands often does not entirely disappear. (After all, Coca-Cola typically sells at higher prices than local brands of soda, based on its brand recognition and not on patents.) In some markets, the first-in and well-promoted generics can themselves establish a significant brand identity as branded generics. These can create variation among generic prices for the same medicine in many markets. In short, even after patents expire, the prices of pharmaceutical products with the same active ingredient do not behave as would be predicted by the model of perfect competition; all sorts of price differentials persist. In addition, debates persist about quality differences that may exist among the originator product (off-patent), branded generics, and nonbranded generics—making it a challenge for government agencies, as well as individual consumers, in low- and middle-income countries to decide which products to purchase at which prices.

Research-based companies use various strategies to minimize the price erosion that occurs when a product goes off patent. The original product can be remarketed in new dosage forms (for example, in slow-release form) or as part of a product with a combination of ingredients. Companies often then seek patents for the new offerings, to extend the product's patent life, in a process known as "patent evergreening" (Kesselheim and Avorn 2006). Another strategic response is for research-based companies to form alliances with generic manufacturers or establish their own generic subsidiaries. The companies then compete with both on-patent and off-patent products, which allows them to continue production of certain medicines after the patent has expired, as branded generics. The expansion of research-oriented companies into generic competition has important implications for low- and middle-income countries because those markets (especially those with economic growth) are potential targets for multinational companies.

As some major R&D firms are diversifying downward into the generic market, some generic firms are diversifying upward. That is especially true of some of the larger producers in the major middle-income countries, such as India, China, and Brazil. Some companies in those countries are increasing their research capacity and their ability to produce new or more sophisticated active ingredients. They do that with the hope not only of offering generic versions of the most sophisticated chemical entities, but also of creating new molecules that can be patented and sold in higher-income markets in the future.

The Role of National Policy

National policy affects the pharmaceutical sector in multiple ways. National policy on patents—especially whether the country protects product patents or only process patents—establishes some basic market rules, which are especially important to multinational R&D-based companies as well as the domestic manufacturing industry. National policy on trademarks and copyright protection is central to determining whether generic off-patent producers promote their branded generics. Government decision making also shapes the distribution chain for medicines. To varying degrees, governments approve products for sale, control import and export, regulate product quality, decide which are covered by national health insurance schemes, decide on prices for retail sales of medicines, control access through prescription standards, and shape the distribution system by licensing pharmacists and pharmacies and other retail outlets. Moreover, many countries operate extensive public health care sectors, so governments are directly engaged in acquisition, supply chain management, and dispensing activities.

The Patent System

The core idea of the patent system is a "deal" with inventors. The system provides a potentially very profitable period of exclusive rights, in exchange for public disclosure of the technology to promote general scientific progress. It provides both an incentive to invest in developing new technology and (through the profits it generates) a source of funds to support such research. This kind of system was first put in place in Venice in the 15th century and was formalized in England under James I, with the promulgation of a Statute of Monopolies in 1632. Patents are a tool of industrial policy, supporting efforts by governments to influence economic or industrial development.

Patent law has always been a matter of national government determination, but with some degree of international coordination. The Paris Convention for the Protection of Industrial Property, a treaty signed in 1883, began the process of coordinating rules across countries. In general, to receive patent protection in different countries an inventor must apply separately to each relevant national authority. However, in 1994, as part of the Uruguay Round of negotiations in connection with the international treaty called the

General Agreement on Tariffs and Trade (GATT), a subsidiary agreement on intellectual property was reached. This treaty is called TRIPS, the Agreement on Trade-Related Aspects of Intellectual Property Rights, and it covers patents, trademarks, and copyright for artistic products, music, and other forms of intellectual property. TRIPS is administered by the World Trade Organization (WTO). The WTO also has some quasi-judicial functions to resolve international trade and intellectual property disputes. Signing on to TRIPS is a precondition for admission to the WTO. Membership in the WTO confers such substantial trade advantages that all nations that can meet the conditions for membership have joined.

In the late 1990s, however, a number of low- and middle-income countries, with support from international AIDS activists, protested against the use of TRIPS to maintain high prices for on-patent medicines, particularly antiretrovirals (ARVs) for treating HIV. They argued that such prices were especially unacceptable in countries where the health consequences would be extremely damaging—for example, in low-income countries with many HIV patients. In response, in 2001 international bargaining produced the Doha Declaration (WTO 2001). The statement clarified TRIPS guidelines with regard to pharmaceuticals. In particular, the Doha Declaration affirms that WTO member states have the "right to protect public health and, in particular, to promote access to medicines for all." The statement explicitly notes that countries have the right to use the provisions in TRIPS that provide "flexibility" to meet urgent public health goals. A key element is the use of compulsory licensing to expand access to medicines still on patent.

The Doha Declaration also extended until 2016 the WTO requirement that the least-developed countries implement product patents for pharmaceuticals. The statement specified that countries can use the mechanism of compulsory licensing to allow domestic production without permission of the patent holder (but with payment of a royalty fee). It also recognized the need to address the problem of countries with insufficient manufacturing facilities to use compulsory licensing. On August 30, 2003, the WTO issued a decision that allowed for an additional mechanism to address this problem by permitting manufacturing to be done outside the country seeking relief (WTO 2003). However, there have been significant problems in implementing this approach.

Not all nations effectively enforce or adhere to TRIPS for pharmaceuticals (or other forms of intellectual property). Nonenforcement can give a country and its domestic industry significant short-term economic advantages. However, in cases of TRIPS violations, the offended nation can take the case to the WTO for arbitration. A number of complex disputes between producing countries and major Indian and Chinese producers over alleged TRIPS violations are ongoing.

Regulatory Roles

In addition to patents, governments use national policy to impose many kinds of regulation on the pharmaceutical sector, addressing product registration, distribution, licensing, and prescribing and dispensing. WHO identifies many areas of activity for a national regulatory authority (WHO 2007), which are discussed in more detail in chapter 10. A few key regulatory roles are the following:

- *Product registration.* Government regulation of safety and efficacy is critical in deciding which products can be legally sold and used within a country. Government policies determine the kinds of documentation and scientific evidence that a manufacturer must submit to have a product approved for use in a country. Policies on rescinding product registration for ineffective or dangerous medicines are also important for protecting consumers.

- *Licensing of importers, exporters, wholesalers, and distributors.* Countries regulate the different middlemen involved in the medicine supply chain and the roles they play. In some countries, a relatively small number of importers and wholesalers dominate the importing and distribution of medicines, limiting competition in the market. Some governments, such as the Philippines, have intervened in this kind of situation to counteract cartel behavior in the distribution chain. In other places (especially in sub-Saharan Africa), some faith-based nongovernmental organizations do their own importing and have their own distribution systems.

- *Licensing of pharmacies and retail outlets.* Governments largely shape the role and functioning of pharmacies and retail outlets in the pharmaceutical sector. In Germany, for example, government policy has prevented the growth of chain pharmacies. In many low-income countries, the final distribution points are numerous and relatively unregulated, as private sellers of medicines proliferate in both the formal and informal sectors. Corruption is a challenge in many countries, as bribes and kickbacks influence the behavior of pharmacy operators, physicians, and health care administrators (Cohen, Mrazek, and Hawkins 2007). The nature of medicines makes effective control difficult: They are portable, high-value products; they can easily be diverted from official distribution channels, particularly at the periphery (where staff have low wages and limited supervision and may be tempted to use or sell medicines privately); and their quality is difficult to ascertain without sophisticated testing facilities and scientific knowledge.

- *Prescribing and dispensing.* Governments also use national policy to regulate who can prescribe and who can dispense medicines. A regulatory agency is also typically responsible for the licensing of pharmacy personnel. Several Asian countries—including Japan; the Republic of Korea; and Taiwan, China—have historically allowed doctors to both prescribe and dispense medicines. In recent years these countries have adopted national policies to separate prescribing from dispensing, with different approaches and consequences in the three (Eggleston 2009).

Broader Health Policy

Broader policy decisions also influence the development and functioning of the pharmaceutical sector. These include trade policy, industrial policy, health insurance policy, and advertising policy. For example, in Japan, reimbursement policy for medicines (by the social insurance system) supported the development of the national pharmaceutical industry, creating a focus more on national than on international markets (Reich 1990). In India, the Patent Act of 1970 denied recognition of product patents but allowed process patents. This drove multinational firms to leave the country and contributed to the development of the Indian generic pharmaceutical industry. That eventually allowed India to become self-sufficient in pharmaceuticals and then a major exporter around the world.

Summary on the Pharmaceutical Sector

This chapter has presented four broad trends in the pharmaceutical sector that shape the context of pharmaceutical policy reform in low- and middle-income countries. Most low-income countries represent a very small share of the global pharmaceutical market, giving them limited leverage in negotiations over prices (when purchasing medicines) and other matters. But the structure of the global market is shifting, and several middle-income countries are enlarging their participation in both production and consumption and in the processes of agenda setting for global pharmaceutical issues. National reformers need to take these broader market factors into account—along with the many substantive challenges of national pharmaceutical policy, especially in the regulatory arena—as they seek to change national policy to improve performance in this sector. The next chapter considers some of the basic strategies of problem definition for pharmaceutical policy reform and the grounding of those problem definitions in different ethical traditions.

References

Atkinson, R. D. 2004. *The Past and Future of America's Economy: Long Waves of Innovation that Drive Cycles of Growth.* Northampton, MA: Edward Elgar.

Attridge, C. J., and A. S. Preker. 2005. "Improving Access to Medicines in Developing Countries: Application of New Institutional Economics to the Analysis of Manufacturing and Distribution Issues." HNP Discussion Paper, World Bank, Washington, DC.

Bale, H. E., Jr. 2001. "Consumption and Trade in Off-Patented Medicines." Working Paper No. 65. Indian Council for Research on International Economic Relations, New Delhi, India. http://www.icrier.org/pdf/bale65.PDF.

Burke, M. A., and S. A. Matlin, eds. 2008. *Monitoring Financial Flows for Health Research 2008.* Geneva: Global Forum for Health Research.

Campbell, D., and M. Chui. 2010. "Pharmerging Shake-up: New Imperatives in a Redefined World." Norwalk, CT: IMS Health.

Cohen, J. C., M. Mrazek, and L. Hawkins. 2007. "Tackling Corruption in the Pharmaceutical Systems Worldwide with Courage and Conviction." *Clinical Pharmacology and Therapeutics* 81: 445–49.

Economist. 2007. "Beyond the Blockbuster." June 28.

Eggleston, K., ed. 2009. *Prescribing Cultures and Pharmaceutical Policy in the Asia-Pacific.* Washington, DC: Brookings Institution.

IMS Health. 2009a. "IMS Market Prognosis." March. Parsippany, NJ.

———. 2009b. "IMS Health Lowers 2009 Global Pharmaceutical Market Forecast to 2.5–3.5 Percent Growth." News Release, April 22. Parsippany, NJ.

IMSIHI (IMS Institute for Healthcare Informatics). 2011. "The Global Use of Medicines: Outlook Through 2015." Parsippany, NJ.

Kesselheim, A. S., and J. Avorn. 2006. "Biomedical Patents and the Public's Health: Is There a Role for Eminent Domain?" *New England Journal of Medicine* 295 (4): 434–37.

Lu, Y., P. Hernandez, D. Abegunde, and T. Edejer. 2011. "Medicine Expenditures." In *The World Medicines Situation 2011.* Geneva: WHO. Available at http://www.who.int/medicines/areas/policy/world_medicines_situation/en/index.html.

OECD (Organization for Economic Cooperation and Development). 2009. "Health-related R&D." In *Science, Technology, and Industry Scoreboard.* Paris: OECD Publishing. http://dx.doi.org/10.1787/sti_scoreboard-2009-21-en.

Okie, S. 2009. "Multinational Manufacturing—Ensuring Drug Quality in an Era of Global Manufacturing." *New England Journal of Medicine* 361 (8): 737–40.

Reich, M. 1990. "Why the Japanese Don't Export More Pharmaceuticals: Health Policy as Industrial Policy." *California Management Review* 32 (2): 124–50.

Seiter, A. 2010. *A Practical Approach to Pharmaceutical Policy.* Washington, DC: World Bank.

Singer N. 2009. "Merck-Schering Merger Awaits Reaction from Johnson & Johnson," *New York Times,* March 13, B6.

SustainAbility. 2009. *Pharma Futures 3: Emerging Opportunities.* London: SustainAbility.

UN Comtrade (United Nations Commodity Trade Statistics) Database. United Nations Department of Economic and Social Affairs/Statistics Division, New York. http://comtrade.un.org/db

Wilson, D. 2011. "Drug Firms Face Billions in Losses in '11 as Patents End," *New York Times.* March 7, A1.

WHO (World Health Organization). 2004. *World Medicines Situation.* Geneva: WHO.

———. 2007. *WHO Data Collection Tool for the Review of Drug Regulatory Systems* (WHO/TCM/MRS/2007.1). Geneva: WHO.

WTO (World Trade Organization). 2001. "Declaration on TRIPS and Public Health" (WT/MIN(01)/DEC/2). World Trade Organization, Ministerial Conference, Doha, November 20.

———. 2003. "Implementation of Paragraph 6 of the Doha Declaration on the TRIPS Agreement and Public Health," Decision of August 30 (WT/L/540). Geneva: WTO.

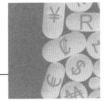

CHAPTER 4

Ethics and Priority Setting in Pharmaceutical Reform

Chapter 2 discussed the need to begin the process of pharmaceutical reform by focusing on where the performance of the pharmaceutical system is inadequate and using those performance failures to set priorities for improvement. We stressed the essential role of both politics and ethics in that process, and indeed throughout the reform cycle. Chapter 6 explores how politics influences the reform process and how reformers can act more effectively in the political realm. This chapter turns to the role of ethics. Let us suppose that reformers want to do not only what is politically attractive and feasible but also what is *right*. How can such priorities and courses of action be identified?

"Benchmarking" is one approach to priority setting that is widely discussed in the quality management literature (Berwick 1989; Bullivant 1996). The core idea is simple. Quality managers often confront questions such as, What rate of defects should we accept? The benchmarking approach counsels that they should aim for a rate of performance (a benchmark) comparable to that of acknowledged industry leaders. The argument is that such a rate of performance ought to be achievable with reasonable effort. Although some have advocated a "zero defects" approach to quality (Crosby 1979), the calculation implicit in most benchmarking efforts is that successive steps in improving performance are likely to be increasingly costly. Economists call this idea "diminishing marginal returns." So rates of performance that others achieve show us what is feasible in both cost and technical terms.

The strategic idea implicit in benchmarking is that it is better for a company (or a country) to focus improvement efforts where it does badly, rather than where it already does relatively well. That approach is often sensible, but not always. Sometimes a company (or a country) should play to its strengths and, even if it is already the industry (or regional) leader in some arena, strive to do even better in that realm. For example, a country with high levels of availability of essential medicines in public clinics in general might want to focus attention on the few medicines that they do not do so well with—especially if those are important for health outcomes. In short, benchmarking can be helpful to assess the feasibility of different goals, but it cannot substitute for an informed and conscious choice of priorities.

Four forms of benchmarking can help policy makers decide on pharmaceutical reform priorities:

- *External benchmarking.* External benchmarking is based on emulating another country. For example, a country could decide to try to reduce the amount of counterfeit drugs in private retail outlets (as determined by an appropriate survey) to the level achieved by the best-performing country in the region. The caveat here is that it makes the most sense to pick a country that is similar with regard to culture, geography, politics, and resources, if a nation wants to use benchmarking as way to test the feasibility of choosing certain goals as priorities.

- *Internal benchmarking.* This approach uses variations in a country's own performance to set benchmarks. For example, a country might try to bring stock-out levels in all rural health centers down to the performance levels of the best districts.

- *Historic benchmarking.* This approach can be useful in postconflict, disaster recovery, or postcrisis situations. The goal is returning the nation to where it was before the adverse events occurred.

- *Ideal benchmarking.* Ideal benchmarking transforms the process from a tool for feasibility assessment to a priority-setting exercise driven by political or ethical ambitions. The experience of efforts to meet the Millennium Development Goals (an example of an ideal benchmark) illustrates such a situation.

This brief discussion shows that formulating national pharmaceutical policy is much more complicated than dealing with quality improvement in a corporate context. A nation trying to improve pharmaceutical sector performance is not like an appliance manufacturer trying to minimize repair costs and improve customer perceptions of quality to maximize profits. Pharmaceutical reformers face multiple possible objectives that are likely to conflict, a variety of complicated processes and subsystems, numerous interest groups, and complex equity considerations. Deciding what to do requires that reformers think carefully about what they care about and what they *should* care about. That brings us to a discussion, first, of the priorities for pharmaceutical sector improvement that often are chosen, and second, to consideration of the role of ethics in that process.

Commonly Identified Pharmaceutical Sector Problems

In our experience, countries often do not formulate their pharmaceutical sector problems in terms of failure to meet the ultimate performance goals discussed in chapter 2. Instead, after a largely implicit diagnostic analysis, they tend to identify certain process issues as "the problem." This section turns to those typical formulations and relates them to the ultimate performance goals that we have suggested and to various ethical ideas that are often assumed or implied in such discussions.

As noted in chapter 1, in low-income countries the bulk of pharmaceutical spending (more than 75 percent) occurs in the private sector, mostly in out-of-pocket outlays by households. Hence reformers concerned about access to medicines often focus appropriately on opportunities to improve performance in both the public and private sectors, as well as on their interaction.

Commonly identified private sector problems involve the products that are provided and the prices that customers pay. These are often linked to the nature of the advice that buyers receive, inasmuch as medicines are often sold in relatively informal settings where dispensers have little or no technical training. On the product side, a number of concerns are frequently expressed. Substandard and counterfeit products may be prevalent in the private sector (see case study G, "Counterfeit Medicines in Nigeria"). Inappropriate use is common. That includes the overuse of unneeded antibiotics and not taking the full course of those medications; the use of injections over oral administration; overuse of psychoactive medicines; and the use of unhelpful elixirs and herbal remedies. Too often dispensers push expensive on-patent or originator-branded products instead of equally effective (and cheaper) generics.

The purchase of needlessly expensive products produces high out-of-pocket spending, which imposes financial burdens on consumers. In many low-income countries, prices are higher than international reference prices, which serve as a benchmark for reasonable price levels. In addition, those prices are high enough, relative to local low-income wages, to pose significant affordability problems (Cameron et al. 2009). One often-cited explanation for those prices is high private sector markups that accumulate as products move through successive stages of the distribution system. Noncompetitive market structures at various points in the production and distribution chain are also blamed for those markups and for high prices generally.

Complaints about poor public sector performance typically focus on availability. Supply chain failures and high levels of stock-outs are a frequently identified problem. Observers also complain about high costs and delays in public procurement and about the poor quality of the products that are acquired. In addition, there is the question of whether governments can afford certain expensive medicines (especially antiretrovirals [ARVs] and artemisinin-based combination therapies [ACTs]), which are effective but whose normal international price puts them beyond the reach of low-income country budgets. The selection of products available in the public sector has also been contentious in some contexts, particularly whether a country's essential medicines list should or should not include new and expensive on-patent products (Heuser 2009) (see case study A, "Defining an Essential Medicines List in Sudamerica"). Less frequently, some countries have focused on inappropriate overuse in the public sector. That is sometimes attributed to the absence of co-pays or to the desire of clinic providers to move patients through as quickly as possible.

Other problems that have been identified are farther up the causal chain; in effect they are explanations of the problems already discussed. For example, some reformers focus on consumers, on their relative lack of information, their irrationality, or their poverty, as the causes of poor choices, and the magnitude of their financial burdens. Others focus on government policies that increase medicines prices. Examples here include retail taxes on pharmaceuticals and efforts to promote domestic producers even at the expense of higher costs (and lower quality). Still others point to general governmental weaknesses (corruption, low salaries, and poor management) as explanations of both inadequate direct provision and faulty regulation of the private sector.

Relating Identified Problems to Performance Goals

How do all of these different problems relate to the ultimate performance goals reviewed in chapter 3?

As figure 4.1 shows, the connections are numerous and overlapping. One way to summarize the preceding paragraphs is to say that reformers tend to focus on four major problems: (1) high out-of-pocket spending caused by high prices and the purchase of inappropriately expensive products in the private sector; (2) poor private sector quality; (3) poor public sector availability; and (4) underuse, overuse, and misuse. As figure 4.1 suggests, all of these problems affect health status, given the potential health benefits of appropriate drug use. Two of the four—high spending due to high private sector prices and poor public sector availability—also affect both satisfaction and financial protection and do so with strong interaction effects. When drugs are not available in the public sector, citizens turn to the private sector, leading to both dissatisfaction and a lack of financial protection. Poor quality of medicines affects both health and satisfaction, although it only decreases satisfaction to the extent that consumers are aware of those failings. Finally, overuse and underuse are mainly problems from a health status perspective. Indeed, such problems may even reflect (or, in a sense, cause) an increase in satisfaction because of actual consumer preferences.

It is also important to address the distribution of these outcomes. In particular, the lack of financial protection caused by high private sector prices disproportionately affects low-income families. Similarly, the lack of availability of medicines in the public sector is likely to be of most concern for those families, since higher-income citizens can afford to purchase private sector medicines. Availability problems are likely to have a geographic as well as an economic dimension. For example, such prob-

Figure 4.1   The Relationship of Pharmaceutical Sector Problems to Ultimate Performance Goals

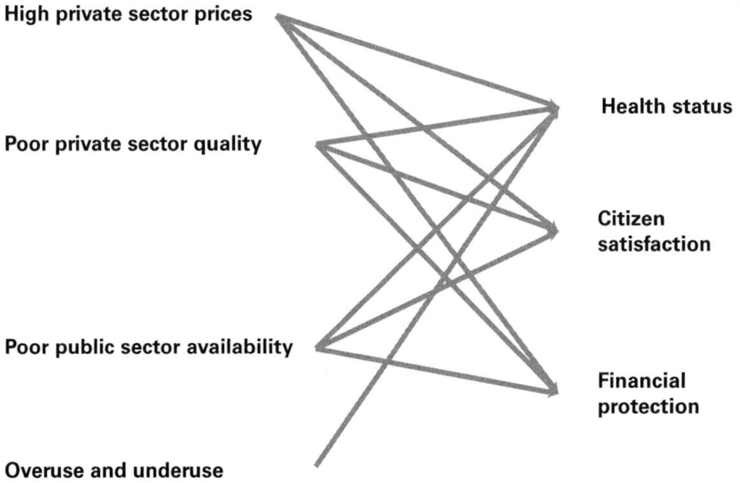

Source: Authors' representation.

lems are often worse in rural areas and at the periphery, where people are also more likely to be poor.

Certain quality problems are also likely to be more acute for particular groups, especially those with less education or income. For example, rural areas often have fewer private outlets, so that the lack of competition limits the disciplining effect of market forces on both quality and price.

Relating Performance Goals to Ethical Perspectives: Utilitarianism

All three main outcomes of the pharmaceutical sector that we have identified are in the spirit of one of the dominant lines of thinking on the ethics of public policy. That perspective, which says that policies should be judged by their consequences, not surprisingly is called "consequentialism." Putting the argument that way, however, only leads to a second question, namely, Which consequences? Here, the answer that has had the greatest impact on European and American thinking, and on policy debates worldwide, is a perspective known as "utilitarianism." Its most influential advocates were John Stuart Mill and Jeremy Bentham, 19th-century British social reformers and moral philosophers (Roberts and Reich 2002).

Reflecting the effects of the Enlightenment and the Protestant Reformation, Mill and Bentham took a highly individualistic approach. They argued that the consequences that should matter were the levels of well-being of all the individuals affected by a policy. Eager to rescue arguments about what was good or bad from religious traditionalists, they sought to make social policy scientifically. So they asserted that the right way to take account of all the effects of a policy was to add up the gains and losses to everyone involved. The right policy, in Bentham's well-known phrase, came from doing "the greatest good for the greatest number."

That leads to a further critical question: How were changes in well-being to be measured and added up? Mill's and Bentham's answer again reflects their goal of empowering ordinary people against self-proclaimed moral authorities from the church or the aristocracy. They argued that each person had an internal level of happiness or well-being that could be measured. And it was that *subjective* state—which they called "utility"—that was to be central for policy making. Hence the name, *utilitarianism*.

This point of view is represented in our framework by including citizens' satisfaction with their access to and use of pharmaceuticals as a performance goal. It is also reflected in much of modern economic theory, which says that the right way to allocate resources is to respond to market demand and give people what they want, as revealed by what they are willing to pay for. Thus economists often advocate for significant co-pays for drugs on the grounds that low or zero prices encourage overuse. By this they mean uses that are not sufficiently valuable to the users because those users do not have to pay prices that fully reflect the costs of producing the goods that they consume (Bator 1957). (Of course, that is not the same as uses that have no medical value.)

However, pharmaceutical policy making illustrates the problems that can arise from taking this kind of utilitarianism too uncritically. Do we really want to formulate policy only to respond to people's preferences, even when they are confused or mistaken about antibiotics or injections, or the efficacy of generics, or the treatment of HIV?

Moreover, how is utility to be measured (assuming that it even exists, which most psychologists doubt)? The economist's answer is to measure utility by determining individuals' "willingness to pay" for various goods. But that approach both reflects and reinforces economic inequalities. Regardless of the value to them, poor people are typically willing to pay less for a good than rich people exactly because they are poor. Thus if we formulate public pharmaceutical policy to respond to willingness to pay, pharmaceuticals will flow disproportionately to upper-income individuals, just as they do in actual markets. And there really are no other practical ways to measure utility that we can use to add up gains and losses across a population.

This original form of utilitarianism is often called "subjective" or "hedonistic" utilitarianism, reflecting its focus on what people feel. A widely used alternative does not focus on people's internal, subjective feelings but on their objective situations. It argues that too many people are too uninformed to know what is really good for them. So instead of decentralizing the process of identifying and assigning value to each individual, as Mill and Bentham wanted to do, objective utilitarians centralize the process. They want a group of experts to construct an index that measures well-being in a way that can be observed and added up. Their approach draws less on economics and more on engineering, as well as on various kinds of operations research and systems analysis done for the military during and after World War II.

Prominent examples of that thinking are the Quality Adjusted Life Years (QALY) and Disability Adjusted Life Years (DALY) indexes that are often used to guide decisions on health policy and resource allocation. They form the backbone, for example, of the work of the National Institute for Health and Clinical Excellence (NICE) in the United Kingdom, which has been very active in advising the National Health Service on which procedures and which pharmaceuticals to provide (Claxton, Schulpher, and Drummond 2002). Similarly, under the national disease management program in Germany, IQWiG, the German equivalent of NICE, establishes expert panels that develop clinical guidelines for drug use. And those panels are explicitly instructed to take cost-effectiveness into account (Drummond and Rutten 2008).

In the Flagship Framework, the prominent role of health status as an ultimate goal is a reflection of the objective utilitarian perspective. Within pharmaceutical policy making, however, tensions have repeatedly arisen between that view and the subjective utilitarian desire to give people what they want. Indeed, it is not just a matter of allowing people to choose drugs that are pleasing to them but harmless. Responding to patient demand may actually do harm. For example, patient-driven polypharmacy (using many different medicines at the same time) can expose patients to adverse drug interactions. The harm can extend beyond the patient to populations, as noted previously. Not taking a full course of antiretrovirals or antibiotics and the inappropriate overuse of antimalaria drugs for nonmalarial fevers all contribute to the development of drug-resistant infectious agents, to the detriment of all.

When making objective utilitarianism operational, countries have to consider whether to make departures from any of the widely used metrics like QALYs or DALYs. Those indexes embody ways of valuing different outcomes that were selected by various experts to allow for worldwide, intercountry comparisons. For national priority setting, however, the weights or values implicit in a particular index might not reflect the ethics, culture, and politics of the country concerned (Musgrove 2000).

For example, both indexes add up the number of years of life saved by an intervention, adjusted for quality of life. This gives greater value to saving the young and healthy, rather than the old and frail, since doing the former produces more (and higher-quality) additional life years. Such an analysis implies that a country should give more priority to providing inexpensive medicines that fight childhood diseases than to providing expensive anticancer agents for older people. We are not saying which is the right answer. Rather we are calling the reader's attention to the fact that all measures of "gain" come with implicit value judgments. Indeed, in practice, many nations allocate significant resources to caring for those with life-threatening illness, even when that is not cost-effective on a DALY or QALY basis (Hadorn 1991).

National decisions about how to quantify health gains for policy purposes are not just technical choices but also value choices. For a policy maker it can be politically helpful, as a way of dealing with pressures from diverse constituencies, to shift responsibility for a controversial priority-setting decision to some expert body. It is not unusual for a political leader to claim, "The numbers made me do it," with regard to a decision such as excluding a product from a nation's essential medicines list. However, when the index used in the analysis was devised by some group of international experts and was adopted without regard to local values and priorities, such claims are an abdication of responsibility. NICE, in contrast, is at pains to make its value assumptions explicit, and it invites public comment on this and other aspects of its work, both before and after any actual analysis is done (see the agency's website at http://www.nice.org.uk).

Relating Performance Goals to Ethical Perspectives: Liberalism

The focus of utilitarians on "the greatest good," based on an aggregate measure of well-being, leads to an insensitivity about the distribution of gains and losses within a population. In particular, strict utilitarians find it ethically acceptable to sacrifice some for the sake of others. Also, in pursuit of the greatest good, objective utilitarianism can easily lead to paternalism (and coercion): "We know what is best for you and will insist on your cooperation, whether it is immunizations, motorcycle helmets, or smoking cessation."

That lack of concern for distribution most often leads to a clash between utilitarians and another school of ethical thought that plays a prominent role in pharmaceutical policy making and in the Flagship Framework. That perspective emphasizes individual rights and is rooted in a doctrine that philosophers call "liberalism."

Like utilitarianism, liberalism is rooted in both the Enlightenment and the Reformation. Liberalism, however, takes as its point of departure the notion that all persons are independent and autonomous creatures, capable, at least potentially, of making their own decisions about how to live their lives. In this view, the role of the state is to provide a framework or context for those individuals. It is there to keep them safe, provide common services, and create a functioning political and legal system. But how people live their lives, where they go, and what they do—these are all up to their individual choices.

If utilitarianism focuses on where everyone ends up (consequences), liberalism focuses on where they start. Each person's claim to freedom and autonomy is embodied in the idea of rights. Rights are restraints against the authority of the state and claims against fellow citizens, which together embody a system of mutual respect. Neither I nor the government can tell you what to do, and vice versa (as long as your actions do not affect me).

One version of liberalism, now called "libertarianism," is characterized by a focus on everyone's *negative* right to be left alone. Those negative rights, importantly, include the protection of my property rights. Libertarianism argues that I cannot effectively exercise my autonomy unless I am secure in my property. (That notion was perhaps plausible in the context of an 18th-century, heavily agricultural society.) Indeed, because taxation deprives me of my property, libertarians argue that government activity should be kept to a bare minimum to avoid, as much as possible, any infringement on property rights. In many upper-income countries today, various center-right "liberal" parties defend some version of that position.

This approach to ethics originally owed much to the Judeo-Christian notion that God endows each human being with an immortal soul. It was the possession of that soul that 18th- and 19th-century writers invoked to justify the claim for universal human autonomy and respect. A famous passage from the U.S. Declaration of Independence illustrates this line of thought:

> We hold these truths to be self evident, that all men are created equal, that they are endowed by their Creator with certain inalienable rights, that among these rights are life, liberty and the pursuit of happiness, that to secure these rights, governments are established among men, deriving their just powers from the consent of the governed.

More recently, liberals have shifted from a theological to a philosophical justification. They now argue that human beings are unique in their capacity for rational thought and planning and in their ability to recognize moral values. That capacity entitles them to mutual respect and to the rights that embody that respect (Scanlon 1998).

The other important development in liberal thought has been to move beyond the focus on autonomy and mutual noninterference. Instead of an exclusive concern with negative rights, many modern liberals also argue for the existence of *positive* rights—to various goods and services such as education or health care (Daniels 2008). This line of thought, known as "egalitarian liberalism," has been strongly influenced by European democratic socialist traditions and finds some of its chief political advocates today in socialist and other center-left parties. The perspective is also reflected in a number of national constitutions that include a specific reference to a right to health. Indeed, in some countries individual patients have used that right to compel governments to provide access to medicines and treatment through legal action (Hogerzeil et al. 2006).

The argument of egalitarian liberals is that protecting negative rights does not ensure that everyone will have access to a fair distribution of opportunity. To ensure that everyone has some minimum level of food, shelter, schooling, and medical care, the government's tax and expenditure systems have to redistribute income and wealth from the top to the bottom of the society. Many egalitarian liberals focus on what they believe to be the illegitimate and unfair basis of the existing distribution of property. That unfairness, they argue, makes redistribution acceptable and ensures that it does not constitute an infringement of the property rights of those who are taxed (Dworkin 2000).

These egalitarian concerns are reflected in the Flagship Framework in its emphasis not just on national average levels of performance but also on the distribution of performance. In our analytical framework, *equity* is not a distinct performance measure. Rather, equity has to be described and analyzed in terms of the distribution of some other performance goal, such as health status or financial protection, among different sectors of a population. In that formulation, every country has to decide if it wants to treat some level of health care and pharmaceutical use, or even of health itself, as a right. Each country must also determine which patterns of distribution, across which dimensions of performance (for example, maternal mortality rate, life expectancy, pharmaceutical spending, or HIV/AIDS infection rates) and which population groups, deserve priority attention.

It should be noted that improving medicine access and health status among the worst-off can sometimes be very cost-effective. Providing basic medicines and primary care to underserved groups can often yield large returns. In those instances, reducing inequities can produce significant gains in population health. But when the worst-off groups are geographically and socially isolated, or resist the use of modern medicines, providing services and supplies to them can be difficult and not especially cost-effective. (In fact, many nations are willing to accept this trade-off and provide such services anyway, based on their egalitarian commitments.)

In many countries, the most cost-ineffective use of health care resources (including medicines) occurs at the top (not the bottom) of the distribution of income and wealth. So policy makers concerned about maximizing overall impact should probably worry less about the high costs of reaching the hard-to-serve poor and more about restraining low-productivity use by the overserved rich. Such efforts would both enhance efficiency and foster a more equitable distribution of resources.

Relating Performance Goals to Ethical Perspectives: Communitarianism

The two ethical views discussed so far are both individualistic. It is individual well-being or individual opportunity that forms the basis of the utilitarian and liberal approaches. But much of the ethical thinking that human beings have done has had a different orientation. It does not focus on where people start (rights and opportunity) or where they end up (well-being and utility). Instead, it focuses on the kind of human beings people are, on whether they have appropriate character and act in a virtuous manner. On a social level, that is expressed as concern for whether individuals behave in ways that allow them to fit into, and help construct, a society that embodies particular virtues. Essentially all of the world's major religious traditions are in this category, which we call "communitarianism."

Communitarianism differs from the other two categories because it is a much larger "box" and holds a much more diverse set of ideas. Indeed, it is not possible to say what communitarians believe. Unlike utilitarians, communitarians have many different definitions of virtuous conduct and many different visions of what makes a good society. After all, this category contains Mao, the pope, Buddha, and Greenpeace. In short, the substantive values depend on the specific communitarian philosophy.

Pharmaceutical policy debates tend to bring out two kinds of communitarian concerns. One of them reflects moral or religious convictions around issues of sexuality and reproduction. For example, a heated debate has occurred in a number of countries over whether to exclude misoprostol (originally a gastric ulcer medicine) from the essential medicines list because, although the product is effective against postpartum hemorrhage (the leading cause of maternal deaths), it can be used to induce abortion (Burns 2005). Indeed, misoprostol was added to the 14th edition (2005) of the World Health Organization (WHO) Model List of Essential Medicines explicitly for use in medical abortions and labor induction. Some countries, however, such as the Philippines (where abortion is illegal), have refused to register misoprostol as a gastric ulcer medicine because of those other uses, even though the product is inexpensively available on the black market and widely used for medical abortions (Juarez et al. 2005) (see case study B, "Registering Misoprostol in Sri Lanka").

A second kind of communitarian concern involves whether to provide very expensive care, such as certain anticancer medicines, that is not cost-effective in terms of dollars per years of life saved. Yet such care can be a patient's only alternative in the face of a fatal illness. The impulse to spend large sums of money on treatments for patients near death has sometimes been called "rescue medicine" (McKie and Richardson 2003). And it can come wrapped in communitarian justifications such as, What sort of country are we that we would let someone die who might be saved? Such arguments are often based on appeals to virtues such as generosity, solidarity, and beneficence rather than on rights or on achieving the greatest good.

No performance measure in the Flagship Framework directly reflects communitarian concerns. The reason in part is that such concerns are so varied—and even opposed to one another—that there is no simple way to incorporate these diverse perspectives into the analysis. Communitarian views would enter, however, when following moral dictates or rescuing terminally ill patients affects citizens' satisfaction. We must acknowledge, however, that many communitarians believe that there is only one right way for society to be organized, a way whose norms should be respected regardless of individual reactions. Illustrative examples include traditional Catholic views on contraception, abortion, and in vitro fertilization.

Not all communitarians are of that universal sort. Some want to allow each society to set its own rules (relative communitarians). But even for them, once a society's norms have been established, they are presumed to have great moral force inside the society. Those who argue that Westerners should not interfere with local policy making on issues such as female genital cutting are clearly in this camp.

Table 4.1 provides a summary of these three ethical perspectives (and the variations within the three broader views), along with a sample application in pharmaceutical policy.

Table 4.1 Summary of Three Ethical Views

Ethical view	Brief definition	Sample application in pharmaceutical policy
Utilitarian	Subjective: Achieve maximum aggregate individual happiness at lowest cost.	Use an assessment of people's preferences to decide which products to place on essential medicines list.
	Objective: Achieve maximum aggregate well-being based on a particular index (such as health status).	Use cost-effectiveness analysis to decide which products to place on essential medicines list.
Liberal	Egalitarian liberal: Emphasize positive rights for individuals, with attention to helping the worst-off.	Design a state-funded program that would provide most-needed medicines to the poorest members of society.
	Libertarian: Emphasize negative rights for individuals, which results in minimal level of state activity.	Let the free market decide which medicines are sold, with minimal state intervention or regulation.
Communitarian	Universal: Emphasize character and virtues as universal traits for deciding on public policy.	Certain pharmaceutical products (such as contraceptives) should not be registered or sold anywhere because they violate universal values.
	Relative: Emphasize a particular set of traits in character and virtue as basis for a single society or for group members.	Community members should not use certain pharmaceutical products, but nonmembers can do so.

Source: Authors' representation.

The Flagship Framework and Economic Development Goals

The Flagship Framework was developed to explore health sector issues. Yet some difficult pharmaceutical policy choices that low- and middle-income countries confront lie at the intersection of health goals and economic development objectives. They require us to consider some questions that prior work on the Flagship Framework has not explored.

Economic development is an obviously valuable goal for national governments to pursue and is generally seen in that way within both utilitarianism and liberalism. Utilitarians recognize that higher levels of per capita gross domestic product (GDP) make possible higher levels of well-being for citizens, whether measured by subjective feelings or objective circumstances. Liberals also generally favor development, as it typically expands individual opportunities. Libertarians focus more on private wealth creation, while egalitarian liberals applaud the increase in government revenues that growth creates, for it makes possible increased funding for redistributive social services such as education and health care. But in general, they are pro growth. Of course, where growth undermines traditional cultures, relative communitarians will dissent, as will some egalitarian liberals if growth is accompanied by increased inequality.

How should pharmaceutical policy makers respond when someone advocates sacrificing pharmaceutical sector performance for growth objectives? Such conflicts arise, for example, in cases of proposed preferential purchasing from local manufacturers when that may increase cost and decrease quality. Other examples include import duties and sales taxes on medicines, policies intended to protect locally based importers, and even decreased quality standards for local firms.

Pharmaceutical policy makers need to acknowledge the obvious reality that health is only one aspect of well-being and opportunity. And one may argue that, in some specific situations, it might be appropriate to make some short-term sacrifice of health goals to achieve large economic development gains. For example, a nation might plausibly decide to reallocate budget resources from health to development projects for a few years to complete vital transportation infrastructure. However, in most national policy-making discussions there will be many growth advocates, including the ministry of finance and the executives of the industries concerned. Given the likely forces on the other side, we suggest that those responsible for the pharmaceutical sector can, quite defensibly, be reasoned advocates for their own activities and responsibilities.

That conclusion suggests that pharmaceutical policy makers take a skeptical attitude toward claims that health status goals should be sacrificed for economic development objectives. The skepticism can take various forms, such as insisting that a careful, unbiased analysis be made of the potential economic effects before policies that decrease access to medicines for economic development reasons are adopted. Or it could involve pushing to make any protections temporary so as to avoid long-term effects on prices and access to medicines.

The International Dimension of Pharmaceutical Policy

No area of health policy making is as international as national pharmaceutical policy. Many developers and manufacturers of medicines are global companies. Many of the intermediaries (brokers, procurement agents, and negotiators) operate internationally. The rules governing trade and intellectual property are embodied in international treaties. Much of the funding—especially for high-value products in low-income countries—comes from bilateral and multilateral donors, and many countries receive significant direct donations of medicines. In addition, international agencies can play an extensive operational role in the pharmaceutical sector, from prequalifying sellers, to inspecting products, to doing their own procurement and importing, to supporting policy development through training, loans, and technical assistance. Many international nongovernmental organizations also are involved in the pharmaceutical supply chain in poor countries, providing medicines for mission hospitals, for treatment of specific diseases (such as HIV, tuberculosis, onchocerciasis, and schistosomiasis), and for government primary care facilities, and carrying out important functions in emergencies.

These developments reflect two important features of the modern world. First, radically decreased transportation and communication costs have created a whole new network of globalized economic, political, and social relationships. Second, this expanding interdependence has led those in the richer parts of the world to feel more responsible for ensuring some minimum level of opportunity worldwide.

Historically, arguments for redistribution have often been communitarian, based on claims of reciprocity and mutuality among the citizens of a nation defined in part by ethnicity. Access to health care or education has been something that Germans owe to other Germans, or Swedes to other

Swedes, as a matter of national solidarity. And national political institutions have largely been organized in precisely that way. Redistribution occurs among the group of citizens who vote in national elections for representatives who raise the relevant taxes and decide on the relevant policies.

But if both negative and positive rights are rooted in each individual's humanity, then why should the recognition of, and the funding for, those rights be limited by national political borders? Indeed, a long-standing internationalist strain is part of the egalitarian liberal tradition, whether the French Republic seeking to foster uprisings against *anciens régimes* throughout Europe, various socialist "internationals" urging transnational class solidarity, or the International Declaration of Human Rights. Indeed, the Australian political philosopher Peter Singer has argued, from a global utilitarian perspective, that individuals in rich countries have a moral obligation to give money to help poor people in poor countries, until the point where it may have negative consequences for their own life (Singer 2009).

Despite the rhetoric of advocates for international positive rights and international obligations, aid-related discussions in donor countries typically invoke less far-reaching claims. Providing foreign aid funds is often justified in terms of compassion or generosity or urged as a matter of national self-interest as a way to open up beneficial trade or political connections or as a route to the development of "soft power" (Nye 2004). Indeed, some critics of the current global scene see international aid and trade policy (including World Trade Organization rulemaking) as excessively driven by the interests of upper-income nations in ensuring raw materials supplies, opening up markets, preventing political instability, and controlling international contagion. To such critics, current aid programs often serve to divert attention from more fundamental questions of global equity.

As recipient countries all too painfully recognize, reliance on international sources also creates vulnerability to international pressures. It is not just a matter of policy conditions attached to World Bank loans or the economic policy constraints pushed by the International Monetary Fund on borrower nations (Stiglitz 2002). For example, when international agencies come into a country and help establish special programs for HIV, malaria, or polio eradication, or press countries to focus on achieving the Millennium Development Goals, the efforts can drain staff and resources from other health and medicines activities. Moreover, donors can seek access to recipient countries at many points in the political structure and can win agreements from presidents or ministers that are not consistent with the orderly process of policy development.

Although nations often resent such external pressures, it is not easy for recipients of aid to explain why those transfers should be unconditional.

As noted above, typically redistribution from rich to poor has been based on the assumption that the two groups are bound together in a broader political relationship that gives rise to their mutual obligations. Once such a relationship is established, political interference is inevitable. For example, is it illegitimate for the Global Fund, or other donors, to seek to control fraud connected with their grants? And how should we react if they temporarily curtail funding in countries where they discover problems, in a way that endangers the continuity of medicines funding? The tricky part is keeping such interventions within limits that are respectful of the sovereignty of those who receive the aid, a line that in practice can lead to much disagreement.

The Importance of Fair Process

Regardless of the philosophical perspective that reformers adopt, they often find that their general ideas are not sufficiently detailed to answer specific policy questions. For example, choosing to follow an objective utilitarian approach does not tell an analyst how to value the impact of providing antidepressants to treat clinical depression against the value of ARVs in extending the life of someone with HIV/AIDS. Similarly, an egalitarian liberal who believes in a right to health care cannot easily move from that position to a decision about which drugs should be made available free in rural health centers.

Given that reasonable and well-meaning individuals can disagree about such matters, how is a society to resolve them? In recent years the philosopher Norman Daniels, among others, has advocated decision processes that meet a test that he calls "accountability for reasonableness" (Daniels 2000). The notion is that decision-making processes should be open and transparent. Decisions have to be reached on the basis of explicit criteria and justified by publicly available reasoning. Affected parties need an opportunity to present their views. The best available scientific information must be relied upon, and policies need to be revised and revisable as evidence of their consequences accumulates.

Daniels's argument for these positions is rooted in liberal ideas. Respect for the rights of those who will be affected by a policy, he maintains, implies that they should have a fair opportunity to influence it. And he points to examples such as NICE in the United Kingdom to show that creating institutions along these lines is possible.

Ironically, accountability for reasonableness is subject to some of the same problems that it is designed to correct. For example, we know from other areas where participatory decision processes have been tried with experts and citizens that careful attention has to be paid to the details of process design (Laird 1993). Otherwise, the most informed or committed interests, or those with the greatest stakes and resources, end up playing an undue role. The history of environmental mediation efforts in the United States, for example, offers ample evidence on this point (Ackerman et al. 1974). But what is "undue" influence? Do we need a process to design the process? An endless regress threatens.

From a practical point of view, the work by Daniels has much to recommend it to those responsible for pharmaceutical policy. It reflects not only an ethical imperative but a political one as well. Carefully designed decision-making processes are essential to enhance both learning and consent, if a society is to develop and implement effective pharmaceutical policy.

Summary on Ethics (and Some Suggestions)

As we have stressed, making priority-setting decisions for pharmaceutical policy is an appropriate function of a nation's political authority. Although the Flagship Framework does not specify the substance of those policy decisions, it provides guidance on how to approach the questions and how to think about the ethical dimensions of priority setting (see table 4.1 for a summary of the three ethical perspectives presented in this chapter). This section goes beyond that summary to offer a set of substantive suggestions about how to set priorities with regard to some of the central performance issues that arise in the pharmaceutical policy arena.

(1) *Begin by trying to improve health status—with significant concern for improving the status of the worst-off groups in the population.* Health status should be the primary concern of pharmaceutical policy making, the basis on which other considerations are judged. This formulation does not say which aspects of health status or which groups should be given priority. But it does highlight the need to address and resolve those equity and detailed priority issues.

(2) *Deal with claims for rescue spending that is not cost-effective by trying to impose budget limits on such funding and by creating an appropriate process.* Experience teaches that it is much easier to impose limits on spending when the decisions are comparative—that is, which patient gets on the ventilator or who gets to go abroad for expensive chemotherapy. Budget limits, established and allocated by an accountability-for-reasonableness process, are one way to handle pressures for high-cost pharmaceutical treatment for a small number of patients.

(3) *Respond in only limited ways to patient demands for therapies that are not cost-effective.* Wasteful spending is just that: wasteful of a nation's scarce resources. Patients who spend their own money on harmless medicines raise the less-problematic form of this difficulty, but they are an appropriate target for efforts to increase rational medicines use. Using public funds for such purposes is more problematic because public sector spending should be easier to control. Even more serious is spending that leads to harm to the patient or to others (for example, by fostering antimicrobial resistance). Political constraints may limit how tough pharmaceutical policy makers can be on these issues. But decreasing wasteful or harmful expenditures is very important for reaching what we believe should be a nation's main goal—a cost-effective pharmaceutical system that maximally, and equitably, improves population health.

(4) *Work to improve the population's understanding of pharmaceutical uses and choices.* This is a long-range but important goal, one that is equally important (and difficult to achieve) in rich countries. Better public understanding helps decrease the tension between wants and needs. Remember, however, that relying on brand identification can be a rational strategy for information-limited consumers and is one that is followed by most individuals worldwide. Deeply rooted cultural norms (such as a preference for injections) are not easy to alter. But moving citizens to a more informed and empowered position, we believe, is an ethical obligation. In addition to being a useful strategy, it strengthens individual autonomy in a way valued by liberal thought.

(5) *Resist efforts to sacrifice health gains for economic development purposes, but do so reasonably and in ways that facilitate accountability and transparency.* This point is discussed extensively a few sections back.

These ideas are proposed as a starting point, to provoke a discussion about acceptable ethical goals of pharmaceutical policy. They are meant not to undermine the moral responsibility of national leaders to make their own choices, but rather to give some guidance on ways to enter that decision process in a constructive manner.

Case Studies for Chapter 4 (Ethics)

Guyer, Anya Levy, and Marc J. Roberts, "Defining an Essential Medicines List in Sudamerica," Case Study A.

Kumar, Ramya, and Michael R. Reich, "Registering Misoprostol in Sri Lanka," Case Study B.

References

Ackerman, B. A., S. R. Ackerman, J. W. Sawyer, and D. W. Henderson. 1974. *Uncertain Search for Environmental Quality*. New York: Free Press.

Bator, F. M. 1957. "The Simple Analytics of Welfare Maximization." *American Economic Review* 47: 22–59.

Berwick, D. M. 1989. "Continuous Improvement as an Ideal in Health Care." *New England Journal of Medicine* 320: 53–56.

Bullivant, J. R. N. 1996. "Benchmarking in the UK National Health Service." *International Journal of Health Care Quality Assurance* 9 (2): 9–14.

Burns, M. 2005. "Misoprostol Use in Obstetrics and Gynecology." *Outlook (PATH)* 21 (4): 1–8.

Cameron, A., M. Ewen, D. Ross-Degnan, D. Ball, and R. Laing. 2009. "Medicine Prices, Availability, and Affordability in 36 Developing and Middle-Income Countries: A Secondary Analysis." *Lancet* 373: 240–49.

Claxton, K., M. Schulpher, and M. Drummond. 2002. "A Rational Framework for Decision Making by the National Institute for Clinical Excellence (NICE)." *Lancet* 360: 711–15.

Crosby, P. B. 1979. *Quality Is Free*. New York: McGraw-Hill.

Daniels, N. 2000. Accountability for Reasonableness. *British Medical Journal* 321: 1300–01.

———. 2008. *Just Health: Meeting Health Needs Fairly*. New York: Cambridge University Press, 2008.

Drummond, M., and F. Rutten. 2008. *New Guidelines for Economic Evaluation in Germany and the United Kingdom*. London: Office of Health Economics.

Dworkin, R. 2000. *Sovereign Virtue: The Theory and Practice of Equality*. Cambridge, MA: Harvard University Press.

Hadorn, D. 1991. "Setting Health Care Priorities in Oregon: Cost-Effectiveness Meets the Rule of Rescue." *Journal of the American Medical Association* 265 (17): 2218–25.

Heuser, S. 2009. "One Girl's Hope, A Nation's Dilemma, A Cambridge Firm's Drug Worked Wonders, but Was Hugely Costly." *Boston Globe*. June 14.

Hogerzeil, H., M. Samson, J. Casanovas, and L. Rahmani-Ocora. 2006. "Is Access to Essential Medicines as Part of the Fulfilment of the Right to Health Enforceable through the Courts?" *Lancet* 368: 305–11.

Juarez, F., J. Cabigon, S. Singh, and R. Hussain. 2005. "The Incidence of Induced Abortion in the Philippines: Current Level and Recent Trends." *International Family Planning Perspectives* 31 (3): 140–49.

Laird, F. N. 1993. "Participatory Analysis, Democracy, and Technological Decision Making." *Science, Technology and Human Values* 18: 341–61.

McKie, J., and J. Richardson. 2003. "The Rule of Rescue." *Social Science and Medicine* 56: 2407–19.

Musgrove, P. 2000. "A Critical Review of 'A Critical Review': The Methodology of the 1993 World Development Report, 'Investing in Health.'" *Health Policy and Planning* 15 (1): 110–15.

Nye, J. S., Jr. 2004. *Soft Power: The Means to Success in World Politics*. New York: Public Affairs.

Roberts, M. J., and M. R. Reich. 2002. "Ethical Analysis in Public Health." *Lancet* 359: 1055–59.

Scanlon, T. M. 1998. *What We Owe to Each Other*. Cambridge, MA: Harvard University Press.

Singer, P. 2009. *The Life You Save: Acting Now to End World Poverty*. New York: Random House.

Stiglitz, J. E. 2002. *Globalization and Its Discontents*. New York: W.W. Norton.

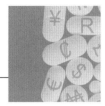

CHAPTER 5

Diagnosing Performance Problems and Developing a Policy Response

We have urged pharmaceutical policy makers to proceed in a disciplined way, to begin by asking which *outcomes*, for which *groups*, are so unsatisfactory as to constitute priority targets for reform efforts. Is it that certain segments of the population lack adequate financial protection because of high out-of-pocket spending in the private sector in the face of poor public sector availability? Is morbidity or mortality for some diseases in some areas higher than it should be? The key message is, The pharmaceutical system is a means to an end, or rather to a set of ends represented by the ultimate performance goals. Setting priorities as to where and how to improve the system is best done by beginning with the goals that a country is trying to achieve.

Once key performance failures are identified, the next step in the reform cycle is to analyze systematically the sources of those failures. This chapter introduces a diagnostic method for doing just that, using an analytical device we call a "diagnostic tree." Only when the sources of performance problems have been identified is it time to proceed to the next stage, namely, developing a policy response.

We urge reformers to go through an explicit, written-down process of diagnosis for three reasons: The first reason is to take into account the variability of local conditions. For example, in some parts of the world poor populations live in dense agricultural settlements, with relatively easy road access (Kerala in southern India, coastal Sri Lanka, some southeastern Chinese provinces). In contrast, in other places physical transport in rural areas is a major concern (for example, in much of rural Africa, the Andean countries, the Mongolian steppes, and the mountainous islands of Indonesia). Equally wide variations exist in social, economic, and political variables, including administrative capacity, per capita gross domestic product, the status of women, and the role of traditional healers. Such conditions can be important causes of variations in national performance in the pharmaceutical sector. They can also be significant constraints on the likely effects of alternative policy initiatives. An explicit diagnostic exercise can identify these conditions and focus attention on how best to respond to them in policy development.

The second reason for undertaking an explicit diagnosis is the way such a process can improve the quality of thinking about pharmaceutical reform. A great deal of evidence points to the value of having a diverse group, with diverse backgrounds, participate in problem solving. All of us are, to some extent, prisoners of our experience (Kuhn 1962). We all have powerful, yet limited, perspectives acquired as part of our cultural backgrounds and professional training. In any discussion of pharmaceutical sector problems, economists, infectious disease doctors, inventory management specialists, and social marketers will have different kinds of experience and think about the functioning of the sector in different ways. An explicit, written framework provides a structured way for diverse individuals to bring their perspectives to bear on the analytical process. By allowing assumptions to be challenged and different experiences to be introduced, it can provide a level of intellectual self-discipline that might otherwise be lacking. Whether the potential advantages are realized, of course, depends on the leadership and quality of the group process.

The third reason for adopting this kind of diagnosis has to do with our concern for transparency and democratic accountability. A diagnostic tree is a conceptual tool that is easy to understand and can be widely shared with interest groups, political leaders, and civil society representatives. It thus can facilitate the process of communicating the analysis to diverse stakeholders and also provide a basis for them to organize their comments and feedback.

A Simple Pharmaceutical Example to Illustrate the Method

The diagnostic tree is a variant of such methods as "fault trees," "fishbone diagrams," and "root cause analysis"—approaches that will be familiar to people who have studied modern quality management (Juran and Godfrey 1999).

- The method begins by asking, What is the performance problem targeted for improvement? What aspects of health status, citizen satisfaction, or financial protection need to be improved, either for specific groups or the population as a whole?

- The next task is to identify the causes of that performance shortfall.

- Then the causes of those causes are identified.

- The step of seeking causes is repeated until the analysis has reached the point where causes have been identified with enough specificity that targeted policy responses can be developed.

As figure 5.1 illustrates, multiple causes can be identified for each problem at each point in the analysis. Moreover, the diagram in figure 5.1 is simplified. It is entirely possible that some causes identified at one stage of the analysis are also causes of other factors identified at the same level of analysis. For example, it might be that lack of artemisinin-based combination therapies (ACTs) in the public sector is itself a cause of high private sector prices. Possibly one cause influences several subsequent effects. For example, ordering, logistical, and theft problems in the public sector might all have poor public sector management as a contributory cause. Nor is the diagram com-

Figure 5.1 Pharmaceutical Performance Diagnostic Tree

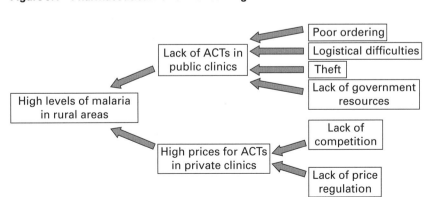

Source: Authors' representation.

Note: ACT = artemisinin-based combination therapy.

plete. A typical country analysis would include two or three more stages of asking, Why? before the process would be complete. And the resulting tree would spread over several large sheets of paper or a large whiteboard.

Figure 5.1, moreover, is just a hypothetical example. The situation in different countries will be different. In some nations, consumers may prefer older and ineffective treatments because they are both familiar and less expensive. Or perhaps ACTs are subject to price regulation, so dispensers push other, unregulated products because they yield greater profit. Also, public sector logistical difficulties may occur because a region is flooded every year in the rainy season, or because corrupt local officials divert the available vehicles for private and political purposes. The appropriate policy response depends on the diagnosis. That is why doing a diagnosis is so important. And the diagnosis will depend on the performance problem that is chosen for attention—that is why the process of problem identification is also so important.

In the course of doing a diagnosis, some causes might appear that policy makers in the pharmaceutical sector cannot address directly. It may or may not be possible to work around, or compensate for, supply disruptions due to natural disaster or armed conflict. Similarly, an analysis may reveal important causes that lie in the health system outside of the pharmaceutical sector, or even causes outside the health system entirely. Such influences on poor outcomes, however important, typically cannot be altered by pharmaceutical policy changes. Pharmaceutical policy makers are likely to have little influence on whether health center staff members in rural areas take up their posts, or whether bridges in flood-prone regions are replaced—never mind influencing the course of armed conflicts. But identifying the part that such causes play in poor pharmaceutical sector performance can call attention to areas where broader health sector reform efforts, or intersectoral action outside the health arena, may be appropriate uses of the energy of those who want to improve the supply of medicines.

It is important to ground the diagnostic process in an honest, evidence-based look at a country's actual situation. It is not unusual for local experts to know more about what really goes on in a nation's pharmaceutical sector than they are comfortable telling international visitors—for example, about how much leakage actually occurs, or whether staff members in remote areas actually appear at their posts. A diagnostic exercise is of little value unless these sometimes uncomfortable facts about the system are acknowledged and incorporated into the analysis.

A serious diagnosis is not a one-hour exercise. Often a series of causes will be proposed for a single problem, but their relative importance will not be clear. That is where evidence-based reform comes into play. Like evidence-based medical practice, evidence-based reform seeks to replace common sense, or "what everyone knows," with systematic empirical data. Just what are the prices in the private sector in different regions? Just what fraction of the stocks purchased show up on health center shelves? A careful look at the available data—or a decision to collect additional data to resolve a critical empirical issue—is part of a well-done diagnostic process.

The Intermediate Performance Goals and Their Role in the Diagnostic Process

The ultimate performance goals are just that—the final outcomes that pharmaceutical reformers need to focus on improving. But other parameters widely discussed in the health sector reform arena are also important in the analytical process, and particularly in the diagnostic exercise. These are "intermediate performance goals." In this section we clarify the terms and discuss their analytical role.

The intermediate performance goals that we have in mind are

- Efficiency

- Quality

- Access

These three goals are *not* ends in themselves. Often, however, they are important causes of variations in performance. Moreover, they are not among the control knobs that were presented in chapter 2 and are explored in more detail in chapters 7 through 11. Instead they are intermediate between policy causes and performance effects. They are also widely and confusingly discussed, with different writers using different definitions. We cannot claim that our definitions are correct. But the formulations we present are ones that we have found to be both clear and helpful in talking about reform efforts around the world.

Efficiency. The core idea covered by the concept of efficiency is a simple one: using resources in the best possible way to reach one's goals. That way of putting it makes clear that to know whether a system is efficient, one needs to specify the goals that it should achieve. To be efficient in this sense, a system has to satisfy two subsidiary conditions:

- Technical efficiency, which requires that all goods and services are produced at minimum cost, and

- Allocative efficiency, which requires that the system or process produces the appropriate set of goods and gets them to the appropriate end users, to reach the goals being sought.

In the pharmaceutical sector, "technical efficiency" means, for example, buying drugs at the lowest possible prices for the public sector and keeping the operating costs of public supply chains as low as is consistent with meeting delivery objectives. "Allocative efficiency" refers to what is provided and to whom. In the pharmaceutical context it means, for example, getting the right products onto the nation's essential medicines list and getting them dispensed to the right patients. It also means encouraging appropriate purchases in the private sector. Clearly judging allocative efficiency depends on how the system's goals are defined. Knowing who are the desired consumers of which drugs depends on a nation's goals and priorities.

Quality. Again, the concept of quality contains a simple core idea, despite widely varying uses in the literature. "High quality" means that a good or service performs in the way that someone desires. So quality, too, is purpose dependent and observer dependent. Different users and producers of a good or service might well have different goals. In part the reason is that quality is multidimensional. Thus one formulation of a drug may be faster acting, whereas another has a longer shelf life. Which is higher quality? The answer depends on a particular observer's priorities.

Following the Flagship Framework, we divide the multiple pharmaceutical sector quality dimensions into two broad groups; we have relabeled them slightly to fit the pharmaceutical context:

- Clinical Quality. In the pharmaceutical context, clinical quality involves the pharmacological activity of the medicines people use and the clinical appropriateness of the treatment regimes they pursue. Thus this category includes the exact levels of active ingredients in medicines and their purity. Substandard and counterfeit medicines are obviously aspects of poor clinical quality. Patients' use of the wrong medicines is also an aspect of clinical quality. Hence misprescribing and antibiotic overuse are aspects of poor clinical quality. But so, too, is the use of needlessly expensive compounds when simpler alternatives will do. When patients purchase an expensive and powerful, branded pain reliever such as Percocet, when all they really need is ordinary ibuprofen, that is a manifestation of poor clinical quality. The appropriateness of the advice patients receive from dispensers (relative to rational drug use standards) is also an aspect of clinical quality.

- Nonclinical Quality. "Nonclinical quality" refers to quality dimensions that do not directly affect clinical outcomes (but that may do so indirectly because of their impact on use). For medicines, the nonclinical aspects include the aesthetics of the drugs themselves, how they are taken (tablet, syrup, or injection and dosage schedule), and their packaging. Another realm of nonclinical quality is service quality in retail locations. Service quality aspects include the way people are treated in dispensing locations, the location and hours of operation of those facilities, waiting times, and the physical environment in the buildings that customers use. From the purchaser's point of view, stock-outs are also an aspect of poor service quality because the medicines the buyer wants are not available.

In pharmaceuticals, as in many areas of health care, patients have a difficult time judging clinical quality. In response, they may use price or brand as a proxy for clinical quality and end up, at best, paying more than they need to, and at worst, with inappropriate medicines. Alternatively, they may make their consumption decisions based on parameters that they can evaluate. Purchasers generally cannot know whether the medicine they acquire at the local drug shop has the full amount of the active ingredient that it should contain. But they can know how it smells and tastes and whether the shop clerk treats them well or badly, compared to the clerk at the drug dispensing window at the local health center. Patients' sensitivity to such nonclinical quality dimensions helps explain why many drug buyers prefer private sector retail outlets and why private clinics and hospitals in many low- and middle-income countries pay attention to service quality.

This multidimensionality shows that managers in the pharmaceutical sector need to develop an explicit quality strategy. They need to consider which dimensions of quality are critical to improved performance (as revealed by their diagnostic tree analysis) and focus on improving those features of the system. In many contexts it is true that better management can improve quality with existing resources, but it is also true that the amount of funds available places limits on the levels of quality that can be attained. Consider a Fiat and a BMW—the latter costs twice as much as the former—and assume that both are manufactured without defects. Under those conditions, the Fiat will not reach the level of performance of the BMW because of the design and quality advantages of higher cost. Similarly, if we spend more to equip, maintain, staff, and supply a local health center, it can potentially offer higher-quality service than a facility with a fraction of that budget.

Access. Access is another concept with multiple definitions. In certain respects it overlaps the domain of service quality. But because access plays such a critical role in many discussions of pharmaceutical policy, we consider it as a distinct intermediate performance goal. Access includes whether customers can easily take advantage of goods and services that they want to consume or that system mangers want them to consume. As with the previous two categories, it is helpful to distinguish two subcomponents:

- Physical availability—whether a good or service is available in a relevant location, and

- Effective availability—whether obstacles such as price, hours of operation, and cultural barriers make it difficult for patients to consume the goods or services that are physically available.

In the pharmaceutical sector, "physical availability" refers to whether appropriate products are on the shelves of a dispensing location (public or private) that customers can reach relatively easily. The overlap here with service quality is obvious, as stock-outs can be viewed either as poor service quality or as a limitation of physical availability and hence a component of poor access. "Effective availability" refers to whether consumers can actually procure the product, if they decide to consume it, or instead encounter barriers such as price, sales practices, or demands for bribes. Again, consumers may perceive the presence of various access barriers as aspects of poor service quality.

It is important to note that access is not the same as use. We use access as a *supply side* concept, whereas use involves a *demand side* as well. So the physical and effective availability of drugs—say, in a well-stocked, nearby public clinic—does not ensure that consumers will take advantage of the products, for example, if they do not believe they are effective. Distinguishing supply-side and demand-side problems through a diagnostic analysis is important and will influence the kinds of policy responses that are chosen.

It is also worth noting that some broader approaches to the concept of access explicitly include attention to the demand side and to processes of adoption of health technologies (Frost and Reich 2008). Those approaches to access are understandable because they focus our attention on the actual use of medicines, which is what is relevant if we are to influence the ultimate performance goals of health status, consumer satisfaction, and risk protection.

Using the Intermediate Performance Measures

Efficiency, quality, and access are not the ultimate goals of the pharmaceutical system. Nor are they features of the system that reformers can directly manipulate to change performance. Rather they are a means to an end. Those categories describe important characteristics of the functioning of various subsystems in the pharmaceutical sector. And that functioning is an

Figure 5.2 Schematic Overview of the Determinants of System Performance

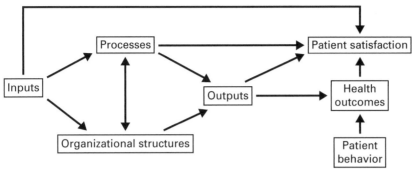

Source: Authors' representation.

important link between policy choices and the ultimate outcomes that the policies produce.

Donabedian's classic analyses of quality improvement efforts distinguished among structure, process, and outcome measures (Donabedian 1988). Figure 5.2 presents a revised and expanded formulation of the determinants of system performance, distinguishing organizational structures from processes, and outputs from two of the outcomes that we focus on: health and satisfaction. Financial protection as an outcome is omitted from this formulation because it is determined by money flows and the diagram only describes physical processes. We also distinguish patient behavior as a causal factor in determining health status outcomes.

If we think about the role of the intermediate performance measures in the context of figure 5.2, it is clear that technical efficiency, many aspects of nonclinical quality, and access are essentially *process* measures. Allocative efficiency, the clinical quality of medicines (including their appropriateness), and the nonclinical characteristics of medicines that patients notice can be thought of as *output* characteristics.

Why should reformers and managers pay attention to these intermediary process and output measures, if it is health and satisfaction *outcomes* that they really care about? The difficulty with some outcome measures, from a pharmaceutical reformer's point of view, is that some time may have to elapse after the implementation of reform before changes in outcomes appear. For example, better supply of chronic disease medications will not show up in changes in life expectancy for a number of years. In addition, assessing health and satisfaction outcomes typically requires expensive and difficult-to-conduct household surveys, which are only conducted infrequently.

In contrast, consider a variety of widely used pharmaceutical sector process and output measures. Examples include the prices paid in the procurement process, stock-out and wastage rates, the percentage of drugs in the market that fail quality tests, the percentage of health centers with trained staff actually in place, and the rate of use of rapid diagnostic tests before malaria medications are prescribed. Many of these metrics can be monitored relatively easily (and inexpensively) using data from routine administrative records. They are thus quite useful for managers and reformers as part of any ongoing system of performance monitoring.

A Systems Approach to Process Improvement

Once reformers agree that they want to improve pharmaceutical system quality (or access, or efficiency), and they have identified process improvement priorities, how should they go about that task? Quality management experts often invoke the idea, "Every system is perfectly designed to produce the results you observe." They mean that achieving quality improvements requires understanding how and why a system is producing unsatisfactory results and then doing something to change the system to obtain more desirable outcomes.

Suppose we observe that a public regulatory agency is doing a poor job of enforcing retail drug price controls, or that the process of restocking medicines in district health centers is crippled by faulty orders and long processing times. An inexperienced reformer might respond by trying to find the "bad guys" who are causing the problem and seeking to get rid of those few "rotten apples." But the system perspective directs our attention in a different direction. If inspectors are not doing their job, then *why* is that the case? If orders take too long to process, rather than criticizing the clerks, can we change the ordering system? Consider the two illustrations of this point

Figure 5.3   The Effect of Alternative Quality Improvement Strategies: The "Rotten Apple" View

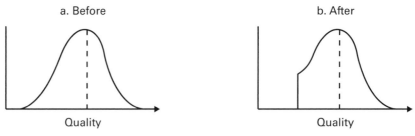

Eliminate the "left-hand tail"

Source: Authors' representation.

Figure 5.4   The Effect of Alternative Quality Improvement Strategies: The Systems View

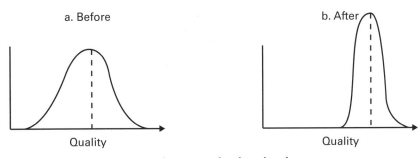

a. Before

Quality

b. After

Quality

Increased mean and reduced variance

Source: Authors' representation.

shown in figure 5.3, which are based on the assumption that we can summarize quality in a single dimension.

Notice in figure 5.3 that removing the few worst performers does nothing to improve the quality experience of most consumers. But if we operate at a system level, as depicted in figure 5.4, then the whole distribution of quality shifts to the right, reflecting an overall improvement for most consumers, and the distribution also shows decreased variation in outcomes.

Developing Policy Responses

Once the diagnosis is complete, where can reformers go to obtain good ideas about policy options, and how should they conduct the policy-making process? On the substantive side, we assume that policy makers have identified the performance problems that they want to fix and have conducted a diagnostic tree exercise, as explained above. They now know which areas of the pharmaceutical system they need to change to improve its functioning.

The first piece of advice we would offer is embodied in the slogan, "Imitate but adapt." There is a rapidly expanding body of international experience in the area of pharmaceutical reform, and using that experience as a source of ideas can be very helpful. Of course a reformer should not assume that a complex reference price regulatory scheme that has worked in New Zealand will necessarily work in Uganda. Reformers need to carefully examine the requirements for successful implementation of a proposed policy in their national context. Does their country have, or can it develop, prerequisites such as the needed data processing capacity, the required number of technically trained staff, or an effective civil law system for settling contract disputes? Thus nations are well advised to look first for ideas from countries that are culturally and economically similar.

Other sources of policy ideas may require greater leaps of faith. Sometimes experience in a different sector can suggest a policy response. The private sector strategy of franchising stores has now moved from fast-food outlets to social purposes and public health. It has become an increasingly popular approach for the delivery of reproductive health and other services in developing countries (McBride and Ahmed 2001; Montagu 2002). Similar approaches are being developed for the pharmaceutical sector (see case study F, "Converting Basic Drug Shops to Accredited Drug Dispensing Outlets in Tanzania").

Sometimes, when a new problem is identified, policy makers have resorted to general theoretical arguments or broad knowledge of a sector to develop a reform proposal. For example, the United States and some European countries have witnessed a big push to change how doctors are paid from salary to "P4P"—pay for performance (Rosenthal 2008). The earliest experiments with this new policy were justified on the basis of general economic arguments rather than any specific prior experience. Similarly, the idea for a global subsidy to support the price of artemisinin-based combination therapies, or ACTs, for malaria emerged from an expert committee at the U.S. Institute of Medicine, headed by economist Kenneth Arrow, who had no prior experience working on that disease and its treatment. The translation of this innovative idea into an implementable initiative required a group of policy champions to guide the process (Frost et al. 2009).

That brings us to the last topic in this chapter, how to construct the process of policy development. We believe strongly that process influences both product and politics. Allowing those potentially affected by a policy to have some input into the policy design process creates opportunities for learning. Of course, interest groups will try to shape a policy in ways that suit their interests. (They are called "interest groups" after all.) But they also have the potential to make substantive contributions to policy development. Interest groups often know a great deal about how various systems and processes operate in practice and what it would take to improve their functioning.

The participation of affected parties can also have a positive impact on the politics of getting a policy approved and implemented. Smart policy designers seek to create "win-win" deals with potentially powerful opponents (Fisher and Ury 1981). Participatory processes can provide information on ways to modify the proposed reform to increase its acceptability without undermining its effectiveness. They can also help each group understand the needs and concerns of the other interest groups that are involved. They clarify for all concerned the diverse objectives and pressures that policy makers have to balance. Participating groups thus get both a hearing and an education. As a result, they may be more likely to accept the final compromise, even if it does not fully suit them. Indeed, even those outside the design process may be more likely to accept the policy proposal if they can be persuaded that the key constituencies have had a reasonable role in its development.

If participatory processes are to produce these gains, they need to be carefully managed. The policy design team has to listen carefully to the less-expert and less-well-resourced voices. It has to make clear that the various interests have a voice but not a veto—to do otherwise would only encourage nonconstructive, even obstructive, behavior. To avoid raising expectations that cannot be met, participants should understand from the beginning that they are acting in an advisory and not a policy-making role. The reform team needs enough resources and expertise to avoid being fooled or outmaneuvered by the other participants—as well as a clear political mandate that allows its members to hold their ground when necessary. But paying attention to process early on can produce significant dividends as a country moves through the reform cycle.

Summary on Diagnosis

In summary, reformers should not assume, when they begin the process, that they already know the causes of poor performance in the pharmaceutical sector. Instead, as many writers on quality management have urged, reformers should first identify which performance problems they most want to improve. Then they need to take a diagnostic journey to discover the causes of that poor performance. The Flagship Framework uses a particular technique, the diagnostic tree, as a way of conducting that analysis, and this chapter has offered some guidance on its use. We have also stressed the importance of open-mindedness and the use of evidence to obtain the maximum benefit from such a diagnostic process.

Diagnosis thus is a critical part of the reform process; it allows reformers to connect the identification of priority problems with the design of proposed solutions. Moreover, we believe that in the course of constructing a diagnostic tree, reformers will often encounter the causal importance of those features of the system's processes and outputs that we have called "intermediate performance measures": efficiency, quality, and access. Readers are reminded that these characteristics of system performance are not ends in themselves and are not self-defining. In particular, allocative efficiency and quality are purpose dependent. They have to do with whether or not a system functions in a way that meets certain goals. Only reformers who explicitly identify their goals are thus in a position to think about allocative efficiency and quality in a sophisticated manner.

Once a diagnosis has been done, it is time to move to the next stage of the reform cycle—developing policy responses using the five control knobs introduced previously. Before turning to the control knobs, however, we must give more attention to the role of politics. For no reform, no matter how elegant, will change performance unless it is adopted and implemented, and adoption and implementation always occur in an intensely political environment.

References

Donabedian, A. 1988. "The Quality of Care: How Can It Be Assessed?" *Journal of the American Medical Association* 260: 1743–48.

Fisher, R., and W. L. Ury. 1981. *Getting to YES: Negotiating Agreement Without Giving In.* New York: Penguin.

Frost, L. J., and M. R. Reich. 2008. *Access: How Do Good Health Technologies Get to Poor People in Poor Countries?* Cambridge, MA: Harvard University Press.

Frost, L., M. R. Reich, B. A. Pratt, and A. L. Guyer. 2009. "Process Evaluation of the Project on *Defining the Architecture and Management of a Global Subsidy for Antimalarial Drugs.*" World Bank, Washington, DC. http://siteresources.worldbank.org/INTMALARIA/Resources/AMFmProcessEvaluation.pdf.

Juran, J. M., and A. B. Godfrey, eds. 1999. *Juran's Quality Control Handbook.* 5th ed. New York: McGraw-Hill, 1999.

Kuhn, T. S. 1962. *The Structure of Scientific Revolutions.* 1st. ed. Chicago: University of Chicago Press.

McBride, J., and R. Ahmed. 2001. *Social Franchising as a Strategy for Expanding Access to Reproductive Health Services.* CMS Technical Paper. Washington, DC: Commercial Market Strategies. September.

Montagu, D. 2002. "Franchising of Health Services in Developing Countries." *Health Policy and Planning* 17 (2): 121–30.

Rosenthal, M. B. 2008. "Beyond Pay for Performance: Emerging Models of Provider-Payment Reform." *New England Journal of Medicine* 359 (12): 1197–1200.

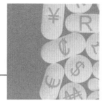

CHAPTER 6

Managing the Politics of Pharmaceutical Policy Reform

Our discussion of the role of politics in pharmaceutical policy reform begins with a brief consideration of the nature of politics and its relationship to policy. That is, what role *does* politics play in policy-making processes, and what role *should* politics play? The chapter offers reformers advice about how to conduct a political analysis and how to design political strategies that can promote their reform proposals. It closes with a discussion of several examples from pharmaceutical politics and policy making.

The Role of Politics in Pharmaceutical Policy Making

First, what do we mean by "politics"? In its broadest sense, the term refers to competition for power and authority among groups and individuals. Usually, but not always, the prize in the competition is control over some decision-making function, one that establishes rules, or allocates resources, or controls the actions of a bureaucracy or organization. In that sense, making reform decisions is political by definition because it involves competition among groups and individuals over "who gets what, when, and how"—the classic definition of politics according to the political scientist Harold D. Lasswell (1936).

But politics also has two narrower meanings. One is shorthand for electoral politics or democratic politics. That usage refers to competition among those who participate in electoral processes. The term "politician" is reserved for those who play a meaningful role in that arena. A second, narrower and more negative meaning of "politics" denotes efforts to influence decision making for personal or partisan gain, to serve certain specific interests, rather than acting to advance broad public interests.

If politics as competition for resources is inevitable in all policy reform processes, politics as competition in elections is equally inevitable in democratic situations. Moreover, electoral politics is both appropriate and desirable, if one believes that democratic government is an important social goal, as we do. As we have seen, any reform program involves value choices. Democratic politics, although imperfect, provides a way to make those choices that is defensible from a number of different—and widely invoked—philosophical points of view.

Because competitive politics, like other human institutions, is imperfect, it is also likely that some of the participants will work to shape what occurs for the benefit of particular interested parties. Someone will always be trying to obtain a contract for a factory in their district or a deal for an importer who has contributed to their political campaign. The issue is one of degree. How far is too far for political actors to go to serve their own interests or a constituent's interests? Because political processes often confer benefits that are eagerly sought, the potential for ethically questionable or even illegal actions is almost always lurking in the political background.

Given that reality, some observers use the word "political" pejoratively—to describe decisions or decision-making processes that they do not particularly like. Thus when they use the term they might mean, "This decision is different from what some technical experts recommend," or even, "This decision is different from what I believe should be done." We believe that such usage is not helpful. In effect, such commentators are trying to present some interests or perspectives (usually their own) as "nonpolitical" and worthy, while suggesting that other, "political" concerns are less legitimate. Yet motivations in the political process are rarely so black and white.

Policy decisions typically involve multiple and conflicting analytical frameworks, stakeholder perspectives, and distributional concerns. For example, suppose that the national pharmacists association calls for higher government salaries to decrease "brain drain" abroad and improve staffing in public health facilities. Similarly, suppose that a local bed net manufacturer argues that public tenders should be based on delivered price, not price at the factory gate, because that is what determines total government outlays. Are these merely self-serving arguments based on interests (pharmacists will get the higher wages, and local manufacturers have lower delivery costs), or do they also embody legitimate, substantive arguments? And if either claim is successful in changing policy, is the result merely "political"?

We do not suggest that arbitrary or self-interested favoritism should dominate policy choices, or that decisions should be left to a no-holds-barred contest among individual and group interests. In many situations, policy decisions involve a choice among alternative principles. For example, a budget decision may involve a choice between the principle that government should spend health dollars to maximize health gains, and the contention that government should spend health dollars for the benefit of the worst-off. Even where the distribution of specific benefits is involved (for example, should active ingredients imported by local manufacturers be exempt from import duties, to give them a competitive edge?), issues of fairness and wider social and economic impact are also at stake.

Priority-setting and distributive decisions inevitably involve value choices. A deliberative political process provides an ethically defensible way to make such difficult social decisions. Pharmaceutical policy reformers need support and training in how to manage such political processes if they are to be effective in pursuing their policy objectives. We turn to these more practical aspects next.

Stakeholder Analysis and Political Context

The first step in analyzing the political aspects of pharmaceutical policy making is to conduct a stakeholder analysis (Brugha and Varvasovszky 2000). This analysis views the political system as a series of actors—they may be groups or individuals—who are competing to push public decision making in the direction they prefer. The actors seek to influence the political process based on their interests, their values, and their perceptions of both problems and solutions.

Those actors have different amounts of various political resources. Such resources can be tangible, such as money, votes, or people willing to work in elections. They also can be intangible, such as expertise, information, access, and credibility. These political resources allow different actors to achieve different levels of influence over the political process and to shape the public debate over important social issues. Various political actors can have dramatically different levels of power in different policy domains. Those with the most influence over higher education spending are likely to be different from those with the most impact on the composition of a nation's essential medicines list.

In debates on national pharmaceutical policy, the major political participants typically include the national medical association, the national and international pharmaceutical manufacturers associations, the generic drug industry, the pharmacists association, different national and international nongovernmental organizations (including civil society groups such as patient associations and consumer associations), national politicians (including the minister of health), and various international agencies and bilateral donors agencies.

As an issue is defined and raised for public action, political actors begin to take positions on the topic and use their resources to influence the process. Their positions may well reflect their narrow interpretations of their own economic interests, but they can also result from other factors. For example, some may be value driven, motivated by philosophy, ideology, or religious beliefs. Or they may be driven by personal experiences. Those concerns can lead stakeholders to advocate views that conflict with their material interests. For example, a minister of health may give priority to access to medicines for a vulnerable group in society (such as the rural poor), even when that policy is opposed by those in the pharmaceutical industry who have been major contributors to his political party's finances. The positions of different actors thus can represent different ethical positions (as discussed in chapter 4). Patterns exist, however, and certain political actors often take similar positions on similar pharmaceutical policies in different countries.

An important aspect of any actor's position is their level of commitment. Actors do not usually deploy all of their resources on each and every issue. The extent to which they do so depends on a variety of considerations. How important is the issue to them? If they do commit fully to a struggle, what is the likelihood of success? What are the implications of the way they deal with this issue for future political battles? In the Republic of Korea, for example, the government implemented a policy in 2000 to separate dispensing from prescribing medicines, and that threatened to reduce the income of physicians. In response, Korean physicians went on strike several times, demonstrating a very high level of commitment on the issue. The government then relented and agreed to change some elements of the reform, including substantial increases in medical fees to compensate physicians for expected income losses (Kwon 2003).

The political game is played within a particular institutional structure, which influences the effectiveness of different kinds of strategies and resources. In a military dictatorship, for example, what usually matters most is personal access to the dictator or key members of his staff or to important officers in the army. In countries where political campaigns are expensive— as in the United States—access to money and to people and organizations with money is vital to political power. In countries where a single political party dominates, as in Mexico under the PRI (Partido Revolucionario Institucional) for 72 years, or in postapartheid South Africa under the ANC (African National Congress), what may matter most is a relationship to the leadership structure of the dominant party. In Bangladesh, for example, in 1983, the country's leader was a new military dictator, who used his substantial political power under martial law to declare a new pharmaceutical policy based on an essential medicines list (Reich 1994). Even that national leader, however, had to contend with intense political opposition from the Bangladesh Medical Association and the multinational pharmaceutical industry.

In some cases, political actors seek to shift the venue for decision making to one that they believe will be more favorable to them. Those who lose in the legislature may appeal to the courts. Those who fear that they will lose at the national level may urge decentralization of a policy choice (or the implementation process) to the provinces, where different political parties may be in power. Decentralization can also create incentives for legislative approval in the policy process. Jason Lakin, in his analysis of the recent health reform in Mexico, argues that "prior implementation [of the reform as pilots] in some states and not in others may have actually helped improve the bill's chances in the legislature by increasing support for the bill among previously excluded states" that wanted similar access to federal resources for health (Lakin 2008, 57).

An important part of any electoral political process is the pattern of competition among a country's political parties. If a group is clearly identified as part of the base of a particular party, its influence will depend on whether that party is in the majority or is part of the governing coalition. Being a swing group can expand one's influence, especially being part of a party that is courted by multiple potential partners to form a coalition government. All of these contextual factors influence how the political process evolves: whether pharmaceutical policy is considered an important item on the public agenda, whether effective policy proposals are developed and debated, whether top leaders take a positive decision on the proposal, and how an adopted policy is implemented in practice.

Moving to Strategy Development

Once reformers have conducted a stakeholder analysis (identifying the key actors and assessing their position and power with regard to the proposed reform), the next step is to design a political strategy to help ensure that the reform will be adopted. The task is to assemble a coalition sufficiently powerful to obtain a favorable political decision. How can reformers turn opponents into supporters, or at least convince them to lessen the intensity of their opposition? How can they mobilize top political leaders (often the minister of health and sometimes the nation's president or prime minister) to support their policy proposals and help deal with political obstacles? The process of developing political strategies requires political skill, which in our view is just as important, if not more important, than political will to policy reformers' success (Reich 1997).

The first set of strategies focuses on influencing various actors to change positions and support the proposed reform. When successful, such efforts can allow reformers to mobilize new groups and individuals, change the political dynamics of the policy debate, and increase the political feasibility of reform. To do that reformers have three broad types of political strategies available to them (Reich 2002).

First are strategies that focus on persuading actors to *change their positions*. That can sometimes be done by modifying the content of the proposal so that it provides some benefits to, or advances the goals of, important political groups or individuals. This change is easiest when the actors in question care about an aspect of the policy that is critical to them but not critical to the overall reform. For example, to convince licensed drug shops to soften their opposition to controls on markups, reformers might agree to exempt various elixirs, over-the-counter preparations, and traditional medicines from the new rules. In this hypothetical example, we can imagine that the reformers' goal is to decrease incentives to sellers to inappropriately push originator brands, and the sellers may accept that if their business in low-end products is left unregulated—a business that reformers may not be especially concerned about.

Another way to influence positions is to offer favors or incentives outside the scope of the proposal itself. Thus reform leaders in parliament might agree to support a new road in a politician's district in return for cooperation on the main policy proposal. Such so-called logrolling is a way of life in the legislatures of all democracies. For example, when the Korean government set out to separate dispensing from prescribing, it changed reimbursement policy under the health insurance system and increased payments to physicians to help reduce their opposition to the new policy (Kwon 2003).

Getting actors to change positions is also possible when those actors do not fully understand their own interests. In those cases, a serious conversation, based on a careful analysis of the implications of a reform, may help a group see common ground or concrete benefits of which they were not previously aware. For example, retailers who fear government interference through anticounterfeiting laws might be convinced that better rules, more effectively enforced, will increase their sales because potential customers will have more confidence in their products.

A second type of strategy focuses on power rather than positions. These strategies seek to increase the resources available to one's supporters and to weaken one's opponents. Friends can be given funding, access, and information; their credibility can be supported in the press; and they can be helped to mobilize their membership more effectively. Conversely, opponents can be cut off from critical decision processes, denied information, and presented in the press as biased or selfish and hence lacking in trustworthiness. These strategies can help readjust the balance of power among groups engaged in a policy debate and help create a more favorable environment for reform. Reformers should bear in mind, however, that such political strategies are likely to generate responses and repercussions from the targeted groups, especially if they are attacked in public. Reformers therefore need to give careful consideration to these strategies, including the potential for counterproductive effects.

The third strategic cluster involves changing the perceptions that both national leaders and the general citizenry have of the issue, including both the problem and the solution. The strategy involves reframing the issue, affecting how it is discussed and portrayed in the public realm and how it relates to broad values held by a population (Lau and Schlesinger 2005). If opponents attack an essential medicines list policy as "restricting access," supporters can portray it as a matter of "using limited funds wisely for greater public benefit" or "providing the most needed medicines for the most common illnesses in the population." Similarly, if opponents of a plan to separate dispensing from prescribing attack it as "undermining tradition," it can be defended as "eliminating long-standing conflicts of interest" and "reducing wasteful and inappropriate use of medicines."

In summary, pharmaceutical policy reformers confront two important political tasks. The first involves understanding, through stakeholder analysis. Reformers need to assess who the players are, what their resources are, and what their positions and levels of commitment are with respect to the policy at hand. The second involves taking action, through strategy design and implementation. Advocates for reform need to devise political strategies that will change the balance of power, position, and perception sufficiently to create a favorable political decision on the policy they are seeking to have adopted and implemented. Policy reform is a profoundly political process, and reformers need to learn that lesson early and well if they hope to succeed in the struggle for pharmaceutical reform. A computer software program for applied political analysis (Reich and Cooper 2009) can help reformers with the tasks of stakeholder analysis and strategy design for specific reform policies.

The Politics of Pharmaceutical Policy Reform—Some Examples

The literature on the politics of pharmaceutical policy reform is not well developed, especially for low- and middle-income countries. Even the literature on the politics of health reform in general in those countries is fairly limited. But a number of case studies have been published, and they suggest certain lessons for reformers who seek to transform national pharmaceutical policies.

An important lesson from the literature is that major pharmaceutical reform is possible under certain political circumstances, despite strong opposition from the international pharmaceutical industry and from rich-country governments. Reich (1995) compared three successful pharmaceutical reforms, in Sri Lanka in the early 1970s, in Bangladesh in the early 1980s, and in the Philippines in the late 1980s. The study concluded that even though foreign pharmaceutical companies dominated the domestic markets in the three countries, major reforms were possible: "For these cases, a strong political base and effective political strategies to manage group competition were more important than the economic structure of the market in determining the feasibility of reform" (Reich 1995, 72). The cases also showed the importance of timing: the chances for reform tend to be better in the early days of a new political regime, whether democratic or not. In all three cases the national physicians associations played a critical role. Because they opposed reform in all three countries, to succeed reformers needed strategies to co-opt or neutralize the physicians association. Another commonality in the three cases was the importance of national political leaders who could invoke broad national values to explain and justify the reform, distinguish the new regime from the old one, and appeal to the majority poor. That illustrates the point that even unorganized members of the population can play a significant political role as a potential source of support and legitimacy for a new regime.

A second important lesson from the literature is that efforts to change licensing and sales policies for medicines depend on the local context and the relative power of the affected stakeholders. Because they involve a substantial redistribution of economic benefits to clearly identified and often well-organized actors, such measures can generate strong opposition from those adversely affected and can produce intense conflicts in a society. Such conflicts can arise, for example, over decisions to introduce an essential medicines list, over the selection of medicines to include on the national formulary, and over decisions to separate prescribing from dispensing by physicians.

An interesting example occurred in Korea in 1993. The Pharmaceutical Act was revised to allow pharmacists trained in contemporary medicine to prepare and sell traditional herbal medicines, and it resulted in a bitter social conflict (Cho 2000). Those medicines, originally brought from China two thousand years ago, developed into a distinct Korean practice known as *Hanbang* medicine with specially trained practitioners known as *hanuisas*. In response to the government's change in policy, the hanuisas organized street demonstrations to protest the sale of herbal medicines by biomedical pharmacists who lacked their special training. When the government moved to require biomedical pharmacists take an exam for handling Hanbang medicines, the pharmacists went on a nationwide strike, with support from the medical association. The conflict continued for several years in the 1990s, as Hanbang medical students organized a strike that lasted two years.

The Korean case also illustrates how economic disputes can easily escalate into broader social struggles, as each side tries to reframe issues to mobilize sympathy from those not directly affected. Opponents of reform invoked "Korean values" as underlying Hanbang medicine, and the developing controversy produced heated attacks and counterattacks about the scientific basis of traditional medicine.

A third important lesson from experiences in pharmaceutical policy is the way that politics can trump science—and not just in low- and middle-income countries. Public health practitioners tend to believe not only that evidence *should* drive policy decisions, but that evidence *does* drive policy decisions. Experience in the real world tells us otherwise. Too often, evidence is shaped and constructed to fit decisions that have already been made by political leaders. It is less, "What does the evidence show us?" than "Find me the evidence to support this."

It is worth noting, from observations of the U.S. political context, that some political leaders are particularly resistant to science and evidence (such as George W. Bush), whereas others are enthusiastic and welcoming to technical expertise and advice (such as Barack Obama). In addition, some policy domains are particularly vulnerable to the politicization of evidence (such as reproductive health and global warming) because they touch directly on core social values. For example, in 2004 the U.S. Food and Drug Administration (FDA) denied over-the-counter access to the emergency contraception medicine mifepristone in the United States. As David Grimes, a leading specialist in obstetrics and gynecology, put it, "Defying the published evidence, the international experience, the recommendation of two FDA advisory committees, and the advice of its own scientific staff, the agency caved in to political pressure" (Grimes 2004, 220). He continued, "The FDA's decision is . . . the antithesis of evidence-based medicine." That example illustrates how the values of political leaders can powerfully drive pharmaceutical policy in ways that may not be resistible or reversible under the existing political regime. Sometimes only a change in leadership can restore evidence-based pharmaceutical policy making.

Summary on Politics

This chapter argues that to be effective, advocates for pharmaceutical policy reform need to engage early and often with political analysis. That engagement has to occur at all steps in the reform process and not just after a policy proposal is formulated. Reformers also need to learn how to create political incentives for leaders and how to deal with political risk. Part of moving reform forward is persuading politicians that the risks of not doing something are greater than the risks of doing something different or new. Such political persuasion requires courage, creativity, persistence, and a capacity to recognize opportunities for change. One of the underappreciated benefits of globalization is that it can sometimes make leaders (and peoples) aware of the advantages of change and reform, that the old ways of doing things are not always the best. Advocates for reforming pharmaceutical policies need to manage the politics of change through hard-nosed political analysis and innovative political strategies.

Case Study on Politics

Guyer, Anya Levy, and Michael R. Reich, "Disentangling Prescribing and Dispensing in the Republic of Korea." Case Study C.

References

Brugha, R., and Z. Varvasovszky. 2000. "Stakeholder Analysis: A Review." *Health Policy and Planning* 15: 239–46.

Cho, B. H. 2000. "The Politics of Herbal Drugs in Korea." *Social Science and Medicine* 51: 505–09.

Grimes, D. A. 2004. "Emergency Contraception: Politics Trumps Science at the U.S. Food and Drug Administration." *Obstetrics and Gynecology* 104: 220–21.

Kwon, S. M. 2003. "Pharmaceutical Reform and Physician Strikes in Korea: Separation of Drug Prescribing and Dispensing." *Social Science and Medicine* 57: 529–38.

Lakin, J. M. 2008. "The Possibilities and Limitations of Insurgent Technocratic Reform: Mexico's Popular Health Insurance Program 2001–2006." PhD diss., Harvard University, Cambridge, MA.

Lasswell, H. D. 1936. *Politics: Who Gets What, When, How.* New York: McGraw-Hill.

Lau, R. R., and M. Schlesinger. 2005. "Policy Frames, Metaphorical Reasoning, and Support for Public Policies." *Political Psychology* 26: 77–114.

Reich, M. R. 1994. "Bangladesh Pharmaceutical Policy and Politics." *Health Policy and Planning* 9: 130–43.

———. 1995. "The Politics of Health Sector Reform in Developing Countries: Three Cases of Pharmaceutical Policy." *Health Policy* 32: 47–77.

———. 1997. "Review of *World Development Report 1993: Investing in Health.*" *Economic Development and Cultural Change* 45: 899–903.

———. 2002. "The Politics of Reforming Health Policies." *Promotion and Education* 9: 138–42.

Reich, M. R., and David M. Cooper. 2009. *PolicyMaker 4.0: Computer-Assisted Political Analysis.* Computer software. Brookline, MA: PoliMap.

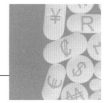

CHAPTER 7

Financing the Pharmaceutical Sector

This chapter starts the second section of the book, which reviews the use of the five control knobs as devices for improving the performance of the pharmaceutical system. Financing is the appropriate place to begin because it involves raising money. It is trivial but true that without money to fund the pharmaceutical sector's activities, the sector would not exist.

Throughout the pharmaceutical sector (and the health care system generally) financing plays a central role in determining who gets what. And because pharmaceutical use has much influence on health status, financing choices have a major impact on that dimension of system performance. When a nation relies heavily on out-of-pocket spending (as is often the case for pharmaceuticals in low- and middle-income countries), purchasers are crucial in who gets what—even if their choices are often influenced by physicians, sellers, manufacturers, and neighbors. When governments use general tax revenue to finance the distribution of medicines through public facilities, government officials make many of the decisions about who gets what. If a nation uses health insurance to cover pharmaceutical costs, decision making is shared. Governments decide what to cover, but patients usually do much of the actual purchasing of medicines from retail outlets.

Financing choices also affect the distribution of the cost burden and whether citizens enjoy any financial protection from pharmaceutical expenses. Relying on out-of-pocket payments—no financial protection—is especially problematic for the poorer people in the population. Such arrangements confront citizens with the need to choose between the medicines they need and other purchases, and that can impose real hardship. It can also lead to significant popular dissatisfaction, in addition to adverse health results. Tax-supported financing, in contrast, provides some risk protection and the possibility of redistributing some of the fiscal burden.

Pharmaceutical Financing and Health Sector Financing

The financing of a nation's pharmaceutical sector cannot be separated from the financing of its overall health care system. The amount of public money available to a country for medicines is the result of a complex mix of forces: its level of economic development, its tax system, and a series of budgetary and expenditure choices. What is the per capita gross domestic product (GDP), and what fraction is in the formal sector? What taxes does the government impose and at what rates? How effectively does it collect those taxes? How much of what it raises does it spend on health care (versus everything else), and how much of that is available for medicines? (Tandon and Cashin 2010).

Especially in low-income countries, needs are great and resources are limited; tax bases are small and collection processes are highly imperfect. Because citizens are often willing to pay out of pocket for pharmaceuticals, it is tempting for governments to allow them to do so. That is especially so because governments often find it difficult to ensure that medicines are available in public facilities, especially in the periphery. The problems of purchasing, distribution, and theft prevention, along with limited capital, are so great that citizens frequently become dissatisfied with the lack of supplies in public facilities. As a result, in many low-income countries we see the paradoxical situation that although medicines are among the most effective forms of health expenditure—and one that citizens care about greatly—they are also an area that governments heavily underfund, so that the greatest part of spending on medicines is left to private, out-of-pocket purchase (as noted in chapter 1).

Sometimes it is possible to change the funding for medicines without changing health sector financing generally (for example, the revolving drug funds supported by the Bamako Initiative). But more usually, the creation of a new insurance scheme or the development of a new tax source involves changes in funding for health sector activities outside of pharmaceuticals. Often it requires the mobilization of a significant support coalition and can lead to complex political negotiations.

In low-income countries, pharmaceutical funding is also entangled with health sector funding through the decision-making processes of donors. Multilateral and bilateral donors that support medicines purchases also often support the health sector generally. So if they spend more on medicines, they may spend less on other health activities and vice versa. Such nonmedicines health funding (and even nonhealth donor support) can, in principle, free local resources for pharmaceutical purchasing. The question is, How do governments choose to use the fiscal space that aid helps to create? At the same time, the conditions tied to donor support can limit the ability of governments to allocate funds to fit their own priorities.

In recent years we have seen a major increase in donor financial aid for medicines for specific diseases (for example, the Global Fund to Fight AIDS, TB, and Malaria; the Global Alliance for Vaccines and Immunization [GAVI]; and the President's Emergency Plan for AIDS Relief [PEPFAR]). Direct donations by manufacturers of drugs for other diseases (such as onchocerciasis, schistosomiasis, and trachoma) have also increased. But these donations are limited in the number of diseases covered and often in the scope of coverage. (For a list of medicine programs supported by pharmaceutical companies, see http://www.globalhealthprogress.org.) As a result, host country funding almost always plays some role in pharmaceutical policy, and it is often the rate-limiting constraint on the scope and composition of public sector activity.

Judging the Distributional Impact of Financing Options

Economists have a particular framework for judging the distributional impact of financing options. They start from a reference point at which all individuals (or families) pay the same fraction of their income to support an activity. Such a burden is said to be "proportional." A financing system in which upper-income people pay a higher proportion of their income is called "progressive," and one in which lower-income people pay a higher proportion of their income is "regressive."

Reformers who care most about increasing equity tend to favor financing systems that are progressive. However, even a regressive system can involve higher absolute (albeit lower proportional) burdens on upper-income households. Hence the combined impact of a regressive financing system (provided it is not too regressive) and a pro-poor distribution of benefits (provided it is sufficiently pro-poor) can, on balance, be redistributive in favor of lower-income groups.

Financing Options

We propose a six-way typology to describe the major options for financing a nation's health system and its pharmaceutical sector.

General Tax Revenue

Almost all nations rely to some extent on general tax revenue for financing pharmaceutical purchases. Which taxes are levied depends on a country's level of economic development. The lowest-income countries, with the smallest formal business sectors, often rely heavily on import duties. The number of possible ports of entry (through which significant quantities of goods can move) is generally sufficiently limited to make enforcement possible. If countries are lucky enough to have minerals, significant commodity exports, or tourist industries, those too are often taxed.

Like taxes on imports, taxes on exports are indirect. Indirect taxes are not directly paid by workers or consumers, but rather by nonretail businesses, and that can make them politically attractive. In practice, however, import duties generally result in higher prices for imported goods. That is one reason why they are often levied at higher rates on luxury goods, such as imported vehicles and imported alcoholic beverages. Export fees are often borne by local producers in the form of lower net incomes, inasmuch as they typically have to meet world prices for their exports.

Once countries attain even a modest level of development, sales and value-added taxes are commonly used. They are easier to implement than taxes on individuals because there are fewer sellers than buyers and hence fewer points of collection. A similar logic applies to certain kinds of business taxes. The conventional wisdom in industrialized economies is that sales and value-added taxes are regressive. Upper-income individuals save a higher proportion of their incomes, and income that is saved escapes such taxes.

In low- and middle-income countries, however, a good deal of economic activity escapes all taxation, for example, subsistence farming and cash transactions in the informal sector. Because a higher percentage of the consumption of upper-income individuals is likely to be subject to tax, the progressivity of retail taxes is increased. That progressivity has been an important consideration in countries, such as Ghana and Colombia, that have chosen to finance social insurance systems for low-income individuals through retail taxes and have used the proceeds in part to provide low-cost medicines in the public sector.

Historically, many low- and middle-income countries have exempted certain commodities from sales taxes. They have even provided subsidies to keep certain prices low in the name of redistributive goals and to increase the political popularity of the regime (bread, rice, gasoline, or housing, depending on the country). Conversely, in many countries some luxury goods are subject to higher sales tax rates (including jewelry, restaurant meals, and automobiles).

The key concept in those schemes is what economists call the "income elasticity of demand." In particular, how does the percentage of income spent on a certain good vary with income? When that percentage rises with income, a tax on the good in question is progressive. When the percentage falls, even if the amount spent rises, a tax on that good is regressive. Taxes on staple commodities, for example, are quite regressive. Yet many countries in recent years have undergone the politically painful process of removing subsidies from basic commodities. Iran, for example, removed subsidies for diesel, gas, and bread in December 2010, with the price of flour jumping 20 times and gas prices rising fourfold (Bozorgmehr 2010). Governments have taken those steps because such subsidies are very costly in budget terms, and much of their benefit goes to people who are not poor.

These conflicting considerations play out in the pharmaceutical sector in debates over whether medicines should be exempt from sales or value-added taxes. With relatively few formal outlets and high sales volumes of a high-value product, pharmaceuticals are a tempting target for tax collectors, who are always short of revenue. And in countries with at least some availability of low-cost medicines in the public sector, private sector purchasers (especially in licensed drug shops) tend to be the relatively better-off. On the other hand, such taxes raise prices, discourage use, and create financial burdens on lower-income families.

Economies that support a significant formal business sector can generally collect considerable revenue through payroll taxes. But the potential contributions from that source depend on the sector's relative importance. Because small farmers and businessmen normally operate on a cash and barter basis, tracking their incomes is effectively impossible. Only industrialized nations, in which almost all producers and financial intermediaries maintain elaborate accounting systems, can implement individual income taxes. Yet only comprehensive income taxes can produce progressive burdens at the top of the income distribution because they are the only taxes that can capture and tax income from investments.

The flexibility of general tax revenue financing is both an advantage and a disadvantage. Because general tax revenues are not tied to a specific activity or area of application, governments can redirect the funds as needs arise or as leaders decide. That, however, makes such revenue an insecure source of pharmaceutical financing, as competing needs, economic difficulties, unforeseen challenges, or political pressures can lead to a loss of funding. In many low-income countries such funding variations have led to procurement difficulties and delays and to serious problems of drug availability in the public sector (see case study E, "Drug Procurement in East Africania").

Social Insurance

As economies have grown in recent years, many countries, from Tunisia to Thailand, have moved to social insurance as a way of financing their health systems (Gottret, Schieber, and Waters 2008). Although the arrangements vary greatly, what we might call the "ideal type" of social insurance system has four features: mandatory contributions by the covered population, funding from dedicated payroll taxes, administration by a quasi-autonomous agency, and fiscal independence. Note that we do not include the direct operation of a tied delivery system as a part of the ideal type, although that is a feature of many systems worldwide.

Compared to general revenue financing, social insurance has some attractive features as a way to finance the pharmaceutical sector. Because the funds are separately administered and held for the purpose of providing benefits to contributors, reformers hope that such a system will be accepted by those subject to the tax, and that tax avoidance and evasion hence will be lower. As a tied revenue source, such financing is also less subject to fluctuations due to the vagaries of national political decision making. Moreover, because membership is mandatory for the covered population, social insurance is an effective mechanism for spreading the risk of illness over that group.

In many countries, such systems began where it was easiest for the government to collect taxes: with civil servants, large industrial concerns such as mining or the railroads, and the security services. With time, a number of middle-income countries have consolidated such separate funds into a national system and extended its coverage, either incrementally or rapidly, into a universal scheme.

Some low-income countries are also introducing this approach, although the traditional route of payroll tax financing is not really available. For example, the largest source of financing for Ghana's new national health insurance scheme has been a dedicated increase in the value-added tax. In addition, social insurance reserves and donors have provided critical support, with little funding coming from contributions by the covered population. It is worth noting that such an insurance scheme is as much a *redistributive* system as a *risk pooling* system—to restate the distinction introduced in chapter 5. In Ghana, nearly 50 percent of the fund's spending has been for medicines, many of which are used to deal with the routine fevers and infections normally seen in a primary care setting. That represents about half of Ghana's total pharmaceutical expenditures. Another 34 percent is funded by out-of-pocket outlays, and 13 percent comes from the ministry of health (Seiter and Gyansa-Lutterodt 2008, 19).

Even in upper-income settings, covering medicines under social insurance has been a challenge for many countries. For an extreme example, the social insurance scheme for elders in the United States—Medicare—only began covering prescription drugs in the last decade (Kravitz and Chang 2005). The main difficulty is controlling the cost of such coverage. Because insured citizens can make medicine purchases without paying the full (or often any) cost, such systems tend to encourage greater use and overwhelm the available funding. This is a pattern that economists call "moral hazard."

To counteract the risk of moral hazard, social insurance systems that pay for drugs often limit the products paid for and the prices that are paid. For example, some plans specify that only certain generics will be funded for patients diagnosed with chronic illnesses. Others adopt "tiered co-payment," meaning that patients have to pay more out-of-pocket for some drugs than others. Or they may use reference pricing (see the next chapter for more details), in which all drugs in a class are reimbursed at the same rate, and citizens have to pay the difference between the reference price and the actual price for more expensive compounds. Where such limits are not in place, drug costs can rise steeply, as they have under the Ghana social insurance plan (see case study J, "Drug Coverage in Ghana's National Health Insurance Scheme"). But trying to limit drug benefits typically produces significant political conflict. The reason is that physicians, manufacturers, and dispensers typically oppose such initiatives vigorously (as the framework on political analysis presented in chapter 6 would predict).

As shown in figure 7.1, population coverage by social health insurance varies significantly around the world, with the highest levels in the established market economies. A broad range of coverage shows up in Latin

Figure 7.1 National Health Insurance Coverage for Countries by Region

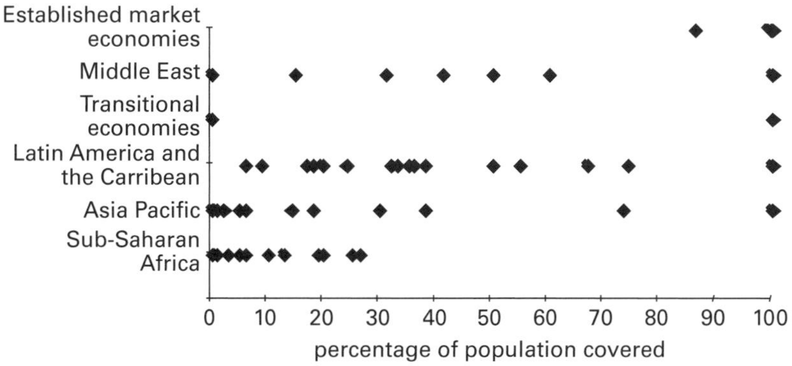

Source: Quick and Tolentino 2000. Reproduced by permission of the publisher.

America and the Caribbean, and the lowest levels are in Sub-Saharan Africa (from zero to 30 percent).

Private Insurance

Private health insurance is the most regressive form of health care financing because it is based on premiums that do not vary at all with the buyer's income level. Hence poorer people, even in upper-income countries, cannot afford such coverage.

Private insurance also confronts a fundamental structural problem in dealing with the health sector. Conceptually, insurance is designed to deal with unpredictable risks. That unpredictability leads a wide variety of purchasers to join insurance plans, thereby spreading the risk of loss over a large number of participants. Yet much of the variation in health care costs across individuals is reasonably predictable. Because of age or chronic disease, some of us are just sicker than others and have higher health care costs, including the costs of medicines for conditions such as hypertension and diabetes.

Faced with that predictability, health insurers have several choices. The most obvious is to charge higher premiums to people who are likely to use more care, or even refuse to cover the sickest individuals. In either case, people who carry the largest financial burdens, and in that sense are most in need of insurance, are likely to be left without affordable coverage. The difficulties caused by predictability only increase as countries move through the epidemiological transition from communicable to noncommunicable disease, as is happening in many low- and middle-income nations.

Alternatively, insurers can charge everyone in a covered population the same rate to encourage widespread insurance purchasing and risk spreading. But then the insurance plan will not be actuarially attractive for the healthiest people with the lowest expected health care costs. The reason is that premiums then have to be set high enough to cover the likely costs of care of high as well as low users. As a result, at least some healthy individuals will decide to take their chances with the costs of getting sick and not buy insurance. As that response continues, insurers are left with a covered group that steadily becomes sicker and more expensive and that has to pay ever-higher premiums. This process is sometimes called the "adverse selection" death spiral.

To counteract such a process, private health insurance is often sold on a group basis (for example, to all the employees in a company), and those in the group are not allowed to opt in or out individually. That allows risk to be spread between the healthier and sicker members of the group, although not between healthier and sicker groups. It is only applicable to relatively large groups of employees in well-organized, formal sector enterprises.

Pharmaceutical Reform

In sum, private insurance is not a viable option for covering the bulk of medicine costs in low- and middle-income countries. Small numbers of multinational, private sector corporations may make group purchases of private health insurance for their executives and white-collar workers. But in general, they are the same people who could and would cover all but the most exceptional medicines costs out of their own pockets without undue economic hardship.

Community Financing

In many low-income counties, even poor rural residents often pay significant amounts for pharmaceuticals out of their personal funds. The question is, Can this willingness to pay be tapped by mechanisms that promote risk protection, more rational use, and the assurance of good quality? In recent years, interest has increased in one possible response, locally controlled, small-scale social insurance schemes that are often called "community financing."

The idea is to get everyone in an area (typically a village or a collection of adjoining villages) to make modest contributions to an insurance fund that can support basic primary care, with local leaders or a local board providing managerial direction. The approach has been especially attractive in providing staff (and funds) to peripheral areas. In some models the fund is supplemented by transfers from higher levels of government, especially for poorer locations.

Experience with these schemes suggests several conditions for success. First, mandatory membership is helpful to counter adverse selection. When only the sickest join, there is less risk spreading, and per member costs become too high. But in many cultures the logic of insurance is not well understood, and it is not easy to persuade citizens to contribute to a fund when they do not immediately need services. The second lesson is the value to the local management group of technical assistance, training, and support. As one might expect, variations in culture (including literacy and sophistication) influence the effectiveness of the management of community funds. Third, the scope of covered benefits has to depend on the size of the group, as well as its income level. To achieve actuarial stability, covering even basic hospital services requires a group so large that the face-to-face accountability of village-level governance can be lost. In addition, in poorer areas residents may simply be unable to afford the necessary premiums, and the managerial challenges grow as well (Carrin, Waelkens, and Criel 2005).

As with social insurance generally, the challenges of covering medicine costs under community financing revolve around cost control. Which medicines are covered, for whom, and with what level of co-pays? The presence of medicine coverage without mandatory membership is likely to exacerbate adverse selection problems. In addition, the promoters of such schemes have to work out how the coverage they provide relates to free medicine distribution that is supposed to occur through the public sector.

One example of a way to deal with these issues is offered by the system of "mutuelles," as community insurance schemes are called in Rwanda (WHO 2008). A basic payment of 1,000 Rwandan francs (about US$2) per person, per year, covers health center services. In terms of pharmaceutical coverage, those health centers only stock basic, generic medicines on the national essential medicines list. (Nonsubscribers have significant co-pays.) Medicines and other costs associated with hospital visits are covered under a separate insurance scheme supported by national government and donor funds, which Rwanda has been fortunate enough to be able to attract in relatively large volume.

Experience with community financing demonstrates a basic truth of all pharmaceutical reform efforts, namely, that "the devil is in the details." How such a scheme operates in practice and its ultimate impact depend greatly on specific features of its design. For example, the Rwandan system has been criticized by some because all participants pay the same fee, regardless of income, and that creates a financial burden on the poorest families. Similar choices include the degree of redistribution from the center to the poorest districts, whether fees are individual or family based, and how pharmaceutical expenses are controlled—including any systems designed to promote appropriate use.

Out-of-Pocket Payment

As we have noted several times, out-of-pocket payment is a major form of pharmaceutical financing in low- and middle-income countries. Because of logistical and managerial failures, and varying amounts of leakage, it is not unusual for significant supply shortages to occur in public clinics and hospitals. That can lead patients and their families to purchase drugs and supplies from the private sector (including, in the case of hospitals, even X-ray film, anesthesia gases, and basic surgical dressings from vendors conveniently located across the street from the hospital entrance).

Payment can also be required in the public sector. A number of poorer countries operate their outpatient public medicine supply systems on a cash-and-carry basis, and patients, health centers, hospitals, and even district stores have to pay for what they take at the time of delivery. The reason is that they cannot afford any other option (as illustrated by experiences in Cameroon and Senegal) (Govindaraj and Herbst 2006).

From an equity or financial protection point of view, out-of-pocket payment is undesirable. As a form of financing it is a source of citizen dissatisfaction and a contributor to poor health outcomes. But as this review of financing options suggests, fiscally hard-pressed governments in low- and middle- income countries do not have many other options to finance the costs of medicines, given citizens' demand for pharmaceuticals.

Out-of-pocket financing for medicines also creates a series of incentives (up and down the supply chain) for inappropriate use. Dispensers have every reason to stock and push more profitable products, including on-patent medicines, well-known originator brands now off-patent, and well-established and branded generics. All are likely to have higher prices and margins, compared to the lowest-priced generics. Another example is customer desires for medicines that are not consistent with principles of rational use. Why not sell a customer less than a full course of antibiotic treatment, if that is what they want or is all they can afford?

Because of the profits to be made, distributors and manufacturers have strong incentives to offer financial inducements to enlist the cooperation of retail sellers to increase the sales of their products. These can be based, for example, on the volume of sales that retailers produce for a wholesaler's product line, or on the amount of visible shelf space they devote to a particular product. The incentives can take the form of rebates, discounts, or cash bonuses—payments that in other contexts might be labeled bribes or kickbacks but which may not be illegal, depending on national law.

In effect, frontline medicine sellers are in the same position as traditional herbalists (and many of their modern medicine counterparts) in Asian countries who both prescribe and dispense medicines and depend on medicines sales for much or most of their income. That situation has led to efforts to separate dispensing from prescribing for physicians in the Republic of Korea; Japan; and Taiwan, China, because of the conflicts of interest inherent when dispensing and prescribing are combined in the same individual or institution.

Studies of cash-and-carry systems in the public sector reveal some of the same tendencies seen in the for-profit sector for dispensers (and central stores managers) to promote high-margin products and the overuse of some medicines to raise total revenue (Govindaraj and Herbst 2006). Similarly, subsidized drugs, which provide little or no profit, can be underused in cash-and-carry public systems, as sellers have no economic incentive to encourage their purchase.

Such questions have been raised about the effect of the new global subsidy for artemisinin-based combination therapies (ACTs) for malaria. These new antimalarials are being sold cheaply in the private sectors of many countries as a result of a carefully constructed system that provides a global subsidy for them. The scheme's creators hope that the subsidized products will displace more expensive and nonsubsidized artemisinin monotherapies (that carry a high risk of fostering antimicrobial resistance) and also displace the inexpensive older medicines (such as chloroquine) that are largely ineffective (Laxminarayan and Gelband 2009).

This approach is not without some risks however. If ACTs are subsidized sufficiently to be competitive with the cheaper alternatives, will private sellers promote the appropriate use of rapid diagnostic tests to confirm malaria infection before supplying ACTs? Doing so might well decrease their sales. Yet the use of such tests is essential to delaying the development of resistance to ACTs. In fact recent studies suggest that even when rapid diagnostic tests are available, in both public and private facilities, the tests are used in less than one-third of the cases where treatment is provided. Instead, most providers still use a symptom-based approach to diagnosis (Uzuchukwu et al. 2010). In addition, how can private sellers be prevented from charging higher prices for the subsidized ACTs and keeping the difference?

Because out-of-pocket financing transfers so much decision making to patients, and because patients are imperfect decision makers, this kind of financing can lead to considerable inappropriate and cost-ineffective use of medicines. That is especially the case in countries where medicines are commonly sold without a physician's prescription. Often they are also countries where many counterfeit and substandard drugs are in the marketplace. In such circumstances consumers are often understandably suspicious of names they are unfamiliar with—especially if the unfamiliar options are relatively cheap. But that response can easily lead them to overbuy based on brand names. (Because of such dynamics, counterfeiters now make great efforts to imitate the packaging of branded products to attract consumers who are seeking good quality.) Similarly, it is inevitable that drug buyers in such settings will gravitate toward products whose look, smell, and taste they find attractive. They will also be attracted to products that produce immediate experiential impact: psychoactive drugs, pain relievers, decongestants, laxatives, and medicines that relieve gastric pain. But do such choices lead to a clinically optimal pattern of use?

In this context we also must note the rise and fall of the revolving drug funds that were established under the Bamako Initiative (named for a WHO regional conference in Bamako, Mali, in 1987) and promoted by United Nations Children's Fund (UNICEF). The initiative in many ways was a precursor to the community financing efforts discussed above. The underlying theory was that decentralization of the primary health care system to the community would improve its performance and effectiveness. The pharmaceutical aspects of the scheme, however, were largely based on out-of-pocket payment, with no meaningful risk-pooling or insurance features. Faced with significant management challenges, including shortages of working capital, many of the funds succumbed to the same revenue-generating incentives that pervade the private sector, behaving in similar fashion (McPake, Hanson, and Mills 1993).

Donor Assistance

As noted above, the pharmaceutical sector is highly attractive for donor assistance. It has become an important source of funding for the sector in low- and middle-income countries. One reason for that pattern can be found in the accountability and governance structures of foreign donors. Donor governments, foundations, and multinational organizations are all under pressure to demonstrate the effectiveness of their funding support in the health sector. The purchase of products such as ACTs or antiretrovirals (ARVs), which promise to do immediate good for poor people in poor countries, provides a tangible result to present to a parliamentary oversight committee or a board of directors. To foster domestic political acceptability, some bilateral donors also place conditions on their funding (so-called tied aid) that require it to be used to purchase goods and services from donor country sources. (Such practices have received more attention in the context of food aid because of their adverse impact on local agricultural markets.) Multilateral agencies also operate within their own accountability structures. Organizations such as the World Bank have to answer to governance boards that ask for proof that money is being well spent. As a result the Bank and other, similar agencies have been criticized for favoring infrastructure over other kinds of projects because of the tangible results such priorities produce (Stiglitz 2002).

This pattern is understandable. We began this book by noting that, when taken properly, medicines can decrease disability and deaths. From the point of view of donors, such aid offers the additional motivational gain that the recipients come close to being identifiable rather than statistical beneficiaries. It is the same motivation that leads many individuals and governments to help those in acute danger without invoking cost-benefit considerations: children trapped in wells, old people in burning buildings, and patients suffering from curable but otherwise fatal diseases (McKie and Richardson 2003). If a donor helps a government in a low-income country reform its health care financing system, on average, some of the latter's citizens will benefit. But exactly who they are and exactly how they gain from the aid cannot be easily known. In contrast, consider the experience of donor representatives on a visit to a primary care center, meeting a young child suffering from cerebral malaria whose life was saved by prompt treatment with ACTs. Such patients call on the moral instinct behind "the rule of rescue," the fundamental human impulse to help a person in danger who is right in front of us (as discussed in chapter 4, on ethics).

Although it is difficult to estimate all sources of donor assistance in a single country, some recent estimates by a consultancy mission (on behalf of the European Commission) to Liberia are illustrative of the patterns of financing for medicines and medical supplies that can occur. Table 7.1 shows the large role of international agencies and nongovernmental organizations and the inability to estimate private out-of-pocket payments.

Table 7.1   Resources for Medicines and Medical Supplies in Liberia, 2007 and 2008

Source	2007 (US$)	2008 (US$)
Government of Liberia[a]	1,000,000	1,000,000
European Commission	0	0
U.S. Agency for International Development	0	0
Global Fund to Fight AIDS, Tuberculosis, and Malaria	1,292,000	2,000,000
GAVI	850,000	2,427,881
UNICEF[b]	2,465,142	1,318,276
WHO[b]	986,336	290,227
United Nations Population Fund	—	—
NGOs[c]	2,840,010	2,840,010
Faith-based organizations	—	—
Revenue (cash sales by National Drug Service)[d]	450,000	450,000
Private out-of-pocket	—	—
United Nations Mission in Liberia	—	—
Commercial (Firestone)	—	—
Total	9,883,488	10,326,394

Source: Osmond, O'Connell, and Bunting 2007.

Note: — = not available; NGO = nongovernmental organization.

a. Based on Ministry of Health and Social Welfare maintaining same level of funding for next year.

b. Figures for vaccines and immunization only.

c. Based on interviews and questionnaire returned by the major NGOs in health and on the same level of funding remaining for 2008.

d. Based on National Drug Service cash sales available for procurement remaining the same.

From a national policy point of view, the chief disadvantage of relying on external sources of financing is loss of control. Donors typically have their own agendas, which may not match national priorities (Périn and Attaran 2003). That problem has been especially troublesome in the HIV arena, as well as in polio eradication, and is reflected in the pressure from GAVI on countries to adopt an expanded set of immunizations. In addition, donors' desire to meet their own accountability requirements can lead to the multiplication of paperwork and the creation of parallel supply chains, all increasing costs. Another challenge is the resistance of many donors to multiyear commitments, making medium-term planning very difficult. The multiple sources of financing thus have real consequences for the structure of the system and can lead to substantial management challenges. The complex map of supply chain routes in Kenya, shown in figure 7.2, is typical of what has happened in many countries as they have responded to these pressures.

Yet donors also can play a positive role. In particular, they can help sincere reformers withstand local political pressures and can support the creation of delivery system organizations with higher levels of professionalism and performance. The Nobel Prize economist Thomas Schelling has explored how in negotiations, not having the power to give in can be an advantage (Schelling 1956). The response, "The donors won't allow that," is one form that such desirable incapacity can take.

Pharmaceutical Financing Choices

As noted at the beginning of this chapter, different pharmaceutical financing strategies have important implications for access, use, and cost of medicines and thereby affect health status, financial protection, and consumer satisfaction. Pharmaceutical policy expert Anita Wagner has compared the advantages and disadvantages of some of the pharmaceutical financing options, with the results shown in table 7.2. Wagner's category "appropriate use" can be considered a process indicator related to our outcome measure of health status, and her subcategory "affordable cost/patient" relates to our category "financial protection."

Focusing on the four options in table 7.2 (out of the six we have discussed) makes sense, given that private insurance is largely irrelevant in low- and middle-income countries and donor financing is outside of a national government's control. Wagner's analysis suggests that keeping down the cost to the state has driven national pharmaceutical funding choices, especially in poorer countries. The relevant question for many nations apparently is whether they can find a way, other than tax-supported financing, to produce additional financial protection for citizens with regard to pharmaceutical

Figure 7.2   Commodity Logistics System in Kenya

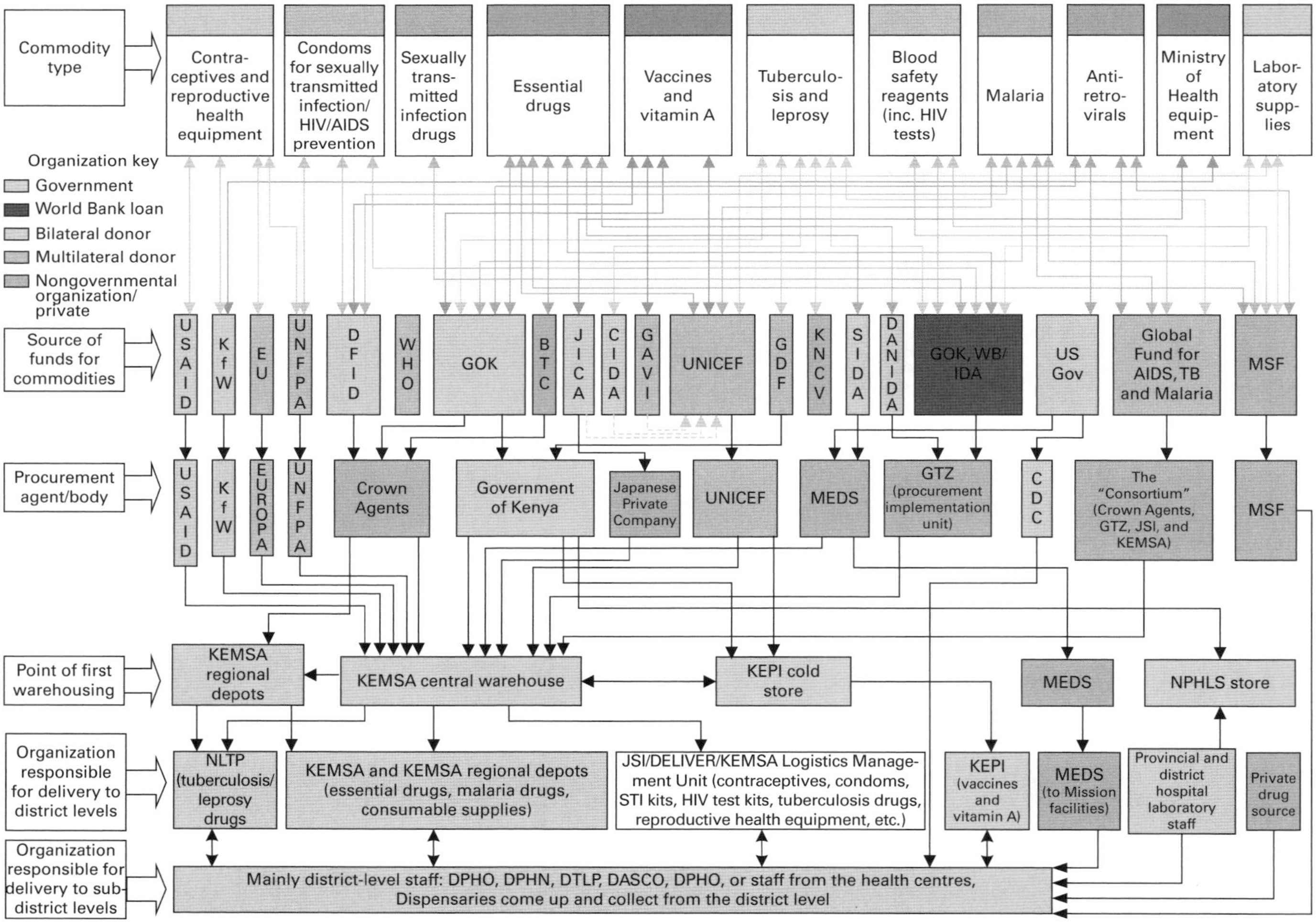

Commodity type

Contraceptives and reproductive health equipment | Condoms for sexually transmitted infection/HIV/AIDS prevention | Sexually transmitted infection drugs | Essential drugs | Vaccines and vitamin A | Tuberculosis and leprosy | Blood safety reagents (inc. HIV tests) | Malaria | Anti-retrovirals | Ministry of Health equipment | Laboratory supplies

Organization key

Source of funds for commodities:
- Government
- World Bank loan
- Bilateral donor
- Multilateral donor
- Nongovernmental organization/private

USAID | KfW | EU | UNFPA | GOK | WHO | DFID | BTC | JICA | GAVI | UNICEF | GDF | KNCV | SIDA | DANIDA | GOK, WB/IDA | US Gov | Global Fund for AIDS, TB and Malaria | MSF

Procurement agent/body

USAID | KfW | EUROPA | UNFPA | Crown Agents | Government of Kenya | Japanese Private Company | UNICEF | MEDS | GTZ (procurement implementation unit) | CDC | The "Consortium" (Crown Agents, GTZ, JSI, and KEMSA) | MSF

Point of first warehousing

KEMSA regional depots | NLTP (tuberculosis/leprosy drugs) | KEMSA central warehouse | KEPI cold store | KEPI (vaccines and vitamin A) | MEDS | NPHLS store | Private drug source

Organization responsible for delivery to district levels

KEMSA and KEMSA regional depots (essential drugs, malaria drugs, consumable supplies) | JSI/DELIVER/KEMSA Logistics Management Unit (contraceptives, condoms, STI kits, HIV test kits, tuberculosis drugs, reproductive health equipment, etc.) | MEDS (to Mission facilities) | Provincial and district hospital laboratory staff

Organization responsible for delivery to sub-district levels

Mainly district-level staff: DPHO, DPHN, DTLP, DASCO, DPHO, or staff from the health centres, Dispensaries come up and collect from the district level

Source: Center for Global Development 2007, 102. Reproduced by permission of the publisher.

116

Table 7.2 Pharmaceutical Financing: Comparing Options

Options	Equitable access	Appropriate use	Affordable cost Patient	Affordable cost State
Tax financing	++	+	++	—
Out-of-pocket payment	—	—	—	++
Donor assistance	++	+	++	++
Social insurance	+	++	++	+

Source: Wagner 2006.

Note: – = not usually achieved; + = potentially somewhat achievable; ++ = potentially quite achievable.

costs. Our review suggests that there is no magic option. The two ways available are either social insurance or community financing. The only other possibility is to continue out-of-pocket payment, with all the inequity and lack of risk protection that that option involves. And if the experience of countries such as Ghana or Colombia is any guide, social insurance for low-income individuals in low- and middle-income countries will have to be supported mainly by general tax revenues, with all the problems of revenue limits and competing claims that such a choice entails (Gottret, Schieber, and Waters 2008).

Readers should note, however, that table 7.2 refers to what is "potentially achievable." Our experience teaches us that the variation in outcomes of the same policy can be as great as the variation between different policies. How a social insurance program that provides some pharmaceutical coverage is implemented will have an enormous impact on the results achieved. For example, how extensive will the benefits be in terms of which medicines are covered? Will high-cost alternatives to effective generics be excluded or discouraged through tiered co-payments? What will that policy do to encourage sellers to push appropriate rather than inappropriate medicines—for example, paying them in the form of a fixed dispensing fee? What will be done, in terms of premiums and co-pays, to expand coverage to lower-income individuals? How can all of that be done without making the cost to the state unaffordable? Those are some of the questions that nations will confront in the years ahead (once our current economic troubles are behind us) if the spread of social insurance continues its recent pace of expansion in the world.

Summary on Financing

There is no simple answer to the dilemmas that low- and middle-income countries face in financing their health care systems in general and their pharmaceutical sectors in particular. The most fundamental difficulty lies in their relative lack of resources. Even so, different financing alternatives can be more or less effective. In particular, financing choices can have a huge impact on the distribution of the financing burden and on the degree of financial protection a country provides to its citizens. However tempting it may be for countries to rely on out-of-pocket payment for medicines, that method does poorly in many respects—especially in equity terms. It creates access barriers, fosters allocative inefficiency, and offers no financial protection, problems that particularly affect low-income citizens. Using general tax revenue, however, is very difficult in a country that lacks such revenue. Classic, payroll-tax-supported social insurance may not be feasible in a nation with a relatively small formal sector. Donor financing also has its drawbacks in the form of added administrative complexity and the external pressures placed on national decision making.

This summary makes it clear that low-income countries, and often middle-income countries as well, will continue to face shortfalls in their systems for financing pharmaceuticals. That realization leads to a number of conclusions. First, regardless of the approach that is adopted, nations need to work to implement their pharmaceuticals financing arrangements in an efficient and corruption-free manner. That means, for example, fighting fraud in claims processing under any social insurance system and putting in place controls and incentives to promote rational drug use (see case study J, "Drug Coverage in Ghana's National Health Insurance Scheme"). We would also urge reformers who move to new financing arrangements to pay particular attention to equity concerns.

Financing, as we said at the beginning of this chapter, is a crucial determinant of who gets what. Any attempt to provide financial protection and diminish access barriers through insurance or community financing requires careful attention to a variety of program design details. Do premiums vary with income? Are special arrangements in place for the poorest citizens? Do remote and backward districts get additional, compensatory assistance? Finally, because funds inevitably are scarce, nations need to pay great attention to using whatever funds are available in the most efficient and effective ways possible. Doing that requires them to pay attention to the operation of the pharmaceutical sector itself—and to the functioning of the other four control knobs, which is the subject we consider next.

Case Study on Financing and Payment

Blanchet, Nathan, and Marc J. Roberts, "Drug Coverage in Ghana's National Health Insurance Scheme." Case Study J.

References

Bozorgmehr, N. 2010. "Iran Cuts Send Diesel Price Soaring." *Financial Times*, December 20.

Carrin, G., M. P. Waelkens, and B. Criel. 2005. "Community-Based Health Insurance in Developing Countries: A Study of its Contribution to the Performance of Health Financing Systems." *Tropical Medicine and International Health* 10: 799–811.

Center for Global Development. 2007. "*A Risky Business: Saving Money and Improving Global Health Through Better Demand Forecasts*. Washington, DC: Center for Global Development.

Gottret, P., G. Schieber, and H. R. Waters. 2008. *Good Practices in Health Financing*. Washington, DC: World Bank.

Govindaraj, R., and C. Herbst. 2006. "Impact of 'Marketizing' Organizational Reform on Public Sector Pharmaceutical Supply in Francophone Africa." Draft, Africa Human Development Department, World Bank, Washington, DC.

Kravitz, R. L., and S. Chang. 2005. "Promise and Perils for Patients and Physicians." *New England Journal of Medicine* 353: 2735–39.

Laxminarayan, R., and H. Gelband. 2009. "A Global Subsidy: Key to Affordable Drugs for Malaria?" *Health Affairs* 28: 949–61.

McKie, J., and J. Richardson. 2003. "The Rule of Rescue." *Social Science and Medicine* 56: 2407–19.

McPake, B., K. Hanson, and A. Mills. 1993. "Community Financing of Health Care in Africa: An Evaluation of the Bamako Initiative." *Social Science and Medicine* 36: 1383–95.

Osmond, B., A. O'Connell, and R. Bunting. 2007. *Review of the Pharmaceuticals Area and Preparation of a Mid-Term Pharmaceuticals Policy and Implementation Plan for the Ministry of Health and Social Welfare, Liberia*. Consultancy on behalf of the European Commission. Draft final report, April.

Périn, I., and A. Attaran. 2003. "Trading Ideology for Dialogue: An Opportunity to Fix International Aid for Health?" *Lancet* 361: 1216–19.

Quick, J. D., and R. B. Tolentino. 2000. *Global Comparative Pharmaceutical Expenditures with Related Reference Information*. Health Economics and Drugs. EDM series No. 3. Geneva: WHO.

Schelling, T. C. 1956. "An Essay on Bargaining." *American Economic Review* 46: 281–306.

Seiter, A., and M. Gyansa-Lutterodt. 2008. "Policy Note: The Pharmaceutical Sector in Ghana." Draft, World Bank, Washington, DC, December.

Stiglitz, J. E. 2002. *Globalization and Its Discontents.* New York: W.W. Norton.

Tandon, A., and C. Cashin. 2010. "Assessing Public Expenditure on Health from a Fiscal Space Perspective." HNP Discussion Paper, World Bank, Washington, DC.

Uzuchukwu, B. S. C., L. O. Chiegboka, C. Enwereuzo, U. Nwoso, D. Okafor, O. E. Onwujekwe, N. P. Uguru, F. T. Sibeudu, and O. P. Ezeoke. 2010. "Examining Appropriate Diagnosis and Treatment of Malaria: Availability and Use of Rapid Diagnostic Tests and Artemisinin-Based Combination Therapy in Public and Private Health Facilities in South East Nigeria." *BMC Public Health* 10: 486.

Wagner, A. 2006. "Financing, Provider Payments, and Opportunities for Change in Insurance Systems." Presentation to the Flagship Course, Washington, DC, World Bank.

WHO (World Health Organization). 2008. "Sharing the Burden of Sickness: Mutual Health Insurance in Rwanda." *Bulletin of the World Health Organization* 86 (11): 823–24.

CHAPTER 8

Paying for Pharmaceuticals

In attempting to understand, and change the performance of, any system of production and distribution, economists give much attention to payment arrangements. That follows from their belief that the incentives that payment systems create greatly affect individual and organizational behavior. Indeed, a current slogan that summarizes that belief is ironically called "the modern Golden Rule": *Whoever has the gold makes the rules*.

Thinking about how changing payment arrangements can influence the performance of the pharmaceutical sector requires that reformers pay attention to three types of transactions:

- Payments made in the course of public sector procurement

- Wholesale payments made by various intermediaries along the supply chain

- Retail payments made by customers at dispensing sites.

In this chapter, under the *payment control knob*, we consider only payments for medicines (and some closely associated services, such as retail consultations). Many other flows of money obviously also occur within the pharmaceutical arena (for example, salary payments to public sector employees); those are considered in the discussion of the organization control knob, in the next chapter.

Broadly considered, every payment system, for medicines or anything else, has three components: (1) the basis or unit of payment, (2) the price paid for each unit, and (3) the method of setting that price. Just noting that triad allows us to see that some issues may need more attention than they generally receive. For example, although the unit question is often discussed when pharmaceutical procurement policy is considered, it receives less attention at the retail level. But there too, as we will see, options exist that reformers may want to consider. Similarly, the strong stakeholder pressures that often swirl around price-setting decisions give countries good reason to consider seriously the design of the institutions and processes that make those choices.

Before we begin our analysis, a word of caution is in order. Reformers need to be aware that the power of the incentives that payment systems generate can lead to significant problems. In practice, it is often not possible to pay for the precise outputs or performance that policy makers want to elicit. As a result, there is always a risk that those paid will respond to the letter rather than the spirit of the system and will do so in ways that suit their own advantage but do not accomplish reformers' objectives. For example, suppose pharmacists receive a fixed dispensing fee for each compound they sell. They might respond by encouraging buyers to engage in inappropriate "polypharmacy," since by selling multiple medicines they collect multiple fees. (Similar issues arise for regulatory constraints, as discussed in chapter 10.)

This chapter first examines the general problem of payment in the context of health sector reform, including the problem of corruption, which affects many processes related to pharmaceutical payment. It then explores the three main categories of payment transactions—customer payments, wholesale payments, and procurement. It concludes with a discussion of the policy lessons related to the payment control knob.

Pharmaceutical Payment Reform and Health Sector Reform

The viability of various pharmaceutical payment options often depends on wider government capacities and performance, both in the health sector and more generally. Do individual delivery institutions have management information systems that allow them to track inventories and expenditures? Are purchasing and regulatory enforcement activities carried out competently and impartially? Do the police and the courts command respect from citizens? All these factors constrain the payment options available to pharmaceutical policy makers.

Changing payment for pharmaceuticals is also intertwined with other aspects of the health system. As a result, achieving such changes often requires the coordinated use of a number of control knobs. For example, suppose a government wants to switch from centralized procurement to allowing district health centers to purchase some medicines from private wholesalers (to decrease stock-out situations). Implementing that change is likely to require giving the district health center director more authority, as well as improving the centers' accounting systems and financial controls. The change also might be more effective if health center directors then had to report their stock-out performance to their superiors (say, at the provincial level) and were held accountable for that performance. These changes are all within the scope of the organizational control knob, as we discuss in the next chapter. Similarly, if private sector payment arrangements are to be changed (for example, by introducing retail price controls), the government typically will have to rely on the regulation control knob to get that job done.

Pharmaceutical Payment and Corruption

In recent years, corruption in low- and middle-income countries has received high-visibility attention from the World Bank and the World Health Organization (WHO) (Cohen, Mrazek, and Hawkins 2007). The attention is illustrated by WHO's Good Governance for Medicines initiative, started in 2004, which developed a tool to assess the vulnerability of a pharmaceutical system to corruption (WHO 2009). While the effectiveness of the tool (and various proposed countermeasures) has not been evaluated, it reflects the growing concern about the need to do a better job of controlling corruption in the pharmaceutical sector, as a core condition of improving its performance.

If pharmaceutical reformers are to control corruption, they need to begin with a clear assessment of how and why such corruption arises. Like other behaviors, corruption emerges from a combination of individuals' internal beliefs and values, on the one hand, and the external opportunities they confront, on the other. On the internal or motivational side, people are corrupt for many reasons: personal gain, political gain for a party or faction, even a sense of obligation to clan and tribe (Smith 2008). Because those motivations are widespread, one should expect corruption to be widespread as well.

On the opportunity side, pharmaceutical payments offer many opportunities for corruption. Particularly at the procurement stage, government decision makers are distributing contracts that create significant profit opportunities for private parties. It is hardly surprising that potential beneficiaries often seek to influence those decisions through corrupt practices.

Putting the matter in that way clarifies the applicability of an old saying in American law enforcement circles about corruption: It takes two to tango. It is also the case that in many countries anticorruption enforcement is weak, inasmuch as the enforcers in turn can be corrupted (see case study E, "Drug Procurement in East Africania"). Corruption can also rise to the highest levels of national leadership in many countries. Readers should remember that former premiers of both Germany (Helmut Kohl) and France (François Mitterrand) were caught up in bribery scandals.

When one looks at motive (self-interest) and opportunity (including low risk of punishment), it is understandable why procurement officials are often tempted to be corrupt. That is especially so when they are paid low wages. It is almost as if governments expect them to be corrupt to have a reasonable standard of living.

To control corruption, reformers need to change both internal motives and external opportunities. On the motivation side, they can appeal to the core values of the responsible officials and urge them to resist corruption in the service of one or more broader ends. (Depending on the national and organizational context, those might include religion, ideology, patriotism, professionalism, organizational loyalty, or concern for clients.) A complementary strategy is to change the payoffs to corruption. For example, reformers could create new administrative arrangements and decision processes that increase transparency and accountability and enhance the government's capacity to impose rewards and penalties through an effective criminal justice system.

Readers should note, however, that increasing transparency and accountability requires political support from the top levels of government (see case study G, "Counterfeit Medicines in Nigeria"). It also requires both effective agency leadership and the kind of widespread social legitimacy that may not be easy to achieve in many low-income countries. In too many of those societies decades of colonialism, military intervention in political life, and poor governance have produced a climate of cynicism about the performance of the public sector that is not easy to change (Smith 2008).

Procurement

Before we discuss procurement in detail, it is worth noting the contrast between the ways in which public and private sector organizations do purchasing, both in general and for pharmaceuticals in particular. Because public purchasing is so susceptible to corruption, the usual response is to create highly formal procedures for making those decisions. Explicit specifications are written, bids are solicited, bids are evaluated, and the purchase is typically awarded to the lowest bid meeting the specifications. Those formal procedures seek to limit the discretion of public officials and thereby limit their opportunities for corrupt behavior.

Moreover, the purchasing cycle in the public sector is often quite fragmented. The necessary functions (authorizing expenditures, forecasting demand, tracking current stocks, reviewing available alternative medicines, preparing tender specifications, evaluating bids, checking deliveries for quality, and disbursing payments) are typically divided among a number of agencies in multiple ministries. Those may include the ministry of finance, an independent drug regulatory authority, the national purchasing unit, the central medical stores, the ministry of health pharmacy division, and others. The result is to add delay and rigidity to the process. It is not unusual for the time between a decision to purchase and the arrival of medicines in a country to exceed six months.

As one review of procurement processes for HIV/AIDS medicines put it, "Regardless of how well organized, planned, and managed the procurement process is, unexpected delays are inevitable" (Chandani et al. 2009). When governments are short of funds, the ministry of finance often will not allow the purchasing cycle even to begin. And some potential sellers, wary of delays in receiving payment, may be unwilling to participate in the tender process. In addition, the use of international competitive bidding processes, which award the tender to the lowest bidder, can sometimes result in contracts for unreliable suppliers. That can lead to delays, stockouts, and confusion, as occurred with antimalarial medicines in Kenya and Uganda in 2008 and 2009 (Tren, Hess, and Bate 2009).

In contrast, private sector purchasing is generally less formal and involves greater interaction between buyers and sellers (Ballou-Aares et al. 2008). The main constraint on corruption in private sector procurement is buyers' strong interest (either as owners or through their incentives) in maximizing their company's economic performance. They know that the ability of their organizations to acquire essential inputs may well depend on the energy, competence, and good will of sellers when unanticipated conditions arise. What will their suppliers do to ensure timely deliveries when confronted with bad weather, materials shortages, labor disputes, or mechanical breakdowns?

Given these concerns, buyers value the creation of relationships of trust and reciprocity with suppliers. A buyer who has had good experience with a seller will often purchase again from that same seller without a formal bidding process. Participants in private sector medicine supply chains routinely consider price-quality trade-offs and the seller's reliability and do not necessarily go with the lowest bidder. They realize that the choice of whether to buy from X or from Y is only part of a larger cycle of activity, and they pay great attention to the processes of contract implementation and monitoring. They know all too well that what happens after the purchasing decision is critically important to their ability to carry out their activities successfully. Moreover, in the context of such relationships, the specifications for what is being purchased are open to discussion. Sellers may offer counterproposals that will lower the price, speed delivery, or improve quality, and the price will be adjusted through negotiation.

It is also true that the procurement process for pharmaceuticals is technically demanding. As a result, governments in low-income countries may be hard-pressed to create and sustain the necessary expertise, given the tendency for their best people to be lured by higher salaries into donor organizations or nongovernmental organizations (NGOs) or to the for-profit sector. In particular, given the variations among potentially competing products from foreign manufacturers, at the molecular level, in dosage forms, and in packaging, deciding on the specifications for a purchase and interpreting bids against those terms can be quite complex.

Examples of such problems include cases in which countries have asked for unusual formulations (for example, pediatric doses) and then found few suppliers, or in which bidders offered a product that did not match bid terms but the discrepancy was not caught until after the product was delivered (for example, suppliers provided loose pills instead of course-of-treatment packaging). Because noncomplying bids may reflect efforts by suppliers to reduce their own costs, and hence increase their profits, purchasers need to examine bids very carefully. Late discovery of problems can cause significant disruptions and stock-outs at various levels of the supply chain if supplies arrive late or must be reordered.

Countries with the most limited expertise in international markets may have to rely on intermediaries to facilitate their purchasing activities (see case study E, "Drug Procurement in East Africania"). In particular, a low-income country tender board is not likely to know, or be in contact with, all the potential suppliers of the various generic medicines it may wish to purchase. That is especially the case in dealings with the many sellers in middle-income countries that purchase active ingredients and then formulate and package final doses. As a result, an international medicines brokerage business has developed, whose participants seek to assemble and aggregate products from a variety of manufacturers, to bid on open tenders around the world.

The difficulty of creating reliable organizations with the necessary technical expertise within the civil services of low-income countries has led some reformers to advocate contracting out those functions. That has been done in a number of countries, such as Zambia. An international entity, such as Crown Agents, then handles a range of procurement and supply chain activities, along with related financial management functions. Governments in low- and middle-income countries have also sought ongoing relationships with an international NGO or government-sponsored suppliers in order to purchase from more reliable sources. Such relationships can take the form of a framework contract within which multiple purchases can occur. In a way, it is an attempt to create in the public sector the kind of buyer-seller relationships that firms cultivate in the private sector.

All these strategies involve changing the unit being purchased from a particular stock of medicines to a combination of technical advice, transaction management, and a series of medicines deliveries. They may also involve a change in the third identified component of any pricing system, namely, how the price is set. Competitive bidding is one such mechanism, but it has disadvantages. A framework contract may change price setting to make it more resemble a negotiation. John Glenn, the first U.S. astronaut to fly into space, was reportedly asked how it felt, and he replied, "How would you like to be sitting on top of a rocket roaring off into space at many hundreds of miles an hour, with thousands of components, all manufactured by the lowest bidder?"

In their review of corruption in the pharmaceutical sector, Cohen, Mrazek, and Hawkins (2007, 447) offered the following specific measures to reduce corruption in procurement:

- Make procurement procedures transparent, following formal, published, written procedures throughout the process and using explicit criteria to award contracts.

- Justify and monitor supplier selection.

- Adhere strictly to announced closing dates.

- Maintain written records for all bids received.

- Provide the results of adjudication to all participating bidders and the public.

- Provide regular reporting on key procurement performance indicators.

The theory underlying those suggestions is that corruption opportunities vary inversely with the transparency of the bidding process. Unadvertised bids allow corrupt officials to reserve opportunities for the well-connected. Explicit criteria and public disclosure of evaluations are designed to make it more difficult for review committees to find technicalities as reasons to turn down less-favored bidders. As the world has moved rapidly into the globalized, Internet age, technological solutions for some of these problems have been developed. The whole bidding process can be carried out electronically, in ways that open it up to much more extensive external scrutiny. Moreover, once a nation has a reputation for fair bidding processes, it is more likely to attract a range of suppliers that have organizational integrity. As long as processes are rigged, suppliers that are not corrupt are more likely to conclude that it is not worthwhile to participate.

Transparency alone, however, is not the whole answer. Those who want to do so can find ways to game the system. For example, they can work behind the scenes to create problems that require "emergency" procurements in local markets (central stores can delay shipments, or sudden stockouts can be reported in facilities). Those responsible for such purchasing can then extort kickbacks from local suppliers. To counter such practices and ensure integrity requires strong managerial leadership from the top that is committed to better performance.

A critical aspect of procurement is the quality testing of what is supplied. Sellers have an incentive to lower their costs by providing products that they can produce or acquire inexpensively. And one way to lower costs is to supply substandard medicines. In some countries, producing for export subjects manufacturers to lower levels of regulatory scrutiny, either officially or because bribe taking is more common in such situations. One West African drug regulator, working undercover, reportedly recorded a conversation with a supplier in which a medicine was offered for sale at several prices, depending on what percentage of the active ingredient (from zero to 100 percent) was actually present.

In these circumstances, much international attention has been given to efforts to improve the promptness, extent, and technical quality of the testing done by national laboratories. One example is the program Promoting the Quality of Medicines, conducted by the U.S. Pharmacopeia and supported by the U.S. Agency for International Development (USAID) since 1992, in more than 35 countries (see http://www.usp.org/worldwide). But again, managerial efforts are required if the laboratories are to function properly and be protected against corrupt influences. In addition, a number of international mechanisms have been established to try to identify reliable sources of supply. They include the WHO Certification Scheme, formal collaboration among countries, and WHO's Prequalification Project, which was set up in 2001 to address quality, safety, efficacy, and good manufacturing practices (GMP) in the production of medicines for HIV, tuberculosis (TB), and malaria (WHO 2004).

Testing is especially important because a low-income country can have difficulty knowing precisely who it is dealing with in the international market, especially when relying on brokers or intermediaries. There are anecdotal reports of countries finding out that they were buying from suppliers connected to the Sicilian or Russian Mafia, or from a company that could no longer be traced (according to one government official in 2008). Those stories underline the inherent difficulty of the procurement process and the need for low-income countries to focus on it if they are to improve the quality and availability of medicines supplies in the public sector while meeting the "technical efficiency" goal of cost control.

Wholesale Payments

Once medicines enter a country, they move through either the public or private supply chains. Private side supply chains vary considerably. Countries may have anywhere from a single importer to 50 or more. Some importers may have ties to particular manufacturers (sometimes in exclusive arrangements), so that significant transactions occur among wholesalers as each seeks to assemble a full product line. Two or three steps may be required to move product from importers to final sellers. The participants might include importers who operate from major port or airport cities, regional intermediaries in provincial capitals, and perhaps district-level distributors as well.

But the full distribution chain is often even more complex. Some larger final sellers also act as wholesalers to smaller or more remote outlets. Indeed, because medicines in many countries are sold by stores with general product lines (as well as by specialized shops), some general wholesalers also distribute medicines to their customers. In other countries, some or all of the major private sector wholesalers are vertically integrated, offering all stages of the process including retail sales.

In many countries, various stages of the wholesale pharmaceutical business exhibit what economists call "high concentration." That is, much of the business is in the hands of a small number of firms. The process of importing and wholesaling medicines enjoys what economists call "economies of scale"; that is, average costs are lower for larger companies. They can order in larger amounts, obtain more favorable terms, spread their administrative costs over larger volumes, and afford more sophisticated inventory management systems. Under such circumstances it is difficult for a new business with smaller volume and higher costs to compete successfully. As a result, smaller countries often have only a few dominant private sector wholesalers. Much the same logic applies at the end of the distribution network. In rural areas and smaller towns, there is often not enough business to support more than one or two retail sellers.

When a few sellers dominate a market, it is tempting for them to collude (either explicitly or implicitly) to limit price competition. They are also tempted to do what they can to deter new entrants to preserve their position. Examples include tying up retailers and manufacturers through exclusive contacts, offering volume discounts to hold onto exclusive relationships, and even threatening would-be competitors (or their customers). Such situations pose problems not only to private sector buyers, but also to public purchasers who are trying to use private sources to fill the gaps in a poorly functioning public sector supply chain (Patouillard, Hanson, and Goodman 2010).

One way to summarize the impact of competition in wholesale markets is to look at how it affects markups—the difference between the seller's cost and the selling price, expressed as a percentage of the seller's cost. Markups vary widely from product to product, from country to country, and with the stage of the distribution system. General economic arguments suggest that the number of sellers competing for business in a market and the degree to which they use price competition as a tool will influence the size of markups. Product-to-product variation is also likely to occur, in part because wholesalers will try to charge higher margins where they believe that retailers will be able to pass on those higher costs to their customers more easily. Price markups from 10 percent to 100 percent—and even more—have been reported. And those are for products that pass through two or three stages between importation and final sale. A survey of medicine prices in Ghana, for example, found wholesale markups of 30 percent to 40 percent, and a similar retail markup, in the private sector. In the public sector, the survey found 20 percent wholesale markups and 10 percent retail markups (Medicine Prices in Ghana 2004).

That markups occur in the public as well as the private sector reflects the fact that a number of low-income countries operate their public distribution systems on a cash-and-carry basis. That is, patients must pay hospitals or health centers for any medications dispensed, health centers have to pay district stores for supplies they receive, and district stores have to pay central stores, just as in the private sector. In part, this practice reflects the lack of funding available to governments and their desire to capture the same willingness to pay that attracts private sector sellers.

In addition, cash-and-carry policies address the pervasive problem of inadequate working capital in the distribution system. Working capital is the money that a wholesale or retail vendor needs to purchase inventory. The larger the inventory, and the more slowly it sells (the "turnover rate"), the greater the working capital needed. If no cash comes in from final sales (either because medicines are free in public settings or because of theft or spoilage), then a government has a large volume of funds tied up in products sitting on shelves at all the stages of the distribution system. And those may be funds that governments in low-income countries simply do not have available.

Determining and tracking wholesale markups at the level of the individual product entail conceptual and practical difficulties. Wholesalers are typically offered complex marketing deals, which they in turn offer to their customers. Those include volume discounts across product lines, the bundling of products into multiproduct purchases, and cross-subsidies across a seller's products. In such contexts, determining the cost of acquiring a particular product, and the revenue derived from its sale, will depend in part on the accounting conventions that are used to make the determinations. In addition, to deflect criticism of their pricing practices, retail pharmacies often report that they "voluntarily" apply a uniform markup to published wholesale prices. It is difficult, however, for investigators to determine what actually happens in the many small shops that are spread over the entire country.

Depending on how the system operates, either the seller or the buyer at each stage pays the transport cost. Frequently it is the seller, who then includes the cost of transport in the delivered price. The seller's markup also has to cover their administrative, warehousing, and working capital costs, as well as provide a profit.

In some cases, sales are FOB (free on board). That means that prices are set at the delivery of the product to a ship or plane in the exporting country, and freight is the responsibility of the customer. Typically, sea transport adds 5 percent to 7 percent, air 10 percent, import taxes 10 percent to 20 percent, and value-added taxes (VAT) 4 percent to 15 percent, depending on the country. When all these charges are considered, retail prices can easily range from one-and-a half to three times (or even four to six times) the manufacturer's selling price for the medicines. Some data on overall markups in the public and private sectors in 11 countries appear in table 8.1.

Table 8.1 Cumulative Percentage Markups in the Public and Private Sectors in 11 Countries

percent

Country	Total cumulative markup, public sector	Total cumulative markup, private sector
China (Shandong)[a]	24–35	11–33
El Salvador[a]	—	165–6,894
Ethiopia[a]	79–83	76–148
India[b]	—	29–694
Malaysia[c]	19–46	65–149
Mali[a]	77–84	87–118
Mongolia[b]	32	68–98
Morocco[c]	—	53–93
Uganda[b]	30–66	100–358
Tanzania[a]	17	56
Pakistan[c]	—	28–35

Source: Cameron et al. 2009, 246. Reprinted with permission of Elsevier.

Note: — = not available.

a. Country surveys of price components using WHO/HAI standard methodology; http://www.haiweb.org/medicineprices/.

b. Kotwani and Levison 2007.

c. Levison 2008.

Although this chapter is concerned with the payment control knob, other control knobs are also needed in efforts to bring down margins in the private distribution chain. And there are no quick and easy solutions. One response is to use legal means (called "antitrust policy" in the United States and "competition policy" in the European Union) to address the worst anticompetitive actions by wholesalers or importers. Another alternative is to create an effective public or quasi-public supply system, which can then exert competitive price pressures on the private sellers. Given the difficulties of operating efficiently in the public sector, the most attractive option may involve the creation of a parastatal or corporatized entity that has public ownership but operates under private sector law and management structure. We discuss the experience of Cameroon in that regard in the next chapter. However, pursuing either course successfully is not easy, given the weak criminal justice systems in many low- and middle-income countries and the significant political power that distributors can mobilize to oppose such measures.

Some groups of end users have tried to deal with high markups in the distribution chain by "backward integration" and creating their own captive distribution system. The distribution system for religious hospitals in Ghana is an example (Seiter and Gyansa-Lutterodt 2008, 16). This approach is easier to propose than to implement. Hospitals and clinics in low-income countries seldom have the logistical, inventory management, and purchasing skills to carry out these functions effectively. As newcomers to the marketplace, they also tend to lack relationships with and knowledge of the international suppliers. Yet it is such knowledge and relationships that allow a purchaser to obtain better terms and find more reliable partners to work with. Moreover, the working capital requirements for such a venture are substantial. Medicines being shipped into low-income countries often have to be paid for months before they arrive, and still more months elapse before they are sold and revenue is earned. All of this increases working capital requirements. The financing difficulties apparently sank the Ghana experiment (Seiter and Gyansa-Lutterodt 2008, 16), although the faith-based-NGO supply system in Uganda, Joint Medical Stores, continues to function quite effectively.

We should also note that wholesalers are not the only agents active in this part of the supply chain. Manufacturers' representatives also push their own products. They may offer sellers bonuses or concessions—such as volume-based kickbacks, or extra discounted (or even free) product to fill up their shelves—to squeeze out competitor brands. Where prescription systems function, manufacturers have every reason to direct significant sales and incentive efforts at doctors. And the experiences of even the most advanced countries indicate that those can have a significant distorting, and cost increasing, impact on a nation's medicines expenditure.

Payments by End Users

Like wholesalers, pharmaceutical retailers typically think about their prices in terms of a markup. Retail markups vary widely, ranging from 15 percent to 35 percent and sometimes even 100 percent to 500 percent (Patouillard, Hanson, and Goodman 2010). Retailers cover their costs (time, working capital, and facilities) and also make their profits out of that margin.

The markup approach to pricing immediately creates an incentive to sell more expensive items because, for the same markup, they offer a larger absolute difference between the seller's costs and the sales price. Moreover, the nonproduct costs that sellers incur vary only modestly with product costs. The time required to maintain the inventory and complete the final sale are likely to be the same for more expensive products, or even less if consumers need less persuasion to buy the brand-name item. Storage requirements are also generally similar. True, slightly more working capital is required to maintain a more expensive inventory, but the costs are not likely to be high, especially if inventory turns over reasonably rapidly at the point of final sale.

In addition, retailers may apply higher markups in *percentage* terms on more expensive options, which provide an added incentive to sell such items. The reason for that practice is that customers who purchase higher-priced goods are often less price sensitive. The key concept again is the "price elasticity of demand." In technical terms, price elasticity is the percentage change in the quantity bought, divided by the percentage change in the price charged. If the quantity change is greater than the price change, the elasticity is greater than 1, and demand is said to be elastic. If quantity changes less than price in percentage terms, demand is said to be inelastic.

When demand is inelastic, smart sellers seek to charge especially high prices. The reason is that increasing the price to price-insensitive buyers does not produce the same reduction in total sales as occurs when buyers are more price sensitive. So the profit-maximizing price is higher. Indeed, a monopolist who could totally control the price would keep raising it until demand became somewhat elastic. For until that point is reached, ever-higher prices continue to produce ever-higher total profits.

The same logic leads international drug companies to set higher prices in higher-income countries. Of course, the existence of health insurance in high-income countries shifts much of the cost of high-priced medicines to third-party payers, so that patients are not very sensitive to the prices. In contrast, the uninsured (in the United States, for example), who pay for medicines out-of-pocket, tend to be more sensitive to high medicine prices, which encourage them to seek lower-priced products in other markets (such as Mexico and Canada, for U.S. patients) and over the Internet.

The ability of sellers to coordinate their behavior to raise prices depends on the number of sellers who are competing in a given retail market. Larger towns and cities are likely to contain a larger number of drug sellers, all of whom have to react to the prices that other sellers are charging. But as population densities go down, not enough business may exist to support multiple sellers in any given location. In the most rural areas there may not be enough business to support even one specialized seller. Instead, drug retailing may be done by a multiproduct, general purpose store. Those situations give sellers, in effect, a local monopoly—and more control over prices (and margins). Their customers would have to travel to another seller (in the closest medium-size town, for example) if they did not like the prices they found in their own village.

An added complexity is that in many low- and middle-income countries, formal sellers of medicines in the larger towns (pharmacies and drug sellers, for example) face price competition at the low end of the product spectrum from stall holders, street vendors, and other informal sellers. That puts pressure on the formal sellers to hold down prices (and markups) for low-end drugs (where there is more competition) or lose that business altogether. That only increases their incentives to promote sales of high-end products, in which they face less competition.

However, data from the WHO-HAI (Health Action International) surveys show that in low-income countries, generics are more widely available than originator products in private retail settings. Presumably the reason is the limited ability of many customers to afford the highest-priced products (Cameron et al. 2009, 243). Figure 8.1 shows the differences between prices for originator brand medicines and those for lowest-priced

Figure 8.1   Private Sector Patient Prices for Selected Medicines in Pakistan Compared to International Reference Prices

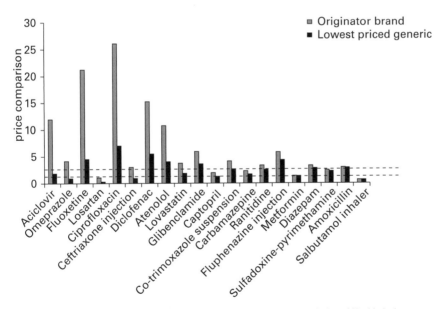

Source: Network for Consumer Protection 2008, 4. Reproduced with permission of Health Action International and WHO Regional Office for the Eastern Mediterranean.

Note: The price comparison figure indicates the number of times more expensive the product is when purchased in a retail pharmacy in Pakistan over the international reference price for the product.

generics in the private sector in Pakistan for different products, compared to international reference prices. For some products, the differences are substantial; for other products, the originators and the generics are priced close to international reference prices.

The standard methodology for studying medicines affordability is to ask how many days of the lowest-paid public sector worker's salary are required to purchase various medicines. That analysis is now done regularly by WHO in conjunction with HAI in many countries around the world, and the method is being used more broadly within the United Nations, as well (MDG Gap Task Force 2008). Table 8.2 shows some recent evidence on affordability of medicines in the Middle East and North Africa region.

All of the options available for making medicines more affordable at the retail level leave something to be desired. One approach is to convince consumers to use lower-priced generics. But doing that successfully is not easy in an environment where substandard or counterfeit products are common and quality concerns are well grounded. As is discussed in chapter 11, effective use of the persuasion control knob has to begin with understanding the beliefs and desires of the target audience—and depicting the desired response as a solution to their decision problems, as they perceive and experience them.

Table 8.2   Affordability of Selected Medicines in the Middle East and North Africa

Illness	Affordability of treatment
Respiratory infection	2.3 days' income to buy a week's supply of originator-branded amoxicillin in Jordan.
Depressive illness	7.7 days' income to buy a month's supply of lowest-priced generic fluoxetine in Pakistan; 36.4 days' income to buy originator-branded fluoxetine.
Ulcer	One month's treatment with lowest-priced generic omeprazole 2.9 days' income in Sudan and 7.7 days' income in Jordan; with originator brand 10.6 days' income in Morocco and 23.7 days' income in Pakistan.
Respiratory infection	2.3 days' income to buy a week's supply of originator-branded amoxicillin in Jordan.
Depressive illness	7.7 days' income to buy a month's supply of lowest-priced generic fluoxetine in Pakistan; 36.4 days' income to buy originator-branded fluoxetine.
Ulcer	One month's treatment with lowest-priced generic omeprazole 2.9 days' income in Sudan and 7.7 days' income in Jordan; with originator brand 10.6 days' income in Morocco and 23.7 days' income in Pakistan.

Source: Mirza 2008. Reprinted with permission of Health Action International and WHO Regional Office for the Eastern Mediterranean.

Another possible response is use public subsidies to lower the prices of medicines considered critical to achieving health status goals. That policy is used by the Affordable Medicines Facility for Malaria to encourage the use of artemisinin-based combination therapies (ACTs). Such subsidies, however, can encourage overuse because consumers do not bear the full costs of their decision making. That risk has led some countries to introduce regulatory constraints (that is, use the regulation control knob) or gate-keeping requirements to limit the inappropriate overuse of subsidized products (see chapter 10).

A more purely payment approach to encourage desired consumption behavior involves *tiered co-payments*. The scheme involves having insured consumers pay lower (or even zero) co-pays for recommended drugs (often generic products) and higher ones for tiers of less-appropriate medicines. That approach has been widely used in U.S. insurance plans and has also been used in the public sector in low-income countries. With tiered co-pays, some medicines are available free, such as those delivered in supervised clinical settings (such as antiretrovirals (ARVs) and TB medicines), and patients pay a flat fee for others.

Another alternative in the insurance context is a mechanism called "reference pricing" (López-Casasnovas and Jönsson 2001). Medicines are sorted into therapeutic classes, and a limit is set on the price that the insurance fund will pay for all the medicines in that class. That reference price may be the lowest price in the group, or it may be set somewhat higher, even up to the median price in the market among all of the relevant medicines. Individuals must pay any difference between the reference price and the retail price. For classes of drugs in which many alternatives exist, the system can have the effect of encouraging manufacturers of the higher-priced options to drop their prices to the reference price level.

Although few low-income countries are considering reference pricing, as middle-income countries expand their social insurance coverage they are increasingly considering such systems. Experience around the world shows the substantial technical and administrative difficulties—and the controversies—that operating this kind of price-setting system generates. Manufacturers have every reason to lobby government officials aggressively over seemingly obscure technical details (such as the size of the classes into which medicines are sorted) to try to maximize their reimbursement.

That calls attention to the third component of pricing decisions: the price-setting process. Operating an effective reference pricing system requires not only technical competence but strong political support, inasmuch as the members of an expert panel set up to insulate decision making from political pressure can be pressured, and even their selection can be influenced by interest groups.

The expansion of social insurance coverage to drug purchases opens up a variety of strategic options for governments (see case study J, "Drug Coverage in Ghana's National Health Insurance Scheme"). But especially where buyers are less sophisticated, reformers need to be aware of the "law of unintended consequences." It suggests that those adversely affected by a reform will try to find ways around the new system and in the process will decrease its effectiveness. That is exactly what happened in Ghana when the national health insurance scheme set price ceilings for products on its essential medicines list. To enforce those prices, it forbade co-payments by patients for those products. In some cases, providers responded by ceasing to carry the inexpensive generic versions on the list and sold patients more expensive brands of the medicine instead. That allowed the sellers to make a substantial profit, while still complying with the rule barring co-payments (Seiter and Gyansa-Lutterodt 2008, 23, 25).

A final set of possible retail payment reforms are directed at the prices themselves. Some have proposed regulating retail margins—insisting on lower percentage margins for higher-priced goods ("regressive margin" rules)—to lessen sellers' incentive to push more-expensive products. Others have proposed trying to do away with margins entirely and having retailers sell at cost plus a fixed dispensing fee. Any of those approaches can encounter the difficulty noted above of defining the cost of individual products. It also is not easy to inspect retail outlets for medicines, because of the large number of outlets and the lack of good record keeping in many countries.

An alternative is simply to regulate private sector prices themselves—if not everywhere, then at least in a limited number of franchised or certified drug shops (see case study F, "Converting Basic Drug Shops to Accredited Drug-Dispensing Outlets in Tanzania"). That gets around the problem of having to inspect records to determine margins, but it raises the possibility of creating serious inequities among shops with different wholesale costs. Requiring such shops to post regulated prices on the wall allows consumers to take on some of the enforcement burden. And because checking prices is technically easier than checking margins, local officials in the district offices of the ministry of health could take on that task. That would greatly simplify the logistics of inspection and enforcement.

Finally, in some settings the government is the seller, not the buyer, most noticeably in its own dispensing activities from government facilities. In those places, governments can control what people pay, and for equity reasons prices are often low—for example, consisting of co-payments that are much less than retail prices. When governments are willing to charge more, they can consider using the equivalent of tiered co-payments to direct patients to the most cost-effective options. And where government supply systems are sufficiently extensive, they could conceivably be used to discipline prices in the private sector.

To be realistic, however, one has to take account of the argument made by the World Bank pharmaceutical expert Andreas Seiter (personal communication 2010). He suggests that the public pharmaceutical sector in many countries is, in a sense, doomed to have insufficient supplies. If it is only 10 percent to 20 percent of the total supply, and offers medicines at lower prices than the private sector, what would we expect to happen? Seiter argues that in such (typical) situations customers, in effect, drain public sector stocks first and then default to the more expensive private sector for the balance of their purchases. When one adds the time lags and the rigidity of public procurement, frequent stock-outs are only to be expected. That suggests that the ability of government to use the prices it directly charges as a policy instrument is limited, exactly because it is not a majority supplier in many areas.

Summary on Payment

Most of the policy initiatives mentioned in this chapter share a feature: They are less about the use of the payment control knob, and more about using other control knobs to modify the incentive effects of the payment system. The following is a partial list:

- Using regulation to control retail prices or margins

- Using organization to improve the functioning of purchasing agencies

- Using regulation to counteract anticompetitive practices in the whole-sale sector

- Using organization to create supply chain alternatives, either quasi-public or private

- Using persuasion to encourage the purchase of lower priced generics.

The point is that government can only use payment directly when it is the party doing either the buying or the selling. This review has identified some areas where that may be applicable. First, governments can change the unit being paid for and use framework contracts. Alternatively, they can contract out certain purchasing functions, to conduct that activity more effectively. Similarly, where the government pays for medicines through insurance funds, it can use tiered co-payments and reference pricing to try to redirect consumer choices to more cost-effective medicines. Government does have control over what—if anything—it charges patients for medicines in government facilities, but for the reasons discussed above, the impact of that kind of intervention is limited.

Case Studies on Financing and Payment

Bannenberg, Wilbert, and Marc J. Roberts. "Drug Procurement in East Africania." Case Study E.

Blanchet, Nathan, and Marc J. Roberts, "Drug Coverage in Ghana's National Health Insurance Scheme." Case Study J.

References

Ballou-Aares, D., A. Freitas, L. R. Kopczak, S. Kraiselburd, M. Laverty, E. Macharia, and P. Yadav. 2008. *Private Sector Role in Health Supply Chains.* New York: Rockefeller Foundation, Dalberg, and MIT-Zaragoza International Logistics Program.

Cameron, A., M. Ewen, D. Ross-Degnan, D. Ball, and R. Laing. 2009. "Medicine Prices, Availability, and Affordability in 36 Developing and Middle-Income Countries: A Secondary Analysis." *Lancet* 373: 240–49.

Chandani, Y., E. Takang, C. Allers, and C. McLaughlin. 2009. "HIV/AIDS Drug Procurement and Supply Chain Management." In *From the Ground Up: Building Comprehensive HIV/AIDS Care Programs in Resource Limited Settings*, ed. R. G. Marlink and S. J. Teitelbaum. Los Angeles, CA: Elizabeth Glaser Pediatric AIDS Foundation Publication. http://ftguonline.org/ftgu-232/index.php/ftgu/article/view/1954/3904. Accessed February 25, 2011.

Cohen, J. C., M. Mrazek, and L. Hawkins. 2007. "Tackling Corruption in the Pharmaceutical Systems Worldwide with Courage and Conviction." *Clinical Pharmacology and Therapeutics* 81: 445–49.

Kotwani, A., and L. Levison. 2007. "Price Components and Access to Medicines in Delhi, India." Unpublished manuscript.

Levison, L. 2008. "Investigating Price Components: Medicine Costs between Procurement and Point of Delivery." Draft report on initial field studies. Unpublished manuscript.

López-Casasnovas, G., and B. Jönsson, eds. 2001. *Reference Pricing and Pharmaceutical Policy: Perspectives on Economics and Innovation.* Barcelona: Springer-Verlag Ibérica.

MDG Gap Task Force. 2008. *Delivering on the Global Partnership for Achieving the Millennium Development Goals.* New York: United Nations.

"Medicine Prices in Ghana: A Comparative Study of Public, Private, and Mission Sector Medicine Prices." 2004. Accra: Ministry of Health and Ghana Health

Service. http://www. fhaiarica.org/index.php?option=com_content&task=view&id=169. Accessed March 15, 2009.

Mirza, Zafar. 2008. "WHO Perspectives on Medicine Prices and Policies." Presentation to the Federal Ministry of Health, Islamabad, Pakistan, November 14. http://www.haiweb.org/medicineprices. Accessed March 14, 2009.

Network for Consumer Protection. 2008. "Medicine Prices, Availability, Affordability, and Price Components, Pakistan." Islamabad, Pakistan: Network for Consumer Protection, HAI, and WHO Regional Office of the Eastern Mediterranean. http://www.haiweb.org/medicineprices/18112008/Pakistan-summary-report-web.pdf. Accessed March 14, 2009.

Patouillard, E., K. G. Hanson, and C. A. Goodman. 2010. "Retail Sector Distribution Chains for Malaria Treatment in the Developing World: A Review of the Literature." *Malaria Journal* 9: 50.

Seiter, A., and M. Gyansa-Lutterodt. 2008. "Policy Note: The Pharmaceutical Sector in Ghana." Draft, World Bank, Washington, DC.

Smith, D. J. 2008. *A Culture of Corruption: Everyday Deception and Popular Discontent in Nigeria*. Princeton, NJ: Princeton University Press.

Tren, R., K. Hess, and R. Bate. 2009. "Drug Procurement, the Global Fund and Misguided Competition Policies." *Malaria Journal* 8: 305.

WHO (World Health Organization). 2004. "The WHO Prequalification Project" Fact Sheet No. 278. Geneva: WHO. http://www.who.int/mediacentre/factsheets/fs278/en/index.html. Accessed July 13, 2009.

———. 2009. *Measuring Transparency in the Public Pharmaceutical Sector: Assessment Instrument* (WHO/EMP/MAR/2009.4). Geneva: WHO.

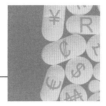

CHAPTER 9

Organizing the Public Sector to Improve Pharmaceutical Performance

The organization control knob brings us face-to-face with the interdependence of pharmaceutical sector reform and health sector reform generally. Some of the key organizations in the pharmaceutical sector, such as a central medicines store or a national quality control laboratory, have specialized pharmaceutical functions. But many relevant organizations (such as health centers that order, stock, and dispense medicines) are part of the general health care delivery system. Their behavior often can only be changed through actions that influence the broader system.

This chapter begins with a general analysis of the roots of organizational performance that uses a set of concepts derived from the Flagship Framework—the "six keys to organizational performance." It then looks at a series of reform options that involve transforming the organizational structure of the pharmaceutical sector in various ways: corporatization, contracting, decentralization, the new public sector management, and franchising. Next we turn to two more specific techniques—essential medicines lists and process improvement. The chapter concludes with a discussion of the managerial challenges of producing change using any of these approaches.

Pharmaceutical Sector Performance: The Six Keys

For a pharmaceutical organization to improve its performance, the people actually doing the work have to perform their tasks more effectively and conscientiously. The central medical store may need better inventory management systems. The quality control laboratory may need more sophisticated testing equipment. But such improvements will only be effective if the workers using those systems want to use them to do a better job.

One way to summarize our approach is through what the Flagship Framework identifies as the "six keys" to improved organizational performance. Figure 9.1 shows the relationship of the six keys to one another and to system performance. The causal path flows through the effects of the six keys on the behavior of frontline workers. It is worker behavior—by stock clerks, pharmacists, delivery drivers, laboratory technicians, and inspectors—that ultimately determines pharmaceutical system performance.

Because worker behavior is critical, we can think of the six keys by working backward from the frontline workers. The first two keys apply directly

Figure 9.1   The Six Keys to Organizational Performance

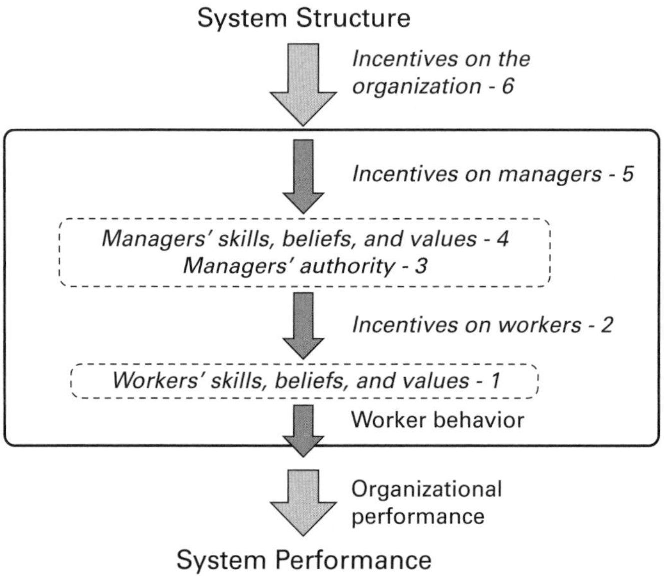

Source: Authors' representation.

to such workers and involve their internal beliefs and values (key #1) and their external incentives (key #2), just as discussed in the previous chapter's consideration of the problem of corruption. But those incentives and, to an extent, those beliefs and values depend critically on managers. Managers not only create incentives for workers but also, through leadership, influence their beliefs and values. Managers' capacity and willingness to do those things depends on their authority within the organization (key #3) and the managers' own skills, beliefs, and values (key #4). But the question also arises of whether managers have any reason to do this work—that is, what are their incentives (key #5)? We also believe that the incentives for managers depend on the incentives for the organization as a whole (key #6), as we explain below.

Pharmaceutical Sector Performance: Workers' Values and Beliefs

In explaining organizational performance, economists tend to focus on incentives. Yet in the management literature equal, if not greater, emphasis is placed on employee motivation as a precondition for the creation of "high-performance organizations" (Lawler, Mohrman, and Ledford 1995). The argument is that incentives only go so far. Many aspects of desirable employee behavior cannot be monitored and rewarded. Employees have to *want* to be conscientious and do a good job. For people to pay attention to detail, follow through, and take responsibility, high-quality work has to be an end in itself, something that staff members strive for out of their own internal motivation (Mills 1986).

What determines the values and beliefs that employees bring to their work? It is in part the culture in which they were raised and their education, especially their professional training. Some is self-selection. Individuals are attracted to organizations whose activities, culture, and rewards they find compatible. Once someone joins a particular organization, they encounter the attitude-forming effects of their work experience. For example, police tend to be cynical about human nature in part because they spend so much of their lives dealing with bad people. There is also some peer pressure to accept group norms. And those who stay and succeed in an organization are, by and large, those who adapt to its culture.

How have those processes affected the public sector workforce in pharmaceutical supply chain activities in low- and middle-income countries? A study of health workers in Mozambique and Cape Verde showed how they struggled with personal conflicts between the norms of public service and using access to medicines as a means for survival (Ferrinho et al. 2004).

Interviews with health workers showed that physicians used their privileged access to medicines to generate additional income. At the same time, the authors reported, "Health workers apparently live a conflict between their self-image as honest civil servant wanting to do a decent job, and the brute facts of life that make them betray that aspiration. The manifest unease that this provokes is an important observation" (Ferrinho et al. 2004, 5).

In many low- and middle-income countries, the health system in general, and the pharmaceutical supply system in particular, function only because many employees work conscientiously despite the difficulties. Some combination of professional pride, national loyalty, and belief in the mission moves these individuals to struggle every day within organizations that are often quite dysfunctional. To improve performance generally, reformers need to redesign critical organizations in the pharmaceutical sector so that reasonable levels of integrity and effort become the norm, not the exception.

Pharmaceutical Sector Performance: Workers' Incentives

Pharmaceutical sector employees in low-income countries are typically paid relatively low salaries, and the level of management attention and supervision they receive can leave much to be desired. Performance-based rewards and punishments are limited, and advancement is not connected to effort, in part because of rigid civil service systems. Suppose that you are a clerk in a district store, responsible for sending in reorder requests based on existing stock levels. If you do not bother to actually check stocks, and instead send in the same reorder requests month by month, it is unlikely that anyone will notice and still less likely you will be disciplined for lax behavior.

The economist Albert Hirschman (1970) wrote that those dissatisfied with their organization had a choice between "voice" (that is, protest) and "exit" (leaving). More recently Peter Gaal, at Semmelweiss University in Budapest, identified a range of behaviors that he calls "inxit"—which stands for "internal exit" (Gaal and McKee 2004). Employees who feel that they are being badly treated, but do not have other options, will stay in an organization but will abuse the system in various ways. They leave early, demand under-the-table payments from patients, steal, and divert patients to their private practices. Everyone justifies the behavior in part by their low pay and in part by the claim that the behavior is so widespread (including among managers) that it is implicitly accepted by the powers that be.

Those patterns are ultimately rooted in the decisions and actions of a country's political leadership. To oversimplify, political leaders have two broad strategies for building political support via public sector activities. First, they can try to satisfy customers and clients—call this the "output" or "good service" strategy. Alternatively, they can seek support from employees and suppliers—the "input" or "patronage" strategy.

The input strategy offers many advantages. Employees and suppliers are easier to identify and organize than customers. Their individual stakes are large, and gains (or losses) that accrue to them are easier to target and adjust. In contrast, attracting political support by, for example, improving the availability of medicines is a difficult, time-consuming, and expensive process. Rather than do such hard work, political leaders can more easily attract campaign funds and political support (not to mention private wealth) by allocating contracts or appointments to those who will pay, or to friends, family, and political allies. As a result, they do not make the commitment to efficiency, service, and minimizing corruption that would lead to an effective system of performance-based rewards and punishments for employees.

Pharmaceutical Sector Performance: Managers

The resulting "poor service equilibrium" both causes and reflects a lack of effective management. Managers who obtain their posts through some combination of personal contacts and political contributions are unlikely to have either much managerial training or much sense of managerial responsibility. In addition, many managers have few tools for doing their job, with little authority over personnel, budgets, purchasing, or policies. Often in a misplaced effort to prevent public sector managers from doing bad things, governments have taken away their authority to do almost anything, good or bad.

The lack of authority is coupled to a lack of accountability, so that future advancement is not tied to managerial performance. Consider what it is like to be the manager of the quality-testing laboratory, the purchasing office, the central warehouse, or the trucking department that delivers to district stores. Usually there is no senior ministry of health official who receives monthly reports on the performance of the facilities under your jurisdiction and whose job it is hold you accountable for that performance. In addition, it is rare for your boss to be a trained and sophisticated manager of managers. Yet that is what is required to put in place an effective combination of support and expectations to improve the performance of lower-level managers. Without such supervision, moreover, it is difficult to create long-run managerial career paths that provide incentives for managerial excellence.

The lack of accountability is typically traceable to the top of the public sector, and that brings us back to overall political leadership. The national political leadership has to want effective public sector services enough to empower the minister of health to ignore political pressure and to hold him or her accountable for actual performance. Only if that happens will the minister have a reason, and the support, to put in place adequate supervisory arrangements. Typically, the minister appoints competent and motivated individuals to senior supervisory roles and holds them accountable for their subordinates' performance.

Yet too often ministers are prominent and politically well connected physicians who lack significant management training and have little experience in leading a complex, large organization that has to serve multiple objectives and constituencies. It is increasingly recognized globally that new ministers of health need new kinds of opportunities to learn how to manage and lead their organizations effectively, especially when their terms in office are likely to be two years or less.

Incentives for Pharmaceutical Organizations

How does the structure of the health care system create incentives for organizations in the pharmaceutical sector, and how, if at all, are those translated into incentives for managers? Organizations acquire their resources in one of three ways: (1) they can sell goods and services, obtaining revenue by pleasing paying customers; (2) they can get their revenue from budgetary processes by convincing the political leadership to support their activities; and (3) they can obtain revenue from donors by convincing them that such support will advance the donors' agendas.

Each way creates its own incentives. Thus in several West African countries in the 1990s, when the central pharmaceutical supply system was converted from a budget-based to a cash-and-carry (that is, market-based) arrangement, its behavior began to resemble that of the private sector sellers whose incentives it now shared (Govindaraj and Herbst 2006). Similarly, as discussed in chapter 5, on financing, foreign donations serve to redirect national government priorities and behavior to satisfy the conditions those donors impose.

Whether or not variations in organizational performance translate into incentives to managers is critical. We noted in the previous chapter that this mechanism is critical to controlling corruption in private sector pharmaceutical purchasing. In the private sector, owner-managers participate directly in an organization's profits. Many companies reward other managers with stock or stock options to create similar incentives, or they give managers bonuses based on their unit's (profit) performance. (Note that such incentives can also have negative effects—for example, encouraging bankers to sell unreliable mortgage-backed securities or pharmaceutical representatives to offer bribes to purchasing agents.) In the public sector such performance-based rewards (especially profit sharing) are much more difficult to implement. But effective supervisory structures, such as performance-based promotions, can still make a difference. Moreover, not all incentives have to be cash. Once a performance monitoring system is operating, congratulations from the minister for producing superior results can have a significant effect.

Although we believe that performance can be improved, it is also true that today, in too many countries, performance in the pharmaceutical sector is far from ideal. Too many employees are happy to do only the minimum and engage in various forms of "inxit"—as discussed above (Ferrinho et al. 1998). As a result a nontrivial percentage of public sector medicines disappears as "leakage," to be resold or used by staff for personal and family purposes. (Indeed, in a good number of low- and middle-income countries, even ministers of health continue their private practices while in office.) In rural areas, where living conditions for staff members and their families are unattractive (and where additional employment opportunities are limited and patients are too poor to provide significant "informal payments"), individuals often find excuses for not taking up their posts or they show up only infrequently. The question we now turn to is, What organizational changes can reformers consider to address this situation?

Autonomy, Corporatization, and Marketization

When reform within the public sector seems difficult or impossible, one alternative is to move some activities (such as purchasing or central supply) partly or wholly outside the public sector. The entities that result are known by a wide variety of terms: parastatal, semipublic, quasi-independent, corporatized, autonomous, or more recently, marketized. Organizations completely out of the public sector are often characterized as "privatized," a term that has been applied to entities with both for-profit and not-for-profit status.

The intent of such reforms is to escape the restrictions on budgeting, purchasing, and personnel policies in the public sector. Frequently, the new entity is required to raise a significant part of its revenue from customers (or if privatized, from investors) rather than through the budget process. It is hoped that the new entity will be more flexible, effective, and businesslike, compared to a pure public sector bureaucracy. Managers will have greater authority over personnel and purchasing. Civil service and public sector union rules will be at least partially sidestepped. But the independence and flexibility given to the new entities vary greatly, and the government typically retains ultimate control.

The history of such activities dates back many decades. In the United States, for example, beginning in the 1930s the government created new entities (often called "authorities") to run ports, highways, public housing, electricity generation, and other activities. In the 1980s and 1990s, the model was applied to hospitals (in New York; Vienna; Melbourne; and Hong Kong SAR, China). Recent governments in the United Kingdom have also pursued this strategy aggressively. A World Bank study examined in detail efforts in Cameroon, Senegal, and Burkina Faso to create new pharmaceutical purchasing and supply organizations partially outside the public sector (Govindaraj and Herbst 2006). A similar organization has also been created in Kenya (see http:// www.kemsa.co.ke).

The arguments for creating new organizations relate to organizational culture—to the views and values of employees and managers—as well as to matters of managerial authority. When donors supported the creation of a new, semipublic medicines purchasing organization in Cameroon, the new management hired a whole new staff, focusing on recruiting individuals who were highly motivated and drawing heavily from the private sector. Initial evaluations suggested that performance improved (Govindaraj and Herbst 2006).

A wide variety of public-private hybrid organizations have arisen in recent years. For example, in Europe a number of governments have taken a controlling interest in private companies and run them under private sector law (for example, the airline Alitalia in Italy). The resulting entities are sometimes called "public corporations." In some cases, previously state-run activities (such as British Rail) have been converted to for-profit corporations.

What can pharmaceutical reformers learn from these efforts?

- Properly done, such reforms can be quite effective. But they require a high level of political commitment to allow the new managers to eliminate patronage, corruption, and favoritism.

- Control over the new entity (that is, its governance) is critical. In Cameroon, the government had only 25 percent of the seats on the governing board, and donors and customers had a voice as large or larger. In contrast, hospital reform in Vienna was hampered when the city council retained control of hospital management appointments.

- The new management has to be given powers broad enough to enable it to operate effectively. The managers do not necessarily need all the powers that private sector managers enjoy, but they do need sufficient authority to move the organization out of the low-performance equilibrium that is typical in the public sector.

- The risk always exists that exposing the new entity to market pressures will lead it to abandon its social responsibility or public mission. To guard against that, the government needs to be prepared to subsidize (or impose requirements for the provision of) worthy but unprofitable activities. Selecting the right board of directors and hiring senior managers with compatible values can also help instill a sense of social mission.

Having listed those difficulties, we still believe that these structural alternatives are worth taking seriously. In Liberia, for example, the ministry has established a chain of three retail outlets that sells essential medicines under its Community Outreach Program (Seiter 2009). It sells compounds in standardized packaging, from a high-quality source, and at prices well below those in the private sector. Its independence from the uncertainties of state budgetary and payment processes has helped the chain establish reasonable commercial agreements with its supplier, allowing the ordering flexibility that minimizes stock-outs. The chain also sells only course-of-treatment packages. It is beginning to develop a noticeable brand identity in the local marketplace, and the government is seeking to expand its role to other areas. This is only a microexample, but it is suggestive.

Contracting In and Contracting Out

Creating a mixed entity on the boundary of the public sector can sometimes be quite difficult. The process can be time-consuming, and the challenges of formulating the needed legal structures can be substantial, depending on the specifics of a nation's legal code. Reformers may believe that they do not have the support for creating an entity that is truly insulated from political pressures. It also may be that the functions in question (transport, warehousing, or laboratory testing) are widely performed in the private sector. In those cases, contracting with the private sector may be a reasonable option.

The pharmaceutical sector around the world offers interesting examples of contracting, particularly ones in which the risks of poor performance are transferred to the contactor. For example, drug transport from the port of entry to district centers can be contracted out, with the transport company being paid only for the drugs actually delivered. That shifts the risks of pilferage, and the incentives to prevent it, to the transporter. In Zambia, privatization of the central medical stores, through an operating contract with Crown Agents, also seems to be working well (see case study D, "Last Mile Logistics for Essential Drugs: The Case of Zambia").

Contracting, however, can carry both performance and corruption risks for public authorities—as the numerous scandals around the world related to such activities suggest. In Mexico, under the national insurance reform, state governments have introduced contracting with private pharmacies to provide medicines to people enrolled in the new program (known as "Seguro Popular"). The state of Jalisco hired a single pharmacy company to provide all such medicines statewide. In 2009, however, questions were raised about the selection of that company, the transparency of financial transactions, and the huge growth in expenditures on medicines that has occurred (Incongruencias en Contratos 2009).

Experience with contracting with the private sector, in many countries and in many functional areas, suggests that reformers need to consider a number of points when pursuing that approach.

- Contracting works better when multiple bidders participate and those bidders do not collude to short-circuit the process. It is generally not a good idea to contract with a private sector monopolist or cartel member because those companies do not have to offer a competitive price, and they do not face the need to perform well or risk losing the contract.

- Contracting works better when the required tasks are sufficiently standardized that they can be specified in detail. That also allows more objective monitoring of performance.

- Agencies writing the contracts need staff members who are trained and experienced in the contracting process. Contracting requires specialized skills and a willingness to be proactive, which can be difficult for an understaffed, undertrained, and undermotivated agency.

- Effective contracting requires meaningful monitoring and enforcement. Those processes work best in nations with an effective civil law system, within which contract performance can be enforced and disputes adjudicated.

Decentralization

Decentralization has been a prominent organizational reform in the government activities of low- and middle-income countries in recent years.

Activities in many sectors, including health, have been decentralized. The general theory is that subnational units of government have both the incentive and the ability to respond to the varied preferences of their local areas whose smaller geographic size allows for greater responsiveness to customers and more effective supervision. In larger countries that already have federal systems, decentralization has sometimes been a way to respond to separatist threats (as in Indonesia and Spain). Where subnational governments already have significant power (as in India), decentralization has sometimes involved the transfer of authority even farther down, to the district or local level.

In the pharmaceutical sector, decentralization has taken various forms. When the health sector has been engaged in a general decentralization, it can have a significant impact on pharmaceutical reform. For example, Ghana's health insurance scheme, which covers pharmaceuticals, has been implemented at the district level. Thus the scheme has not produced nationally uniform results. In other countries, such as Ukraine, procurement has been decentralized to the provincial level. When countries undertake community financing efforts, decisions on and responsibility for medicines supply can be pushed even farther downward. Current community financing schemes for general health care are widely viewed as having been inspired by the Bamako Initiative. As mentioned in chapter 7, that initiative involved a set of programs undertaken after an agreement among West African health ministers in Bamako, Mali, in 1987. A key element of the strategy, which emphasized local community participation and primary care, was the establishment of self-financing, revolving drug funds at the village level (Hanson and McPake 1993).

What has been learned from experiences with decentralization?

- Decentralization can involve many different dimensions of a "decision space," such as purchasing, budgeting, and control over personnel. The effect of decentralization is highly dependent on the details of exactly what authority managers have and which functions are decentralized (Bossert, Bowser, and Amenyah 2003).

- Within the pharmaceutical supply chain, some functions are more appropriately decentralized than others. For example, Bossert and colleagues found that centralizing inventory management and reporting requirements improved performance. However, giving districts more capacity to reallocate budgets in response to budget cuts also improved performance (Bossert, Bowser, and Amenyah 2003). A reasonable conclusion is that in some areas uniformity is valuable and in other areas it is not.

- The effect of a given pattern of decentralization depends on the context in which it occurs, including aspects of political accountability, technical skill, and cultural norms. As a result, the same reform can produce different results in different countries.

- When functions are decentralized, it is important to match capacity development with responsibility transfer, so that the decentralized units are able to carry out their expanded responsibilities.

- Decentralization is not a cure-all for a public sector dominated by patronage and corruption. Instead, as decentralization shifts the locus of decision making for particular activities, it can even lead to more corruption in less-supervised units in the periphery.

The key step for a reformer interested in decentralization is to analyze how the proposed structural changes will affect workers' behavior. That can be done by examining the impact of the proposed reform on each of the six keys to organizational performance. For example, in Kerala, India, the power to hire health center doctors was decentralized to the village level. That apparently improved service quality and physician attendance because village leaders knew whether the doctor showed up and provided good service. Moreover, those leaders cared a great deal about such performance and were prepared to act on that information when the time came to make hiring decisions (former governor of Kerala, personal communication 2008).

A related set of issues revolves around the economies of scale in a production process. If costs are lower for large-scale activities, then centralization has advantages. When large-scale production leads to higher costs (so-called diseconomies of scale), the opposite is true. For information and reporting systems, strong arguments exist for the uniformity that centralization can produce. But once again implementation matters. To ensure reliability and comparability over space and time, centrally specified reporting systems must be conscientiously implemented by lower-level workers. When that does not occur, the ability of managers to use the systems to identify and correct poor performance is compromised.

Social Franchising

An alternative organization reform strategy, rather than making public activities more like private sector ones, does the reverse: it seeks to move parts of a delivery system away from independent, for-profit operation to some level of social responsibility or public sector connection. That strategy, known as "social franchising," tries to replicate the relationship between some private sector retail outlets and brand-name chains (Bishai et al. 2008). Operators have *franchises*, that is, reciprocal agreements that govern their relationship to the brand owner. Retailers agree to meet standards of training, facility design, product mix, and service organization. The chain (such as McDonalds) supplies inputs, equipment, and even loans to individual operators. But the local owner has much greater incentive than a hired manager would have to oversee operations and make the outlet successful.

In social franchising, a nongovernmental organization (NGO) or a public agency takes the role of the brand owner—training staffs and supervising activities at individual outlets to guarantee quality and control price. In return, the individual operator may use the brand name. The hope is that growing brand recognition will lead to increased sales, making the added effort required to be a branded outlet worthwhile, as shown by the HealthStore franchise approach in Kenya (Fertig and Tzaras 2005) (see also case study F, "Converting Basic Drug Shops to Accredited Drug Dispensing Outlets in Tanzania"). A prominent example of social franchising is the Indian NGO Janani, which operates in three of the country's poorest states (Bihar, Jharkhand, and Madhya Pradesh). Janani began in 1996 with a social marketing program focused on family planning that was designed to reach underserved areas. The organization has since expanded into a network of franchised rural clinics. A unique feature of Janani is its affiliation with DKT International, a Washington-based social marketing NGO (http://www.janani.org).

In some middle-income countries, for-profit private entrepreneurs have taken a similar approach, as illustrated by the retail chain of drugstores Farmacias Similares, in Mexico (Hayden 2007). In India, the pharmacy chain MedPlus began operations in 2006, providing consumers with "quality, convenience, and low prices"—but seeking especially to assure consumers that its products were not fake medicines, to "take the risk out of buying medicines" (see http://www.medplusindia.com). This firm reflects a much broader expansion of private sector retail pharmacy chains in India, including pharmacies affiliated with private hospital chains, such as the Apollo Pharmacy, which promises "genuine medicines," that it is "open around the clock," and that it has "international quality certification" (Lowe and Montagu 2009; see http://www.apollopharmacy.in). The approach is now moving back to the public sector, as the Indian government is seeking to encourage reputable Indian pharmacy chains to open outlets in African countries (such as Nigeria) to counter the negative image created by fake medicines labeled "Made in India"—compounds that the Indian government claims are actually manufactured in China (Shankar 2009).

Using the New Public Sector Management

In recent years, a good deal of attention has been directed by the World Bank and other bodies toward the "new public sector management" (Shaw 1999). This reform movement began with an analysis of the deficiencies of public sector organizations, similar to the one we have offered above. The movement proposes to put in place managerial and incentive reforms designed to transform public sector organizations to produce significantly improved performance. The menu of reform proposals is extensive, including the following:

- Performance-Based Budgeting. Under this system, organizations are not guaranteed funding based on past support levels or some other simple formula, such as their authorized manning table. Instead, budgets are adjusted up or down based on a measure of performance. It is designed (in our terms) to operate on the broadest of the six keys: incentives on the organization.

- Global Budgeting. Many public sector organizations operate with very restrictive "line item" budgets, in which funds are segregated into specific categories. That limits managers' ability to change the allocation of resources in ways that improve performance. The process can be reformed by acting on the "managerial authority" element of the six keys and giving mangers a budget to spend as they see fit. As an intermediary step, the budget can be divided into a small number of large categories, with flexibility inside of each.

- Performance Personnel Management. The goal here is to decouple retention and promotion from simple seniority rules. Instead, the goal of this and the next proposal is to act on the "incentives to workers" element of the six keys. Under performance personnel management, personnel are subject to periodic evaluations, and their career paths are based on the results.

- Merit Pay and Pay for Performance. As a complement to an evaluation system, employee pay is made more flexible. Annual increments are made dependent on performance evaluations, and some component of compensation is made dependent on volume or quality performance.

- Management Development and Accountability. A key step is putting in place a system for simultaneously evaluating managerial performance, giving managers training opportunities to, and promoting them in a systematic way based on their performance, skills, and training. Such a program acts on both "incentives to managers" and "managers' skills, attitudes, and beliefs."

An underlying feature of the list of reform proposals is its focus on managers. The idea is to change the system so that managers both have more authority and are more accountable. It is hoped that when managers have more authority, they will then create incentives for workers and help alter workers' views and values through recruitment, selective retention, and influence. Providing training and increasing their incentives should help managers use their expanded authority effectively.

In some countries, managers have gotten around at least some public sector rules, in the spirit of these reform ideas, to increase their ability to enhance organizational performance. For example, in certain hospitals in Saudi Arabia, Egypt, and the Philippines, some staff have been hired as contract employees—not under civil service rules. That gives managers more flexibility with regard to levels and terms of compensation, as well as the ability to decline to rehire when performance is unsatisfactory. Similarly, money from co-payments and user fees, or from private donations, can be retained by the organizations that collect them and deposited in separate "foundation" accounts, from which managers can spend without restrictive purchasing approvals. In other contexts, however, the laws governing the civil service and public budgeting and contracting need to be amended if the new public sector management is to be put into action. That, however, is often far from easy, given the complex politics of such major reforms.

Essential Medicines Lists

We view essential medicines lists (EML) as a policy tool to guide the operation of the public sector pharmaceutical supply system (WHO 2007). The literature on such systems is extensive, covering both substance and process (Laing et al. 2003; Reich 1987). How should drugs be added to the list, and how should they be removed when better alternatives exist? How and when (if at all) should exemptions be made? In the construction of the list, what roles should be played by carefully controlled clinical research, expert opinion, and consumer preferences? How important is it to consider incremental costs and benefits in adding new drugs, when less-expensive products are already available? Those are only some of the many questions that have to be answered in making an EML policy effective. Moreover, answering many of the questions requires more than just technical analysis. Each involves value trade-offs and ethical priorities of the sort discussed in chapter 4. Based on the literature, we would suggest that reformers pay attention to the following:

- If an EML is to be an instrument for maximizing health gains from limited national resources, the list must use cost-effectiveness as a major consideration both within and across medicine classes.

- In making decisions on which medicines to include in, or remove from, an EML, priority attention needs to be given to well-designed clinical trials that rely on objective end points. The experience of many countries shows that the promotional efforts of pharmaceutical manufacturers can have a large impact on both expert (physician) opinion and popular attitudes, in ways that are not consistent with the best evidence.

- Because inclusion and exclusion decisions are controversial, it is important to construct open, participatory processes based on explicit criteria and analysis. The process should meet the standard of "accountability for reasonableness" discussed in chapter 4. Nations can look to the National Institute for Health and Clinical Excellence in the United Kingdom (http://www.nice.org.uk) for ideas on these procedural points.

- Every rule will provoke claims for exemptions and special treatment. In many countries exemption processes are highly informal. (For example, who has the social, political, or economic status to gain access to the minister of health? And who, in turn, has enough influence to convince the minister to give a patient access to a medicine not on the EML?) The requirements of fair process imply that instead, a formal committee needs to be appointed, with explicit criteria and explanations for its decisions. Moreover, the experience with rationing processes suggests the value of establishing in advance a budget for the total costs of any exemptions—to limit the claims that can be made and hence limit the government's overall expenditure (Calabrese and Bobbitt 1978).

The Potential Contribution of Process Improvement

In recent years a great deal of attention—often led by international donors and consultants—has been directed at *process improvement* in public sector pharmaceutical supply chains. The intellectual roots of the approach lie in operations research and quality management. Such efforts typically begin with a detailed analysis of work flows, followed by an analysis of where, why, and how faults and failures occur. Experienced consultants then work with local experts and workers involved in the process to develop and recommend changes in work flow, decision rules, task assignments, equipment, and monitoring procedures to correct the flaws and improve performance.

Although such efforts can be valuable, we urge reformers to remember that new processes and procedures will only have the desired effect if employees implement them conscientiously. For example, suppose a country wants to move beyond an inflexible "push" inventory management system, based on periodically sending every health center a prescribed package of drugs. A consultant could come in and, depending on the patterns of medicine use and the country's administrative resources, recommend one or another kind of "pull" system based on orders from the periphery (for example, a so-called two-bin system, or a fixed reorder date system) (Muller 2003). But if peripheral sites overorder (to have more supplies to divert into the private market), the new system will not work as planned. Similarly, a new electronic, open bidding system can be undermined if officials threaten some potential suppliers with retaliation (such as the loss of a business license) if they enter competitive bids. Process improvement thus has to be joined to other kinds of managerial reform for the expected benefits to be realized. And as part of such reform, the way in which workers are involved in developing the new routines is critical. Effective participation both taps local knowledge and builds acceptance of the new ideas.

A second and related point is that because new processes are not self-implementing, it is not enough just to purchase or install new computer systems or new software. Staff must be trained in their use, a task that produces fewer photo opportunities for donors than ribbon-cutting ceremonies on the delivery of new equipment. Thought also needs to be given to staff retention because, once they acquire new skills, employees are likely to enjoy enhanced opportunities in the private sector. Similarly, the recent debate on "human resources for health" has tended to focus on physicians and nurses, but the performance of the pharmaceutical sector depends critically on other, less-visible staff, such as pharmacists, supply chain managers, and lab technicians. And they are in especially short supply in many poor countries, as shown in table 9.1.

Finally, it may be helpful to think of the supply chain as an assembly line, requiring a sequence of repetitive tasks to produce any output. In such a process, overall performance is constrained by the weakest link, the slowest or worst-performing subprocess. Improving the weakest link, therefore, can improve system performance. For example, a recent analysis of the causes of stock-outs at health centers in Zambia found that the system worked reasonably well to the point of delivery to district stores

Table 9.1 Limited Human Resources in Low-Income and Other Selected Countries

	Pharmacists	Physicians	Nurses
Angola (1997)	0.00	0.08	1.15
Bolivia (2001)	0.55	1.22	3.19
Botswana (2004)	0.19	0.40	2.65
Brazil (2000)	0.30	1.15	3.84
China (2001)	0.28	1.06	1.05
France (2004)	1.06	3.37	7.24
India (2005)	0.56	0.60	0.80
Sweden (2002)	10.24	3.28	0.66
United Kingdom (1997)	0.51	2.30	12.12

Source: World Health Report 2006, 190–98.

Note: Density per 1,000 population.

and then broke down when it came to deliveries from those stores to the health centers (Ballou-Aares et al. 2008). Once the weakest link is fixed, however, the amount of improvement will be limited by the level of functioning of the next-weakest link. And improving a process that is not the weakest link might have little or no impact on overall performance, until the malfunctioning of the most troublesome stage is addressed. For example, it will not do much good to bring more medicines into the country if the distribution system fails to ship supplies to the periphery.

The Challenges of Change

Regardless of which strategy a country chooses to pursue, managers who want to facilitate change have to address two sources of resistance. One is *psychological*: the fear of newness, anxiety about the unknown, and the comfort of familiar routines and relationships. Workers may also take pride in past accomplishments and resent the criticism implicit in the claim that change is required. The other source of resistance is *practical*: a desire to avoid any loss of status, income, and influence that change may bring. That can also be joined to a desire to avoid expending the time and effort required to learn new roles, methods, and technology. Of course, the practical issues also have psychological dimensions, as workers may fear that they will not be able to perform the new tasks—for example, that they will not be able to master a new computer-based inventory management system.

Sophisticated change managers respond to both sources of resistance. They communicate the need for change, explaining that new pressures are making the old ways unsustainable. (A crisis can thus be useful in making the need for change evident to employees.) Such managers also try to respond to workers' legitimate interests, ensuring that competent and conscientious staff have a role in the new arrangements. Good change managers also make an effort to communicate frequently with workers. In the absence of information, fear and rumor will fill the gap and typically create more resistance. Managers also need to be sympathetic toward workers' fears and anxieties. They need to work to make change seem like birth rather than death—a beginning not an ending.

Managers should make an effort to appeal to the values and commitments of those employees willing to be a part of a new and better way. They should seek to connect with those employees' capacity for pride in their work and their feelings of satisfaction from providing good service. After all, making the pharmaceutical supply system work better has much positive social value. Such an approach takes advantage of the fact that most human beings desire to feel valued and valuable in their work. Indeed it is exactly that process of helping employees see their jobs in a new light that the contemporary management literature talks about under the headings "vision," "mission," "values," and "leadership" (Senge 1990).

Summary on Organization

Our review of initiatives using the organization control knob has often come back to offering the same advice: Performance will not change unless the behavior of people doing the work changes. Behavior will not change unless changes occur in the six keys. The external opportunities and incentives, and the internal beliefs, skills, and values of the organization's managers and workers must change. Any proposed change—whether decentralization, privatization, corporatization, or internal management reform—needs to be tested against these criteria.

By the same token, reformers need strategies to promote the implementation of new systems and processes. Reformers must be able to tell a plausible story, to themselves and others, about how and why the proposed changes will lead to better results. The story has to make sense in the social, cultural, and political context of the country and the organization. Using the organization control knob is not rocket science, but it also is not for the fainthearted or those who refuse to honestly confront organizational realities.

Case Studies on Organization

Kopczak, Laura Rock, Prashant Yadav, and Marc J. Roberts. "Last Mile Logistics for Essential Drugs: The Case of Zambia." Case Study D.

Ervin, Tory, and Marc J. Roberts. "Converting Basic Drug Shops to Accredited Drug Dispensing Outlets (ADDOs) in Tanzania." Case Study F.

References

Ballou-Aares, D., A. Freitas, L. R. Kopczak, S. Kraiselburd, M. Laverty, E. Macharia, and P. Yadav. 2008. *Private Sector Role in Health Supply Chains.* New York: Rockefeller Foundation, Dalberg, and MIT-Zaragoza International Logistics Program.

Bishai, D. M., N. M. Shah, D. G. Walker, W. R. Brieger, and D. H. Peters. 2008. "Social Franchising to Improve Quality and Access in Private Health Care in Developing Countries." *Harvard Health Policy Review* 9: 184–97.

Bossert, T. J., D. M. Bowser, and J. K. Amenyah. 2003. "Is Decentralization Good for Logistics Systems? Evidence on Essential Medicine Logistics in Ghana and Guatemala." *Health Policy and Planning* 22: 73–82.

Calabrese, G., and P. Bobbitt. 1978. *Tragic Choices.* New York: Norton.

Ferrinho, P., W. V. Lerberghe, M. R. Julien, E. Fresta, A. Gomes, F. Dias, A. Gonçalves, and B. Bäckström. 1998. "How and Why Public Sector Doctors Engage in Private Practice in Portuguese-Speaking African Countries." *Health Policy and Planning* 13: 332–38.

Ferrinho, P., M. C. Omar, M. D. Fernandes, P. Blaise, A. M. Bugalho, and W. V. Lerberghe. 2004. "Pilfering for Survival: How Health Workers Use Access to Drugs as a Coping Strategy." *Human Resources for Health* 2: 4.

Fertig, M., and H. Tzaras. 2005. *What Works: HealthStore's Franchise Approach to Healthcare.* Washington, DC: World Resources Institute.

Gaal, P., and M. McKee. 2004. "Informal Payments for Health Care and the Theory of 'Inxit.'" *International Journal of Health Planning and Management* 19: 163–78.

Govindaraj, R., and C. Herbst. 2006. "Impact of 'Marketizing' Organizational Reform on Public Sector Pharmaceutical Supply in Francophone Africa." Africa Human Development Department, World Bank, Washington, DC.

Hanson, K., and B. McPake. 1993. "The Bamako Initiative: Where Is It Going?" *Health Policy and Planning* 8: 247–54.

Hayden, C. 2007. "A Generic Solution? Pharmaceuticals and the Politics of the Similar in Mexico." *Current Anthropology* 28: 475–95.

Hirschman, A.O. 1970. *Exit, Voice, and Loyalty: Responses to Decline in Firms, Organizations, and States.* Cambridge, MA: Harvard University Press.

"Incongruencias en Contratos del Seguro Popular en Jalisco." 2009. *El Informador* (Guadalajara, Jalisco, Mexico). http://www.informador.com.mx/jalisco/2008/64632/6/incongruencias-en-contratos-del-seguro-popular-en-jalisco.htm. Accessed March 17, 2009.

Laing, R., B. Waning, A. Gray, N. Ford, and E. 't Hoen. 2003. "25 Years of the WHO Essential Medicines Lists: Progress and Challenges." *Lancet* 361: 1723–29.

Lawler, E. E., S. A. Mohrman, and G. E. Ledford. 1995. *Creating High Performance Organizations*. San Francisco: Jossey-Bass.

Lowe, R. F., and D. Montagu. 2009. "Legislation, Regulation, and Consolidation in the Retail Pharmacy Sector in Low-Income Countries." *Southern Medical Review* 2 (2): 35–44.

Mills, P. 1986. *Managing Service Industries: Organization Practices in a Post Industrial Economy*. Cambridge, MA: Ballinger.

Muller, M. 2003. *Essentials of Inventory Management*. New York: AMACOM, American Management Association.

Reich, M. R. 1987. "Essential Drugs: Economics and Politics in International Health." *Health Policy* 8: 39–57.

Seiter, A. 2009. "Liberia Mission Report, Update on Pharmaceutical Sector Governance and Management Issues." World Bank, Washington, DC.

Senge, P. M. 1990. *The Fifth Discipline: The Art and Practice of the Learning Organization*. New York: Random House.

Shankar, R. 2009. "Govt Begins to Establish Indian Pharmacy Chains in Africa to Counter Issue of Fake Drugs with 'Made in India' Label by China." Pharmabiz. com, September 21. http://www.gnaipr.com/Articles/govt.pdf. Accessed November 18, 2009.

Shaw, R. P. 1999. *New Trends in Public Sector Management in Health: Applications in Developed and Developing Countries*. Washington, DC: World Bank Institute.

WHO (World Health Organization). 2006. *World Health Report 2006: Working Together for Health*. Geneva: WHO.

———. 2007. *WHO Model List of Essential Medicines, 15th List*. Geneva: WHO.

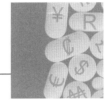

CHAPTER 10

Improving Pharmaceutical Sector Performance through Regulation

The kinds of market failures discussed in chapter 2 are all too common in the pharmaceutical sectors of low- and middle-income countries. Limited competition often leads to high prices. Deceptive trade practices lead to unreliable quality. Dispensers' incentives combine with consumers' lack of information to encourage overuse and misuse. Those problems, in turn, contribute to poor outcomes. Citizen satisfaction and financial protection decline. Quality and access difficulties, along with misuse, decrease health status. Yet medicines of uncertain quality continue to be purchased, as citizens take their chances in the hopes of bettering their health, rather than simply suffering.

Despite these difficulties, significant interest exists around the world in making better use of the private sector to improve pharmaceutical performance. In many nations, of course, much of the supply of medicines and the large majority of medicine purchases are in the private sector. The question that governments then face is, What can they do to reshape those activities to better advance public goals? This chapter reviews our answers to that question. Under the heading of the regulation control knob, it covers various interventions that governments can undertake to address private sector market failures.

For the purposes of our discussion, again as noted in chapter 2, we use the term "regulation" to mean actions by the state that rely on coercion to change behavior. (Incentives were covered in chapter 8, and efforts to persuade actors to change behavior are covered in the next chapter.) Thus regulation inherently deals with a certain degree of conflict and resistance. The reason is that those subject to regulation typically do not want to change their behavior. If they did want to change, they could have done so, and the regulatory effort would not be necessary.

In some cases, however, some of the regulated may welcome, or even propose, certain regulations as a competitive strategy. For example, pharmacists and larger medicine shops might favor requiring all medicines sellers to employ pharmacists. Similarly, international companies may favor more demanding drug registration requirements because domestic and generic competitors are less likely to have the expertise to comply with the new rules. In such cases, those disadvantaged by the new rules are the ones that regulators most need to worry about.

As illustrated in figure 10.1, pharmaceutical regulation involves a series of tasks in the regulatory cycle. Many of the tasks require significant technical expertise and administrative effort. First, governments have to decide to regulate. Then they have to write the rules. For example, as part of a reference pricing scheme, price regulators must decide which compounds are in each "therapeutically equivalent class." That can be both technically difficult and controversial, as the term "therapeutically equivalent" is subject to interpretation. Similarly, once rules have been communicated to those being regulated, instituting an effective inspection and enforcement regime requires expert and committed management to counteract the risks of corruption and subversion. It is also likely to require significant resources—for example, adequate laboratory testing equipment and personnel to test for substandard medications. Imposing sanctions also may not be easy. Often the police and the courts are not fully cooperative and reliable (see case study G, "Counterfeit Medicines in Nigeria"). Finally, designing and implementing a sophisticated evaluation of a regulatory initiative will require resources and foresight, as well as statistical sophistication.

Because some or all of those being regulated are likely to be unhappy with the regulatory regime, they may try to resist at every stage of the regulatory cycle. They may seek to discourage the initiation of regulation; try to influence legislation and rule writing, to make requirements less stringent; and undermine enforcement by limiting budgets or corrupting inspectors (and even judges). Indeed, examples exist around the world of those being regulated actually "capturing" the regulatory agency by placing sympathetic people in key management roles (Stigler 1971).

Figure 10.1 The Regulatory Cycle

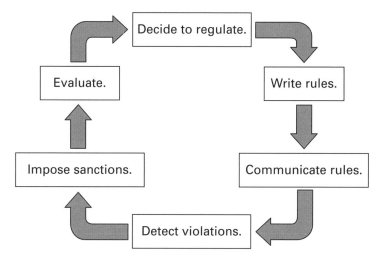

Source: Authors' representation.

The Conditions for Successful Regulation

All regulatory efforts confront some basic difficulties. First, the language that people use to describe reality is generally much less complicated than the world itself. For example, a regulation might require manufacturers to avoid "unsafe" levels of contamination in filler materials in preparing medicines. But what levels of contamination, with what substances, are "unsafe"? Similarly, if a country's pharmacovigilance program requires hospitals to report all "serious drug-related morbidity and mortality complications," what does "serious" mean in that context? What does it mean to require retail shops to display price lists for subsidized commodities on posters that are "clearly legible and prominently displayed"?

We do not want to overstate the point. Not all cases are ambiguous. Death is a "serious" complication, and a poster in the supply room is not "prominently displayed." But it is also easy to give examples of cases that are not black-or-white, in which the words in the rules do not resolve the relevant ambiguities.

In addition to linguistic ambiguity, regulators often confront procedural ambiguity. In testing for contamination in medicines, exactly which machine or laboratory procedure should be used, with what degree of reliability? If an inspector is unhappy with a factory's level of compliance with good manufacturing practices, at what point does he decide that enough is enough and order it closed down for major repairs?

These pervasive and unavoidable ambiguities imply that, within some limits, regulators have substantial *regulatory discretion*. They can, indeed must, decide what the law and the rules require in each case and what consequences to impose when violations occur. As a result, the details of how a regulatory regime is implemented are crucial to the outcomes it produces. That in turn implies that agency leadership and management are critical to what actually happens, as only competent and committed managers can make sure that the discretion we are discussing is used appropriately.

These same ambiguities also leave room for the regulated parties to comply with the letter, but not the spirit, of the law. Regulation-induced distortion in behavior and the unintended consequences that it can produce are a constant risk. Limit prices on essential medicines, and retailers may respond by not stocking them. Require pharmacists to attend continuing education courses, and in response, drug companies may offer such courses and turn them into sales pitches for their products. Similarly, some countries have used regulation to create a protected window for the first generic competitor to enter the market after a patent expires, to encourage competitive entry. Yet in some cases the original patent holder has taken advantage of that window. As a result, the patent holder's own "branded generic" has become established and able to command a price differential, decreasing rather than increasing long-run competition (Reiffen and Ward 2007).

As these examples suggest, designing a successful regulatory regime requires sophistication about the likely responses of those being regulated. It also requires a willingness to learn from both national and international experience and to readjust policy in response to countermoves by the regulated players. That is why the process appears as a cycle in figure 10.1.

Regulatory agencies also must be prepared to deal with deception by the regulated to avoid compliance. For example, manufacturing records or internal testing results can be falsified. Cost accounting reports designed to facilitate margin regulation can be manipulated. The opportunities to avoid regulation through deception are many. Such deceptions can be difficult to detect, and their rewards if successful (in the form of higher profits) can be substantial.

Regulators therefore need to consider which data will allow them to monitor compliance and whether those data are available. They need to consider the costs and reliability of alternative monitoring approaches and how strenuously those being regulated will resist any proposed data collection process. For example, do the regulated firms have to collect the relevant data for their own purposes? Would violations be easy to notice (for example, a failure to post required notices about prices) or expensive to detect (such as substandard levels of active ingredients in some packages)? All of those considerations need to be part of a regulator's analysis before a regulatory program is embarked on.

How can governments resist the likely counterpressures from those being regulated? The conditions for successful regulation are based on answering that question. Aggressive action in five areas can help to create the conditions for successful regulation:

- *Political support.* A regulatory agency is part of the bureaucratic apparatus of government. Unless political leaders want the agency actually to have an impact, it will be difficult for the agency to function effectively. Political leaders affect agency performance through the managers they appoint, the resources they provide, and the support they give for agency actions that generate resistance.

- *Agency leadership.* Effective regulatory agencies must have a competent, committed—sometimes even a courageous—person as their head. Only with capable leadership can regulatory agencies develop an organizational culture committed to professional integrity and a shared sense of mission. Political leaders need to find and appoint such individuals and give them support, rewards, and recognition based on their performance.

- *Adequate resources.* Carrying out difficult regulatory tasks requires resources—inspectors, prosecutors, experts, testing equipment, and an information system. An agency without adequate resources cannot establish effective rules or mount a credible deterrent through enforcement.

- *Technical competence.* Many regulatory activities require high levels of technical expertise, both in writing the rules and in carrying them out. Individuals with the necessary knowledge and experience are not easy to hire into government jobs in low- and middle-income countries because of low salaries and poor working environments.

- *Social legitimacy.* Enforcement influences compliance when potential violators believe that the probability of being apprehended and punished is reasonably high. But that probability becomes quite low if everyone breaks the rules. Then there are not likely to be enough enforcers to punish a significant fraction of the violations. But lowering the number of violations depends on some level of voluntary compliance. Many of the targets of regulation are just citizens trying to get ahead as best they can. If they believe that the rules are reasonably fair and serve legitimate social purposes then some of them at least will conform to regulatory requirements. Then the rate of violations will be low enough that the risk of being caught becomes a meaningful deterrent. The same kind of social legitimacy that promotes such compliance also helps motivate inspectors, prosecutors, and judges to enforce the rules energetically.

This review indicates that effective regulation is not always easy to achieve. Moreover, establishing regulations that are not, or cannot be, enforced has adverse consequences. It breeds cynicism about all regulatory activities and produces a culture of regulatory noncompliance: everyone knows that government rules are not to be taken seriously and hence can be safely ignored.

Those lessons imply that pharmaceutical sector regulation must be used strategically. Reformers need to ask themselves, Where can we use regulation effectively? Where does our country have the necessary expertise? Where can we obtain the necessary resources, political support, and social legitimacy? With this in mind, we believe that regulators should focus first on "the low-hanging fruit." Those are the regulatory targets whose behavior can be successfully influenced at the lowest cost (including economic, social, and political costs) and with the most public support. That approach can lead to some initial regulatory successes, increasing public acceptance and reinforcing political support. Those in turn can help to increase agency resources and morale and make more ambitious regulatory interventions possible in the future.

From that point of view, pharmaceutical policy makers are fortunate in that some pharmaceutical regulations can generate strong popular support. Except among the sellers and their suppliers, little support is likely to exist in society for the sale of worthless counterfeit drugs or for manufacturing facilities whose products contain unhealthy contaminants. That is a lesson that the Chinese have learned recently with some clarity (Yardley and Barboza 2008).

Regulating Product Quality

A core market failure that occurs throughout the pharmaceutical sector involves buyers' inability to judge the quality of what they are buying. (That can be the case at various points in the supply chain—not just with the end consumer.) Because of that inability, for many public health professionals the argument for regulating medicines is simple. For them, the goal of pharmaceutical policy is to improve health status, and therefore ensuring the safety and efficacy of medicines is an obvious regulatory aim because it helps minimize harm and wasted resources and produces maximum health gains.

We should note, however, that for some economists, as well as for some philosophical liberals who want to respect consumer choice, the issue can be more complicated. As discussed in chapter 4, those perspectives focus either on increasing citizens' happiness (rather than their health) or on respecting their right to choose whatever they want in the marketplace. From either of those points of view, why not just let citizens buy what they want?

We believe that one argument for regulating pharmaceutical product quality that should appeal even to free market advocates lies in the twin issues of *mistake costs* and *transaction costs*. Mistake costs are the losses that citizens suffer when their purchases turn out to be unsatisfactory. Transaction costs are the time and effort that citizens devote to purchasing decisions to try to minimize mistake costs.

Regulations that bar unsafe or ineffective products, which few or no citizens would knowingly choose, allow everyone to select from what is available with less concern. Buyers then expend less effort in guarding against mistakes, lowering total transaction costs. Buyers also make fewer mistakes—despite their reduced effort—thereby lowering mistake costs. When regulators eliminate contaminated insulin or understrength antibiotics, it is hard to see how anyone is made worse off, and many are saved the largely impossible task of checking product quality on their own. (Indeed, the difficulty of doing that gives rise to consumers' reliance on brand names as a purchasing guide.)

But not all regulation to limit product variety in the pharmaceutical sector is so straightforward. First, it may not be clear which strategy will maximize health status gains. For example, suppose a country raises educational requirements for medicine sellers. That may improve the quality of the advice given to buyers. But it also could lead to fewer sellers and decrease access. Just how should the balance be struck, in any particular case, between the two effects?

Moreover, tensions may arise between policies directed at health status and those aimed at citizen satisfaction. Some consumers—even with full knowledge of what they are buying—may desire items that regulators would prefer to exclude from the market, such as traditional herbal medicines. In such cases, should government give people what they want (subjective utilitarianism) or what experts believe will best contribute to their health (objective utilitarianism)? The tension between wants and needs, between the view of economics and the public health view, is a continuing source of disagreement in the field of pharmaceutical regulation.

At the same time, purchasers of lower-priced options generally want effective quality regulation for the products they buy, especially if it can be done in a way that does not significantly raise prices. They are hardly looking to spend their money on medicines contaminated with harmful substances, or counterfeits with little or no active ingredients. Indeed, from an equity perspective, it is particularly important to guarantee the quality of low-priced products exactly because they are more likely to be chosen by those who are already marginalized, socially and economically.

However, suppose the question is, Should a licensed drug shop be allowed to sell an herbal tonic that is mainly beer and honey? Or suppose the medical society proposes regulatory action to limit the activities of traditional healers—as Western-trained doctors did some years ago in Hong Kong SAR, China. Then the appropriate regulatory policy may not be as clear as it is in cases where few or no customers would knowingly prefer the product that regulators propose to eliminate. In response to such issues, quite a few Asian countries have training and licensing requirements for practitioners of traditional Chinese herbal medicine, and similar requirements also exist for practitioners of Ayurvedic medicine in India (Chopra 2003; WHO 1998; also see case study C, "Disentangling Prescribing and Dispensing in the Republic of Korea").

Concerns about quality arise at many points: at the time of registration, at the time of production or importation, at the point of government purchasing, and throughout the public and private supply chains. If less-regulated, lower-priced, and lower-quality products flow into the system at many points, their increased availability can lead to broader quality problems in the market. Such availability, for example, can create an environment in which manufacturers have a disincentive to invest in good manufacturing practices, as their higher production costs can be undercut by those offering lower-quality alternatives.

Such an overview allows us to identify the main regulatory tasks that are involved in ensuring product quality for pharmaceuticals:

Deciding which medicines can be sold in the country. Logically, registration is the first function that any nation's pharmaceutical regulatory system has to perform. For a poor country, that can be a daunting task. It often involves the review of conflicting scientific opinions about the benefits and side effects of a new medicine. It also involves complex policy decisions—balancing the good and bad consequences against each other and comparing them to the results from medicines already on the market. Those are difficult decisions even for well-funded agencies such as the U.S. Food and Drug Administration (FDA).

For poor and small countries, various shortcuts and cost-saving options are available. Can they take at face value data submitted to the FDA or to its counterpart in Australia, Japan, or the European Union? Can they find an industrialized country whose decision-making process—in terms of the balance it strikes between risks and benefits—seems to mirror the nation's own policy preferences? Can they pool scarce technical expertise and act collaboratively with their neighbors, to go through the process only once for a number of jurisdictions? As with all regulatory activities, to be an effective quality filter, registration activities require agency leadership, adequate resources, technical expertise, and, when controversies arise, a meaningful level of political support.

We should note that in many countries the registration process is funded by fees on the applicants as occurs, for example, in Ghana (Seiter and Gyansa-Lutterodt 2008, 6). That creates an obvious arena of vulnerability to corruption that needs to be counteracted through transparency and accountability. Meetings must be open, decisions explicitly justified, and reports easily available. Such requirements are easier to satisfy in the age of the Internet than they were even a relatively short time ago, although limits exist on what can be released in many countries because of confidentiality agreements with manufacturers.

Ensuring that medicines are manufactured appropriately. Such a require-ment is applicable both to imported supplies and to those manufactured locally, whether purchased by the public or the private sector. For the public sector, prequalification of bidders (for example, by the World Health Orga-nization [WHO]) is one option. Another is purchasing through a govern-ment or nongovernmental organization intermediary that undertakes the function of ensuring good manufacturing practice by suppliers. We should note, however, that "good manufacturing practice" is a somewhat slippery term, and although WHO has made an effort to promulgate clear require-ments, in practice that standard is neither defined nor applied in a uniform way around the world (Cohen, Mrazek, and Hawkins 2007). Whether an importing country can rely on the inspection regime in a source country will of course depend on the regulatory regime in the latter, its technical capac-ity, and its level of corruption. Few low- and middle-income countries are large enough to be able to support their own overseas offices to view manu-facturing firsthand—although Nigeria has moved modestly in that direction (see case study G, "Counterfeit Medicines in Nigeria").

For most low- and middle-income countries, local production is limited to the manufacture of simple medicines or to formulating and packaging with imported active ingredients and other materials. However, regulation of even these less-complex production facilities is technically challenging. Where manufacturers genuinely accept the regulatory regime, inspection can take on a more supportive function. However, where relationships are adversar-ial, inspections should be periodic and unannounced to generate the appro-priate deterrent effect. As in the case of registration, only an agency that is well managed, has adequate resources, and is imbued with a strong sense of mission can withstand the temptations that such inspections produce.

Testing products to verify quality. Product testing is an important part of any regulatory regime that aims to ensure the quality of a nation's pharmaceutical supply. It has to occur at multiple points along the supply chain—not just at the port of entry or the factory gate. Counterfeit products do not typically come in through authorized channels and therefore do not pass through those screening points. It is also true, especially in tropical climates, that improper storage and handling can cause product degradation that cannot be caught by screening that takes place at the beginning of the supply chain.

The issues described above, in connection with registration and the regulation of manufacturing practices, are also relevant here: the need for technical expertise, the potential for corruption, and the difficulties of maintaining an agency's mission orientation. Given these difficulties, various options discussed in the previous chapter for creating technical expertise and protection from political influence (including using contract employees outside the civil service system or corporatization of national testing laboratories) need to be considered. Similarly, it may be sensible to explore the possibilities of regional cooperation for product testing.

One way to enhance the social legitimacy of anticounterfeit efforts, and to supplement limited agency resources, is to involve consumers in the processes of identifying substandard and counterfeit medicines. An example of such a system is the Drug Quality and Information Program (DQI) in Ghana, which has been supported by the U.S. Pharmacopeia (a nonprofit scientific organization) with funding from the U.S. Agency for International Development (U.S. Pharmacopeia 2009). The DQI set up five sentinel sites in Ghana to which citizens can bring suspicious medicines for quality testing. The program recently identified a fake sample of the Novartis Coartem antimalarial product (an artemisinin-based combination therapy [ACT]), which led to government seizure of the counterfeit product from wholesale and retail pharmacies and an information campaign to warn consumers.

Ensuring quality at retail outlets. Quality regulation at the retail level requires enforcers to deal with a large number of small, widely dispersed entities. Inspectors making the rounds of such sites are themselves difficult to supervise, even as they are subject to repeated efforts to deflect their attention, greatly increasing the opportunities for corruption.

One approach to the problem is development of a system of government-accredited private medicine shops (see case study F, "Converting Basic Drug Shops to Accredited Drug Dispensing Outlets in Tanzania"). That strategy is a way of upgrading existing private sector outlets in rural areas and ensuring that people living outside of urban areas have access to an expanded list of good quality prescription and nonprescription medicines. The approach was developed by Strategies for Enhancing Access to Medicines

(SEAM), a project supported by the Bill and Melinda Gates Foundation and implemented by Management Sciences for Health, a consultancy based in Cambridge, Massachusetts. The project includes a strong enforcement component. However, because all owners of accredited shops benefit (via a shared reputation for quality) from a system that operates with integrity, the confrontational nature of standards enforcement is somewhat softened.

Thinking about what it is like to work as a drug shop inspector leads to a paradoxical realization about the enforcement process. One might think that compliance-through-deterrence is best accomplished by imposing large penalties even for small violations, but that is not the case. Enforcement is a human process, and disproportionate penalties that seem unfair to inspectors and judges only lead to violations' not being reported or penalized. That is so especially if imposing large penalties has social costs, such as closure of the only medicines supply point in a rural area.

This point is even more important if regulators want those regulated to self-report minor rule violations, as occurs, for example, in some manufacturing regulatory regimes. Such reporting is obviously unlikely to occur if the penalties for self-reported transgressions are large. Instead, the punishment should fit the crime. Penalties for small infractions should be modest enough to encourage accurate monitoring and enforcement.

Ensuring accurate labeling and branding. The process of quality testing needs to be complemented by a process for ensuring that branding and other aspects of labeling are accurate. Labeling integrity involves a strong convergence of the interests of governments and those of the major international manufacturers, who would like to minimize their victimization by counterfeiters.

Here again, some potential technological fixes are available. Devices such as bar codes and holograms are already being used—the latter because they are difficult for low-budget counterfeiters to copy. RFID (radio-frequency identification) tags—tiny radio transmitters contained in labels that emit identifying signals—are also attracting increased interest. Because most consumers are interested in getting what they think they are paying for, consumer information campaigns and hotlines for buyers to call with inquiries about suspect products are useful complements to such strategies (as were implemented in Azerbaijan) (Cohen, Mrazek, and Hawkins 2007). The widespread diffusion of cell phones is making it much more feasible for consumers to undertake this kind of inspection function. As always, however, the introduction of new technology needs to be accompanied by efforts to educate and mobilize consumers.

Nigeria's experience with anticounterfeiting regulation shows what is possible (Raufu 2006). In the 1990s, the new director of the National Agency for Food and Drug Administration and Control (NAFDAC) led an aggressive effort to attack drug counterfeiting. Inspections at ports and airports increased. Unauthorized imports were seized. Raids were conducted on the large urban drug markets, and large quantities of unregistered materials and fake medicines were burned. Community mobilization efforts included school-based organizations. Ultimately, legitimate sellers turned on the illegal importers and helped to identify them to the regulators. All of that occurred because of high levels of political support, dedicated agency leadership, additional technical resources, and support from the donor community. As a result, the prevalence of counterfeiting (which by some estimates had reached 80 percent of medicines sold in some Nigerian markets) decreased significantly (see case study G, "Counterfeit Medicines in Nigeria").

Yet real difficulties also arose. The regulatory pressures put NAFDAC staff in some personal danger. Assassination attempts were made against the director, and various offices were burned down. Corruption in the police and the judiciary also undermined efforts to punish major counterfeiters. Only about 50 successful prosecutions occurred over a decade, and the large drug markets were only closed for six months each, reopening later and flourishing once again.

Regulating Use

Worldwide, the accumulated evidence shows a great deal of overuse and misuse of medicines. The pattern is complicated by the fact that in low- and middle-income counties, controls on use through prescription requirements are rarely enforced. Although the situation varies by a country's level of economic development, many medicines sellers are not registered or regulated, even those that operate formal shops. And even within a country, central urban areas are less dominated by informal supplies than are periurban slums or rural areas. Given the variations, using regulation to change the ways people use medicines can face formidable difficulties. Restrictions on citizens' free access to private sector medicines often do not have a high level of social legitimacy and hence tend to be unattractive politically. It is one thing to use regulation to ensure that consumers get what they think they are paying for. It is quite another to use regulation to prevent them from getting what they want, especially when they are willing to pay for it.

Three kinds of regulatory initiatives are widely employed in high-income countries to influence use of pharmaceuticals:

Facility licensing. Licensing involves limiting which organizations can perform which functions at various stages in the supply chain. Most industrialized countries limit the sale of certain medicines to pharmacies and have requirements (including staffing requirements) for licensing such premises. Although similar legislation exists in many low- and middle-income countries, it is rarely effectively enforced, and medicines are widely sold on the street and in local markets, as well as in more organized outlets, and often by staff with little or no formal training.

Professional licensing. Professional licensing rules limit who can perform certain functions, based on education and, in some cases, separate examinations. It should be noted that in many low- and middle-income countries professional pharmacy training is a relatively difficult-to-achieve and high-status professional qualification—one well beyond the reach of most retail sellers of medicines.

Prescription requirements. In those low- and middle-income countries where prescription requirements are in place, they often are not effectively enforced. And in areas without physicians, enforcing such rules would deny people access to needed medicines. It is also true that in public clinics in many middle-income countries (as well as in some high-income countries) visit times can be very short, and multiple prescriptions are often provided at each visit. This pattern is particularly likely to develop when low-cost medicines are available with a prescription from public suppliers or are eligible for insurance reimbursement. That suggests that physicians in those counties are doing little effective gatekeeping with respect to pharmaceutical use.

The difficulty of implementing any of these general approaches suggests to us that regulators trying to deal with overuse, underuse, and misuse need to follow more selective and targeted strategies. That means focusing on those specific conditions and compounds where problems are likely to be most serious. One such approach involves limiting the terms and conditions under which particular medicines are sold. Requiring directly observed treatment for access to tuberculosis medications or a prior diagnostic test for access to subsidized ACTs are examples. Another alternative is to limit the form in which some medicines are sold—for example, requiring course-of-treatment packaging. A third strategy is to limit who can dispense certain medications. Some nations, for example, only dispense selected high-cost medications with authorization from (or, in the case of Rwanda, only at) the district hospital. Similarly, some countries only allow selected retailers—typically those with higher levels of training—to sell a list of restricted compounds.

All of these efforts, however modest, face enforcement difficulties. They may only be feasible because they do not try to do too much—compared to an attempt to impose universal prescription requirements. In addition, to be accepted such efforts will almost certainly have to be complemented by efforts at public education and behavior change (which are discussed in chapter 11).

Regulation Directed at Controlling Prices

Two broad regulatory strategies can influence retail prices for medicines. The first focuses on increasing competition by changing the structure of a market and the conduct of the sellers in that market. (Here "structure" means the number of competitors and competitive products and their relative market shares.) This approach is typically called "antimonopoly" or "competition policy." The second approach seeks to regulate prices and margins directly.

Antimonopoly policy has not been widely used in the pharmaceutical sector in many low- and middle-income countries. An exception is South Africa, where the Competition Commission became an important force in the struggle for expanded access to AIDS medicines in that country (Commission Questions Conduct 2003). As noted in chapter 8, in small countries, economies of scale limit the number of sellers at the wholesale level. The same forces also constrain retail competition in all but the larger urban areas. Where competitors engage in blatant anticompetitive behavior (such as bid rigging and threatening would-be newcomers), some opportunities for regulatory intervention may exist. But major supply chain firms are often economically significant and politically well connected. So regulators are well-advised to make sure that they have appropriate political support before embarking on such actions. Regulators also need to make sure they have an adequate legislative basis for such initiatives, because the required statutory framework is quite sophisticated and may not be present in all situations.

Regulation of prices and margins can be accomplished in various ways. Sometimes it takes the form of price regulation for some or all products on the essential medicines list. Sometimes it takes the form of setting maximum prices that public insurance funds will pay. Sometimes it has involved regulating the margins between the prices paid to wholesalers and the prices charged at the retail level. Recently, interest has increased in a particular form of this regulation, called "regressive margins." It allows higher percentage margins on lower-priced products, as a way to counteract retailers' incentives to push higher-priced and higher-margin products on customers.

Absent a comprehensive and sophisticated price control system—which is difficult to implement even in an advanced economy—regulators have to expect that distortions will occur with any price or margin control regime. In low- and middle-income countries, where many retail outlets are small and lack sophisticated records (and most transactions are in cash), inspection and enforcement of margin controls are especially difficult. As discussed in chapter 8 on payment, the most successful efforts have been targeted ones—for example, requiring sellers of subsidized products to post, and comply, with prices for those items. That allows customers to participate in enforcement in an arena where seller behavior is far easier for buyers to monitor than product quality, as discussed above.

Another strategy is to use social franchising or accreditation initiatives, which may permit slightly higher prices that are justified by guaranteed quality (of product and service). Two examples are the ADDO (accredited drug dispensing outlet) shops in Tanzania and the Green Star network in Pakistan. (For more information on these alternatives, see the SEAM project, at http://www.msh.org/seam, and case study F, "Converting Basic Drug Shops to Accredited Drug Dispensing Outlets in Tanzania.")

Summary on Regulation

Regulating the pharmaceutical sector in low- and middle-income countries is not easy. Assembling enough skilled personnel, ensuring political support, developing a suitable statutory framework, and conducting corruption-free inspections are all challenging activities. All of the recommendations from chapter 9 on the organization control knob, concerning what it takes to create an effective public sector organization, apply here with great force. That is why, for some regulatory tasks (such as running a testing laboratory), corporatization or contracting out merit consideration. No matter what form the regulatory agency takes, pervasive problems of regulatory discretion and opposition by at least some of those regulated will occur. That means that effective agency leadership and high-level political support are essential for success.

To point out these difficulties is not to suggest that nations should avoid medicines regulation. To restate an earlier point, we urge a strategic approach to pharmaceutical regulation, starting with the low-hanging fruit. As some of the examples discussed suggest, political and popular support is obtainable for certain kinds of regulatory efforts, especially those directed at counterfeit and substandard drugs. Effective action on those problems can produce meaningful gains in both health status and citizen satisfaction. Unenforced regulations, however, only breed contempt for the rule of law and for government action generally. The regulatory enterprise is difficult enough without having to contend with such a self-created burden.

Case Studies on Regulation

Ervin, Tory, and Marc J. Roberts. "Converting Basic Drug Shops to Accredited Drug Dispensing Outlets in Tanzania." Case Study F.

Moore, Eric O., Michael R. Reich, and Marc J. Roberts. "Counterfeit Medicines in Nigeria." Case Study G.

References

Chopra, A. S. 2003. "Āyurveda." In *Medicine Across Cultures: History and Practice of Medicine in Non-Western Cultures*, ed. Helaine Selin, 75–83. Norwell, MA: Kluwer Academic Publishers.

Cohen, J. C., M. Mrazek, and L. Hawkins. 2007. "Corruption and Pharmaceuticals: Strengthening Good Governance to Improve Access." In *The Many Faces of Corruption: Tracking Vulnerabilities at the Sector Level*, ed. J. E. Campos and S. Pradhan. Washington, DC: World Bank.

"Commission Questions Conduct of Anti-Retroviral Companies." 2003. *Competition News, The Official Newsletter of the Competition Commission*, edition 14, December, 1–2. http://www.compcom.co.za/resources/Comp%20Com%20 News%20(Dec)2003.pdf. Accessed March 16, 2009.

Raufu, A. 2006. "Nigeria Leads Fight against 'Killer' Counterfeit Drugs." *Bulletin of the World Health Organization* 84: 690.

Reiffen, D., and M. R. Ward. 2007. "'Branded Generics' as a Strategy to Limit Cannibalization of Pharmaceutical Markets." *Managerial and Decision Economics* 28: 251–65.

Seiter, A., and M. Gyansa-Lutterodt. 2008. "Policy Note: The Pharmaceutical Sector in Ghana." Draft, World Bank, Washington, DC.

Stigler, G. 1971. "The Theory of Economic Regulation." *Bell Journal of Economics and Management Science* 2: 3–21.

U.S. Pharmacopeia. 2009. "Counterfeit Antimalarial Drug Discovered in Ghana with Aid of USP Drug Quality and Information Program." Press Release, July 22. U.S. Pharmacopeia, Rockville, MD.

WHO (World Health Organization). 1998. *Regulatory Situation of Herbal Medicines: A Worldwide Review*. Geneva: WHO.

Yardley, J., and D. Barboza. 2008. "Despite Warnings, China's Regulators Failed to Stop Tainted Milk." *New York Times*, September 27, A1.

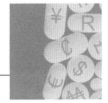

CHAPTER 11

Using Persuasion to Influence Pharmaceutical Use

Persuading citizens to change how they buy and use pharmaceuticals—and convincing doctors and medicines sellers to interact differently with patients and customers—is not easy. Public health has a long history of unsuccessful attempts at changing individual behavior, attempts often driven by the mistaken belief that simply providing better information will produce the desired change. In fact, behavior reflects the influence of many more forces than just the information someone has about a situation. The good news is that when the full range of causal factors is considered and acted on, behavior *can* be changed, as illustrated by public health successes on tobacco control. This chapter first discusses some of the motivations that drive all human behavior, including pharmaceutical use. It then explores some general lessons from the field of social marketing about what it takes to influence behavior. Next those lessons are applied to changing the behaviors that are important to pharmaceutical sector performance in low- and middle-income countries.

Elements of Human Decision Making

Several aspects of human decision making are particularly relevant to patients' choices about pharmaceutical use: the limits on our analytical capacities, the role of decision rules in light of those limits, and the role of emotion and instinct.

In fact, human beings are not very good at weighing diverse consequences to make even moderately complicated decisions. Our analytical capacities are actually quite limited. It is not easy for us to compare outcomes that have multiple dimensions—especially when one option is better in one way and another option is better in a different way. When the relevant outcomes are not fully known or are uncertain, our ability to make careful comparisons is rapidly overwhelmed

Consider the decisions that medicine buyers in low- and middle-income countries face all the time. They go to a retail outlet to purchase a particular medicine and find that they have three choices: the high-price originator brand; a midprice branded generic; and a low-price, unbranded generic. Such buyers face many questions. Is it worthwhile to save money by purchasing the unbranded generic that may—or may not—have different pharmacological qualities and, at first glance, looks less attractive? Alternatively, is the higher-price, brand-name generic likely to be of better quality, and if so, how does that potential but uncertain benefit compare to the price difference? Finally, is it worthwhile to play it safe and pay even more for the originator brand, or is that option more likely to be counterfeit?

Formal methods exist—known as "decision analysis"—for making such complex choices. But they require a great deal of time, effort, and sophistication, as well as a good deal of difficult-to-obtain data. Even a simplified analysis of the kind of decision just described would make for a good term paper in a graduate course in this subject. Thus although the formal methods may be helpful to a university-trained, large-volume, professional buyer making an important decision, they are of no practical use to individual consumers purchasing retail medicines.

How do real people make such decisions, when a full, "rational" analysis is beyond their capacity and they have only a few minutes to devote to the purchase? One common way is to use "decision rules" or standard operating procedures. Over time, people tend to develop relatively simple approaches to certain classes of repeated decisions, and they follow their approach without thinking much about it. A pharmaceutical example might be, "Don't buy either the least expensive or the most expensive option, but look for an option in-between that has a recognizable brand name and comes in packaging that doesn't look too scruffy or like a fake." Notice that that decision rule may not be fully conscious. To the customer it is likely to seem that what they are doing is making a reasonable compromise.

Patterns of choice that are so routinized that customers are barely aware of them can be thought of as habits. We necessarily rely on habits to guide much of our daily behavior. They allow us to get on with our life and reserve our scarce attention and conscious decision-making capacity for those instances where they are really needed.

Brand loyalty is an example of such a habit. If a particular brand name is known and familiar, consumers often choose that product more-or-less reflexively. It is a way of making choices (partly based on one's own experience and partly based on reputation, which is reflective of other people's experience) without expending a lot of decision-making effort. In many low- and middle-income countries, many relatively established generic products, in addition to the originator brands, have developed a substantial level of what marketers call "brand identification."

Over time, consumers may readjust their decision rules if they don't lead to satisfactory results. The Nobel Prize–winning economist Herbert Simon (1956) called that process "satisficing." If I get richer or poorer, or if I have a bad experience with some choices, or if I impulsively make an exception and it turns out well—any of those can lead me to change my decision rule.

In any one area of life, at any one time, my decision rules are not likely to give me the best possible results. In contrast to the assumptions of the normal economic model, I am not "maximizing" my gain. But the rules that I use yield results that are satisfactory enough that I spend my time doing something else besides trying to improve them. I spend a few minutes in the drug shop and make my purchase; I don't spend all day at it. Instead, I go on my way—to work or to do more shopping—or I go home and make dinner for my family. If I face what seems like a big decision—on a cancer drug instead of cough syrup—I may put my decision rule to one side and give the options additional consideration and analysis.

An individual's specific decision rules are shaped by their more general system of ideas, theories, and approaches. I cannot, every time I have a decision to make, go back to first principles and re-ask basic questions such as, "Do I believe that illness comes from evil spirits, so that I should consult the local shaman, or do I accept the germ theory of disease, which means that I should go to the drug shop?" Instead, my more specific decision rules—when a child has a fever, go and get medicines—are likely to reflect the implicit answers I give to those more general questions. Here is another example: Do I presume that a medicine that looks, smells, and tastes good will be good for me, as is presumed in many cultures, or bad for me, as is presumed in a few? (Think of the reliance in 18th- and 19th-century Europe and America on foul-tasting doses of castor oil.) We all have an extensive set of beliefs about how the world works, and those beliefs provide a basis or framework for much of what we do in our daily activities.

These beliefs are transmitted by many mechanisms: families, schools, religious institutions, peers, and the mass media. Different aspects of our belief systems carry different labels: religion, ideology, science, tradition, and social norms. Whatever they are called, those basic beliefs can be powerful determinants of individual choices. Reformers who want to persuade citizens to alter their pharmaceutical consumption patterns must be aware of those beliefs and of their persistence, if they want to be effective in changing behavior.

Finally, individuals are also heavily influenced by emotion and impulse—especially in decisions that are made quickly or in difficult and emotionally charged situations. Since Darwin, scientists concerned with evolution have argued that those impulses have become hard-wired in the human brain because of their survival value during earlier periods of human existence. Much of human behavior around basic needs and drives, from mating and parenting to social cooperation and reactions to danger, reflects these forces. They show themselves in our immediate and instinctive reactions and in the strong feelings we experience in certain situations.

Recent research has also shown that among these reactions, human beings have a set of what some scholars call "moral impulses" (Buss 2005; Hauser 2006). They include, among others, a willingness to help those in distress, a sense of fairness, a respect for hierarchy, a sense of group identity, and a deep revulsion for some practices seen as "unnatural" or "unclean." The way they are expressed at any time is deeply influenced by the culture in which a person has grown up. For example, is someone of another racial or ethnic group seen as a "person" in need of rescuing? But these and other basic impulses, however modified or shaped, are always operating.

Those emotions and impulses need to be taken into account in efforts to influence pharmaceutical purchasing behavior. For example, when a child is sick, emotions may take over. Even poor parents might decide to purchase the expensive, brand-name version of a medicine. The reason is that, given their general ideas about illness and treatment, they believe that the expensive medicine is likely to be more effective, and they want to do all they can to save their child. This is a natural, common, and powerful human response.

Using Persuasion: The Lessons of Social Marketing

In recent years, a large literature has appeared that draws on the lessons of commercial advertising and marketing to shape public persuasion activities. The approach, known as "social marketing," has been applied to many areas of behavior change in public health, including HIV prevention (Lamptey and Press 1998), tobacco control (Müller-Riemenschneider et al. 2008), and diet (Walsh et al. 1993). The insights of social marketing have important implications for efforts to improve the performance of the pharmaceutical sector by altering behavior through persuasion. In part, social marketing approaches to medicines use are designed to counteract the powerful commercial marketing of the pharmaceutical industry (Angell 2004). And in part, the social marketing approach for medicines has learned from the methods of commercial marketing to work toward different goals, illustrated by the practice of academic detailing (Soumerai and Avorn 1990).

First, because basic behaviors are difficult to change, social marketing tells us that persuasion efforts must be carefully designed and go beyond just presenting data, if they are actually to influence people's choices. Because of the power of habits, broader beliefs, and decision rules and the roles of instinct and emotion in choice, just giving the target audience new information is unlikely to have much impact. Commercial marketing rarely relies on only providing information. Similarly, social marketing designed to shape behavior in the pharmaceutical sector must use the full array of persuasion methods.

A second conclusion of the social marketing literature is that successful marketing begins with product design. In the case of pharmaceutical reform, the "product" is the behavior that reformers hope to influence people to adopt. That product has to respond to the motives, ideas, and beliefs that members of the target audience already hold. Asking the target audience to do something that they are emotionally unwilling or habitually reluctant to do is not an effective basis for exerting influence. Effective persuasion requires the social marketer to present the desired behavior as the solution to a problem from the customer's point of view—as a way to achieve the customer's goals. A successful campaign to reduce drunk driving used the slogan, "Friends don't let friends drive drunk" (Smith 2006). That campaign was organized by the Ad Council and the U.S. Department of Transportation (a public-private partnership) to shift the intervention focus from the drinking person to the nondrinking friend—who became known as the "designated driver"—and who provided a safe ride home (NHTSA 2011). The shift gave people a concrete action they could take, rather than trying to get them to stop drinking. Targeted at teenagers, the campaign was based on research showing that young drivers cared greatly about their peers and were most likely to respond to suggestions from those same individuals. The campaign has gained widespread acceptance around the world.

Second, as the last example suggests, effective social marketing requires a sophisticated understanding of the target audience to create the right kind of promotion. That means doing market research and dividing the target audience into "market segments," that is, distinct groups of people who share certain beliefs and values. Those distinct market segments need to be separately understood and addressed in the effort to promote the product. For example, in addressing overprescribing of antibiotics, analysts need to give separate attention to physicians and to patients, and their interactions, to understand how to change their expectations and behaviors (Hamm, Hicks, and Bemben 1996). Patients who differ in age, income, education, or illness are likely to have different beliefs about and use of antibiotics. And such differences in turn will require distinct behavior change approaches (see case study H, "Changing the Use of Antibiotics in Peru").

A third important lesson from social marketing involves the place where the message is delivered. Here we note the importance of "life path points," that is, how members of the target audience move through their day and where messages can be placed to reach them. The organization Grassroot Soccer, for example, observed that African youths are heavily involved in playing and watching that game. So it uses "the power of soccer" to develop life skills and knowledge about HIV prevention to help them live HIV free (see www.grassrootsoccer.org).

The same logic applies to selecting a mass media approach and a spokesperson. If the target audience does not have television, maybe radio can be used. If they do have TVs and watch certain soap operas, it may be possible to build the key message into the scripts. If you want to reach teenagers, use rock stars or sports figures. A famous American antidrug campaign featured Nancy Reagan, the president's wife, and the message, "Just say no!" Although the "no-use" approach became very popular for both government and nongovernmental programs in the United States, a systematic review of studies in 1991 concluded, "There is no evidence that the no-use approach is more successful than alternative approaches, or even successful in its own right" (USGAO 1991, 44).

The fourth important lesson from social marketing involves the question of price. A simplistic view is that a low or even a negative price—that is, a subsidy—is the best way to encourage use. In some cases that may be true. Some studies of bed nets for mosquito control to prevent malaria, for example, suggest a sharp decline in purchases with even modest price increases, especially among the lowest income groups (Cohen and Dupas 2010). But other examples show that a simple product donation program, without additional components, is unlikely to achieve success. To achieve its success, for example, the Mectizan Donation Program has evolved into a complex effort at community-directed treatment that includes major efforts in community mobilization and education, combined with significant national and regional organizations implemented through the African Program on Onchocerciasis Control (Hodgkin et al. 2007).

In other cases, low prices can even be counterproductive because they signal low quality to customers, or they encourage inappropriate use or hoarding. Using market research to identify and understand the likely responses of distinct market segments, and tailoring the campaign to those different segments, is as important in price setting as in other elements of persuasion. (Note that consideration of price as part of persuasion efforts can also be understood as moving reformers in the direction of using the payment control knob, and the incentives that it can create, as a way to change behavior.)

These four lessons of social marketing reflect the four key components of a marketing effort—product, promotion, place, and price. Social marketing can be particularly important when introducing a new kind of product in public health, such as microbicides for prevention of HIV infection in women (see case study I, "Preparing for Microbicide Introduction in South Africa"). Finding the right combination of the four elements is critical to successfully influencing the behavior of the key actors in the pharmaceutical sector, especially physicians and patients, as we discuss next.

Changing Behavior in the Pharmaceutical Sector

This brief review of human decision making and social marketing allows us now to consider three areas where changing behavior is important to the performance of the pharmaceutical sector in low- and middle-income countries (and in many high-income countries as well). The areas are treatment-seeking behaviors by patients, health professional behaviors around prescribing and dispensing, and patient compliance behaviors.

Treatment-Seeking Behaviors

Having decided to seek treatment, someone who feels ill must then decide where to go for care. In low- and middle-income countries the choice is likely to be between the public sector and the for-profit private sector. Perhaps a faith-based facility or a secular nongovernmental organization is also available. In many low- and middle-income countries, poor quality in the public sector encourages patients to go elsewhere, even if the cost of doing so is higher. In Pakistan, for example, treatment in the public health system is free, "but due to insufficient supply of medicines and lack of laboratory equipment and medical staff, these government-owned hospitals and health facilities fail to provide adequate medical care to consumers." As a result, in Pakistan private practice has become "the backbone of the health care system" (Nizami, Khan, and Bhutta 1996, 1133).

Once consumers decide to seek treatment in the private sector, those at the lowest income level often decide to purchase medicines directly from private drug sellers. That allows them to avoid paying a consultation fee in either a public or a private health clinic in addition to the cost of the medicine. Consumers who take this option often ask medicine sellers for advice, even if the person is not a trained pharmacist. Poor customers frequently end up purchasing medicines from small or informal sellers, who are often the only venders available in rural areas or periurban slums. These informal sellers offer advice, providing an informal diagnosis and suggested treatment, even though they typically have little technical background beyond what they have picked up on the job over the years. It is not a situation designed to foster rational medicines use.

One study of medicine purchases in shops in Nigeria found that most of the interactions (about 70 percent) involved simply selling the requested products. However, 20 percent to 30 percent of the interactions involved exchanges about which medicines to take, how to take the medicine, and questions about the illness (Brieger et al. 2004). As the researchers concluded, most of the customers in these shops "know what products they want to purchase in advance." But they also see the shops as a source of advice and information about illness and treatment. That latter role has encouraged public health professionals to look at the shops as places for behavior change interventions (Goel et al. 1996).

How do consumers select a medicine to purchase? First of all, as discussed above, consumers in all countries are influenced to some extent by brand loyalty. If they have had good experience with an imported, brand-name antibiotic in the past, and it has a good reputation among their friends, why not buy it again? For nonbranded, generic medicines, consumers may rely on observable characteristics, such as taste, smell, appearance, packaging, and price. Such behavior reflects the belief that on average, better packaged and more attractively presented medicines probably have been produced to more exacting standards. Nor is that a foolish decision rule. Although the correlations between external packaging and internal quality are not perfect, they also are not zero. As noted in chapter 5 in the discussion of quality, reliance on aspects of "service quality" as an indicator of "clinical quality" is a pervasive feature of many health care markets.

When poor people spend their hard-earned money for medicines, it is not surprising that they prefer products whose impact is directly apparent to them, such as pain relievers, antihistamines, antidepressants, and antibiotics. Those perceptions are typically joined to a variety of preferences and beliefs about various forms of treatment: preferences for antibiotics over oral rehydration salts for treatment of diarrhea; preferences for antibiotics for treatment of colds and respiratory infections; preferences for injections rather than pills; and preferences for antimalarial pills for the presumptive treatment of fevers.

In that context it is important to remember the well-documented power of the placebo effect—in which belief in the effectiveness of medicines shapes the symptom relief that a patient experiences (Beecher 1955). Thus patients who believe that injections "work better" are likely to have that belief confirmed by their own experience. Given all these factors, one review about the purchase of medicines in developing countries concluded, "A large proportion of patients are spending scarce resources on medicines that will do them no good, and may cause them harm, or may contribute to antibiotic resistance in human pathogens" (Trostle 1996).

What can be done to change any of these behaviors? Social marketing interventions targeted at consumers need to be designed in ways that complement other reform efforts. For example, quite a few countries have been trying to use social marketing to promote the use of rapid diagnostic tests (RDTs) before offering customers artemisinin-based combination therapies (ACTs) for possible malaria cases, to counteract the development of antimicrobial resistance. And in fact, asking mothers to get an RDT before purchasing ACTs for a child with a fever has the advantage of potentially producing some cost saving if the test comes back negative (indicating the child does not have malaria). But then the pharmacist has to have something else to offer the mother (and the feverish child) if the package of behavior change interventions is to fully respond to her motivations (Gordon 2010). As this example suggests, changing patient behaviors is complicated by the need also to change the behaviors of health workers, physicians, pharmacists, and medicine sellers.

Health Professional Behaviors

Health professionals, as well as the many nonlicensed practitioners who sell medicines, have much influence over how patients use pharmaceuticals. Their influence is exercised not only through consultations, care giving, and prescribing practices, but also in the form of advice giving in the course of sales transactions. It is important to recognize that dispensing medicines serves multiple purposes for the health workers. As Trostle noted, "Biomedical practitioners use pills to heal, but they also use them to signal the end of a therapeutic encounter, create additional income, maintain professional prestige, and increase patient loyalty" (Trostle 1996, 1117). To be successful, interventions intended to change provider behavior must take account of this complexity.

Many interventions have sought to change the prescribing and dispensing patterns of health workers in low- and middle-income countries. An intervention in Indonesia, for example, aimed to reduce the overuse of injections in public health facilities (Hadiyono et al. 1996). The study reported that 60 percent of patients at public health facilities received an injection as part of their treatment. The intervention sought to reduce injections for reasons of clinical risk as well as economic cost. Patient-provider group discussions were used to challenge prescribers' assumptions about patient beliefs, to present scientific information about injections, and to establish peer norms about correct behavior. The randomized trial in 24 public health centers produced significant reductions in injection use and in the average number of drugs per prescription for the health centers in the intervention. Although such interventions can be effective on a small scale, two major challenges are scaling up the behavior change efforts to a systemwide level and maintaining the effects over time, so that the changes persist and the original patterns do not reappear.

The structure of a health system can provide powerful incentives for physicians to prescribe, or overprescribe, certain kinds of medicines, especially when physicians are also allowed to directly dispense, as they are in many Asian countries. In response, a number of efforts have been made in recent years to separate prescribing and dispensing in those nations. The goal has generally been to remove the financial incentive to prescribe higher-priced medicines and larger volumes of medicines (see case study C, "Disentangling Prescribing and Dispensing in the Republic of Korea"). But in practice, the consequences of such legislative changes have been mixed. According to one study, for example, in Taiwan, China, separating the two functions reduced the probability of receiving a prescription during a clinic visit by 17 percent to 34 percent, and reduced spending on medicines by 12 percent to 36 percent per visit, but did not reduce the overall expenditure per visit to the clinic (Chou et al. 2003).

Patient Adherence Behaviors

An aspect of consumer decision making on pharmaceuticals that greatly frustrates public health professionals is widespread lack of patient adherence to recommended doses and uses. Two examples are especially salient: The first involves antibiotics that are discontinued prematurely or are taken when not needed. The second concerns patients who stop taking their chronic disease medications or take smaller doses.

Those decisions often seem justified from the patient's perspective. Chronic disease medications may be expensive and may also have side effects. That can be all the more aggravating when the medicines seem not to be having an effect, perhaps because the patient was asymptomatic to begin with. Similarly, once an antibiotic has eliminated evident symptoms, why bother with the troublesome need to remember to take it several times a day? That can seem especially appealing because unused pills can be stored for future use, saving the trouble and expense of obtaining additional medicine when antibiotics are again needed. Moreover, the effects of early termination on the development of drug resistance are consequences external to the patient who is stopping the treatment.

Medication adherence by chronic disease patients is a problem found around the world. In developed countries, adherence to long-term therapy for chronic diseases such as diabetes, hypertension, and heart disease is estimated to average about 50 percent. In developing countries, the rates are even lower (Sabaté 2003). Problems of adherence are also critical for infectious diseases that require long-term treatment, such as HIV/AIDS and tuberculosis. And the development of antimicrobial resistance is a serious problem for many critical conditions worldwide, as illustrated by the decision to dedicate World Health Day in 2011 to that issue (WHO 2011).

One approach for encouraging behavior change among patients is to use community-based group processes. Group discussions, guided by a trained facilitator, can help to create new norms for participants and to motivate changes in behavior related to particular medicines or conditions. Interactive group discussions were used in Indonesia, for example, to teach groups of mothers how to review drug package inserts and make informed decisions when purchasing over-the-counter medicines. Those efforts led to changes in how the mothers purchased medicines, reducing the number of duplicative products and also monthly purchases of brand-name products from 5.3 to 1.5 per month (Suryawati and Santoso 1997).

Another example of a comprehensive community-based approach is an effort to ensure adherence to HIV treatment through the mobilization of *accompagnateurs* (community health workers) in rural Haiti (Koenig, Léandre, and Farmer 2004). Organized by Partners in Health, that program used daily visits by the *accompagnateurs* to provide integrated prevention and treatment for HIV, tuberculosis, and sexually transmitted diseases in the homes of patients. The care combined medical treatment with social support, coordinated by the community workers who link the villages, the families, and the clinic. The use of home-delivered persuasion by community members resulted in high levels of adherence to treatment regimens and undetectable viral load levels in 86 percent of a tested subsample of patients. The success of this approach contributed to a global shift in attitudes about HIV treatment in poor countries in the 1990s.

Summary on Persuasion

This chapter has shown the importance of using persuasion to change behavior in the pharmaceutical sector in order to improve system performance. The relevant behaviors include how and where people seek treatment, how health professionals (and others) prescribe and dispense medicines, and the extent to which patients follow recommended regimens for taking their medicines. In short, persuading individuals to change their behavior is a central task that pharmaceutical reformers often confront.

The chapter also shows how efforts to change behavior through persuasion often require the use of other control knobs discussed in this book. For example, the payment control knob needs to be addressed when considering how prices affect consumer behavior, or how reimbursement rates or profit margins affect prescribing behavior. In examining how a change in rules (such as banning the sale of certain medicines at retail shops without a trained pharmacist) might be enforced, use of the regulation control knob and the challenges of enforcement are relevant.

Proposals to change behavior of specific groups can also raise political and ethical dilemmas. Efforts to change the behavior of physicians, for example, by separating prescribing from dispensing functions, often confront political opposition from the medical association as it seeks to protect the interests of its members. And plans to offer cash payments conditional on implementing certain home-based behaviors (for example, nutritional standards for infants) can raise ethical questions about whether certain levels of payment verge on coercion for very poor people and whether those kinds of pressures are ethically acceptable. In short, use of the persuasion control knob illustrates how issues raised at different points in this book interact and must be considered together in seeking to achieve improvements in the performance of the pharmaceutical sector.

Case Studies on Persuasion

Guyer, Anya Levy, and Michael R. Reich, "Changing the Use of Antibiotics in Peru." Case study H.

Guyer, Anya Levy, Michael R. Reich, Marc J. Roberts, and Pamela Norick. "Preparing for Microbicide Introduction in South Africa." Case study I.

References

Angell, M. 2004. "Excess in the Pharmaceutical Industry." *Canadian Medical Association Journal* 171: 1451–53.

Beecher, H. K. 1955. "The Powerful Placebo." *Journal of the American Medical Association* 159: 1602–06.

Brieger, W. R., P. E. Osamor, K. K. Salami, O. Oladepo, and S. A. Otusanya. 2004. "Interactions between Patent Medicine Vendors and Customers in Urban and Rural Nigeria." *Health Policy and Planning* 19: 177–82.

Buss, D. M., ed. 2005. *The Handbook of Evolutionary Psychology*. Hoboken, NJ: John Wiley and Sons.

Chou, Y. J., W. C. Yip, C. H. Lee, N. Huang, Y. P. Sun, and H. J. Chang. 2003. "Impact of Separating Drug Prescribing and Dispensing on Provider Behaviour: Taiwan's Experience." *Health Policy and Planning* 18: 316–29.

Cohen, J., and P. Dupas. 2010. "Free Distribution or Cost-Sharing? Evidence from a Randomized Malaria Prevention Experiment." *Quarterly Journal of Economics* 75 (1): 1–45.

Goel, P., D. Ross-Degnan, P. Berman, and S. Soumerai. 1996. "Retail Pharmacies in Developing Countries: A Behavior and Intervention Framework." *Social Science and Medicine* 42: 1155–61.

Gordon, M. 2010. "Diagnosis in the AMFm." Presentation at the Fourth Meeting of the Case Management Working Group, July 6–7. Geneva: AMFm. http://www.rbm.who.int/partnership/wg/wg_management/ppt/4cmwg/20MGordon.pdf. Accessed March 4, 2011.

Hadiyono, J. E. P., S. Suryawati, S. S. Danu, Sunartono, and B. Santoso. 1996. "Interactional Group Discussion: Results of a Controlled Trial Using a Behavioral Intervention to Reduce the Use of Injections in Public Health Facilities." *Social Science and Medicine* 42: 1177–83.

Hamm, R. M., R. J. Hicks, and D. A. Bemben. 1996. "Antibiotics and Respiratory Infections: Are Patients More Satisfied When Expectations Are Met?" *Journal of Family Practice* 43: 56–62.

Hauser, M. 2006. *Moral Minds: How Nature Designed Our Universal Sense of Right and Wrong*. New York: HarperCollins.

Hodgkin, C., D. H. Molyneaux, A. Abiose, B. Philippon, M. R. Reich, J. H. Remme, B. Thylefors, M. Traore, and K. Grepin. 2007. "The Future of Onchocerciasis Control in Africa." *PLoS Neglected Tropical Diseases* 1 (1): e74. doi:10.1371/journal.pntd.0000074.

Koenig, S. P., F. Léandre, and P. E. Farmer. 2004. "Scaling-Up HIV Treatment Programmes in Resource-Limited Settings: The Rural Haiti Experience." *AIDS* 18: S21–S25.

Lamptey, P. R., and J. E. Press. 1998. "Social Marketing Sexually Transmitted Disease and HIV Prevention: A Consumer-Centered Approach to Achieving Behaviour Change." *AIDS* 12 (Suppl 2): S1–9.

Müller-Riemenschneider, F., A. Bockelbrink, T. Reinhold, A. Rasch, W. Greiner, and S. N. Willich. 2008. "Long-Term Effectiveness of Behavioural Interventions to Prevent Smoking among Children and Youth." *Tobacco Control* 17: 301–12.

NHTSA (U.S. National Highway Traffic Safety Administration). "What Is a Designated Driver Program?" http://icsw.nhtsa.gov/people/injury/alcohol/DesignatedDriver/intro1.html. Accessed February 26, 2011.

Nizami, S. Q., I. A. Khan, and Z. A. Bhutta. 1996. "Drug Prescribing Practices of General Practitioners and Paediatricians for Childhood Diarrhoea in Karachi, Pakistan." *Social Science and Medicine* 42: 1133–39.

Sabaté, E., ed. 2003. *Adherence to Long-Term Therapies: Evidence for Action.* Geneva: World Health Organization.

Simon, H. A. 1956. *Models of Man.* New York: John Wiley.

Smith, W. A. 2006. "Social Marketing: An Overview of Approach and Effects." *Injury Prevention* 12: i38–i43.

Soumerai, S. B., and J. Avorn. 1990. "Principles of Educational Outreach ('Academic Detailing') to Improve Clinical Decision Making." *JAMA* 263: 549–56.

Suryawati, S., and B. Santoso. 1997. "Self-Learning for Self-Medication: An Alternative to Improve the Rational Use of OTCs." Paper Presented at ICIUM Conference, Chang Mai, Thailand, April.

Trostle, J. 1996. "Inappropriate Distribution of Medicines by Professionals in Developing Countries." *Social Science and Medicine* 42: 1117–20.

USGAO (U.S. General Accounting Office). 1991. *Drug Abuse Prevention: Federal Efforts to Identify Exemplary Programs Need Stronger Design.* GAO/PEMD-91-15, p. 44. Washington, DC: USGAO.

Walsh, D. C., R. E. Rudd, B. A. Moeykens, and T. W. Moloney. 1993. "Social Marketing for Public Health." *Health Affairs* 12: 104–19.

WHO (World Health Organization). 2011. "World Health Day – 7 April 2011." http://www.who.int/world-health-day/2011/en/index.html. Accessed February 27, 2011.

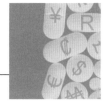

CHAPTER 12

Conclusions

Reforming the pharmaceutical sector is usually a difficult and demanding task. But we believe it is a task well worth doing. As we argued in chapter 1, modern medicines have great potential to improve the health status of millions of people around the world. The problem in many countries is that the complex set of institutions that make up the pharmaceutical sector do not do a particularly good job of getting the right medicines to the right people in a way that does not impose substantial financial burdens on them.

Thinking about Pharmaceutical Systems

Pharmaceutical systems are overlapping and intersecting mixtures of public and private production and purchasing, extensive government regulatory activities, a multiplicity of widely dispersed supply chains, complicated international and domestic markets, strong cultural patterns among consumers, and a bewildering array of bilateral and multilateral donors. Add in international nongovernmental organizations, faith-based health care systems, civil society organizations, professional associations, and training institutions, and the complexity can be overwhelming.

Moreover, within this complexity different players have different goals and interests. Private sector businesses focus mainly on profit—but typically compete with each other, so that more profit for some means less profit for others. Public agencies have social missions, but they also often compete—for funding, authority and political support. Even the donors have their own particular concerns and troubles—serving the visions of their governing boards or responding to the priorities of their sponsoring national governments.

The individuals in all these organizations (both public and private) also worry about their own economic and career interests. Many of them may be committed to certain social goals—such as providing buyers access to medicines or promoting the nation's purchasing rules for the public sector. But they can face great temptation and frustration in pursuing those ends. And those temptations and frustrations can lead to behavior that makes it less likely that the right medicines will in fact get to (and in turn get into) those who will most benefit from them.

Those who are sick—and their families—want their government to ensure their access to the medicines that will alleviate those illnesses. Moreover, they want access without major financial burdens. Of course, those would-be consumers care about the quality and price of what is offered in the marketplace. But given their beliefs and circumstances, they may not be enthusiastic about efforts to change their behavior to comply with what some technocrat defines as "rational use."

Despite this daunting complexity, we firmly believe that the performance of a nation's pharmaceutical system can be improved by well-designed and effectively implemented public policy. Designing a good reform package requires both disciplined thinking and a deep understanding of the particular system being reformed. That is why we have stressed the value of using the Flagship Framework as a method for developing effective reform ideas—even as we have also stressed the essential role that local knowledge must play in the process.

Before reviewing what the framework teaches, we remind readers of a sobering point. We understand that producing a good reform is very difficult. That may discourage many from attempting such an effort. However, failure to engage in reform will only perpetuate poor performance, with all the potentially avoidable suffering that implies.

Steps in the Process

- *Clarify your goals.* As you embark on the process of reform, remember that the pharmaceutical system is a means to various ends and that those ends can conflict. That is why reformers need to begin by clarifying their goals. They need to identify how the performance of the system is deficient and which of those deficiencies to choose as priorities for improvement. Is it health status, or financial protection, or citizen satisfaction that is animating the reform process? And which aspects of those goals, and for which groups, will you select as the test for indicating a successful reform? Moreover, we urge you to be self-reflective about the role that political realities and ethical concerns play in your thinking and your choices.

- *Carry out an honest diagnosis.* Once key performance problems have been identified, go on a "diagnostic journey." As Ishikawa advises, "Ask why five times." Do a careful diagnostic tree and explore the causes of poor performance, and the causes of those causes, until you have laid out the functioning of the system. Be evidence based, and as we said, ask, don't assume. Defend yourself against all the "policy advocates" who are going to tell you what you should do without a deep understanding of your country's situation, by developing such an understanding yourself.

- *Develop a plan that can work in your national context.* Countries vary in size, epidemiology, levels of social cohesion and economic development, administrative competence, the sophistication of their private pharmaceutical sectors, and the population density in rural areas. Reforms need to be designed in a way that reflects that context. How many pharmacists do you have? How reliable is cell phone coverage? Will public sector workers show up regularly? Are district administrative structures relatively competent? Because the devil is in the details, when it comes to reform, picking a broad approach is the beginning, not the end, of the policy design process, and those details (as well as the broad strategy) need to be chosen in a context-sensitive manner.

- *Embrace politics.* We have argued repeatedly that pharmaceutical sector reform is necessarily and appropriately a political process. For believers in democracy, the only legitimate way to settle the value questions inherent in any reform effort is through an appropriate political process. Even in contexts without competitive elections, political processes within bureaucracies will determine whether reformers' ideas are accepted and implemented. That means that reformers need political skills and must be willing to act politically. Those who want to produce real institutional change need to perform a stakeholder analysis and develop an explicit political strategy. And remember, the time to think about the politics of a reform is while that plan is being developed. Moreover, how a plan is developed (and especially how key stakeholders are involved) will significantly influence its political prospects.

- *Focus on implementation.* It is no use having a great plan if the plan cannot be implemented effectively. Again, the time to start worrying about implementation, like the time to start worrying about politics, is in the design phase. That is one reason why worrying about the details is so important. But plan design is not the only set of variables affecting implementation. Political leadership, competent agency management, and sufficient resources are also key. And notice that management and resources are likely to depend in part on leadership. We cannot stress too strongly that agencies carrying out both service delivery and regulatory functions need to be designed, organized, and managed with attention to the six keys to organizational effectiveness. Technological solutions and sophisticated processes are not self-implementing. Any reform ultimately depends on the behavior of frontline workers. And their behavior, and hence successful implementation, depends critically on the quality of the managers who are entrusted with making the reform a reality.

- *Learn from your mistakes.* The complexity of the pharmaceutical system that we sketched at the beginning of this chapter suggests that reforms will rarely turn out exactly as their designers anticipated. Many of the actors in the sector will defend their own interests, acting and reacting in unanticipated ways. That has two implications. First, it is necessary to put in place a serious and honest evaluation mechanism. Too often evaluations are designed to justify government action or to shield it from scrutiny. But true transparency requires just the opposite. Moreover, how can one learn from mistakes if no process is in place for learning what they are? Second, reformers should be prepared to fail, at least partially. That is, they should expect to find that performance on some goals is not up to expectations and that further reforms and adjustments are required. That is the somewhat world-weary implication of the fact that health sector reform is a cycle; and indeed, as we all know, today's solutions are the source of tomorrow's problems.

Final Thoughts

Finally, why is the work of pharmaceutical reform potentially so challenging, so rewarding, and so important? We argued at the beginning of this book that pharmaceuticals can make a genuinely important contribution to the well-being of citizens. So those who work to improve the functioning of the sector are doing genuinely important work. Second, providing effective access to medicines to those who are most vulnerable is, in terms of our own ethics, an especially urgent and praiseworthy task. The distribution of well-being and opportunity in the world is noticeably unequal. And we believe that those of us (like the writers and readers of this book) who do relatively well in terms of that distribution should consider seriously what they can do to improve the lot of our fellow human beings who suffer from real deprivation. Third, for all of its difficulty and frustration, pharmaceutical sector reform is an arena that can offer great personal satisfaction. It is work in which intelligence, passion, imagination, and critical thinking can all make a real difference. Doing this work requires an appreciation of many aspects of a very complex system—from politics and economics, to social and cultural beliefs, to biological processes, organizational dynamics, and philosophical commitments. It offers opportunities for leadership and craftsmanship, for learning and creating in the process of doing work that is truly worth doing. And that cannot be said of all forms of work in the world.

Unfortunately, we cannot offer a simple, cookie-cutter solution to the political, ethical, and practical dilemmas that reformers will confront. Nor do we have a single formula for how to adjust the control knobs to achieve the greatest improvements in pharmaceutical sector performance. We do believe, however, that explicit discussion of the problems and public deliberation about the issues involved can assist reformers in reaching good decisions, as well as satisfying the conditions for democratic accountability.

Ultimately, reformers need experience and practice in using the control knobs, and that is why we have included the cases in the book. Stories are an important mechanism for capturing and conveying knowledge, and we hope readers may be moved to reread some of them as they go forward with their reform efforts. But studying any book on how to do reform—even this one—can only take you so far. In the end, the question is, How can you apply these ideas in practice, in your particular social, economic, and political context? On that score, we hope that our advice and ideas are helpful. We wish you courage and good luck on your path to reform and improved performance and equity in the pharmaceutical sector.

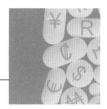

Defining an Essential Medicines List in Sudamerica

Questions to Consider while Reading This Case

This case relates to issues of ethical analysis presented in chapter 4.

- To what extent should decisions on an essential medicines list (EML) be guided by "objective utilitarian" concerns of cost effectiveness and need, as opposed to a "subjective utilitarian" policy of giving people what they want? How would these alternatives affect decisions in Sudamerica?

- In considerations of potential gains, should all citizens count equally, or is it more important to follow "egalitarian liberal" principles and give priority to improving the well-being of the poor and marginalized? If the latter, how would that influence EML decisions?

- What should a country spend on "rescue" cases, in which medicines are very expensive but are the only alternative for an otherwise fatal disease?

- What role should traditional cultural ideas play in the decisions?

- How is the minister doing from the point of view of "accountability for reasonableness"? What else should she do once a decision has been reached on the new list?

This case was prepared by Anya Levy Guyer and Marc J. Roberts. It is intended as a basis for class discussion rather than as an illustration of either effective or ineffective handling of an administrative situation.

Introduction

The minister of health of the fictional Sudamerica, Susana Medina, M.D., sat back and pondered the article she had just read. A former classmate from her time studying in the United States had e-mailed her an article from the *Boston Globe* about a child in Costa Rica who had Gaucher's disease, a rare and fatal condition that can only be controlled with indefinite treatment using a newly developed and extraordinarily expensive biotechnology medicine (Heuser 2009). The article explained how, with help from the manufacturer, Genzyme, the girl's parents were suing the Costa Rican government under the human rights provisions of that country's constitution to provide the treatment.

The minister felt only limited sympathy for her counterparts in Costa Rica. Theirs was a smaller, more homogeneous, and richer country than Sudamerica. She had to deal with a large, mountainous country, balancing the needs of often-isolated indigenous populations in the backcountry who felt, and in fact often had been, exploited by the urbanites of European descent living in the major cities. Despite serious efforts by recent progressive governments, including the one in which Dr. Medina served, the indigenous groups still lagged well behind their urban counterparts on most social, economic, and health indicators.

Inasmuch as Genzyme was looking for other countries to pressure into buying its treatments, she realized, Sudamerica might be next, especially because the nation's constitution contained human rights language similar to that of Costa Rica's. Dr. Medina worried that such claims might divert funds from the ministry's efforts to improve services in rural areas, including significant outlays for new "hardship location" bonuses for medical staff serving in remote regions. The best way to deal with such issues, she decided, was a systematic and rational discussion—in advance of any actual challenge—of which drugs government programs would cover. Then any denials could be put in the context of, and defended by reference to, that process.

With a sigh the minister picked up her mobile phone and dialed the head of the Pharmaceuticals and Consumables Division (PCD) of the ministry. When he answered, she said, "I just read an article about Genzyme's efforts in Costa Rica. I think it's time to update the essential medicines list." The minister knew that the public system only provided about 30 percent of the country's drug supply and that the EML was not used to restrict private sector production and imports. But that 30 percent was especially important to lower-income groups and rural residents.

Essential Medicines Lists

"Essential medicines" are defined by the World Health Organization (WHO) as "those that satisfy the priority health care needs of the population." The responsible health authorities have to define "satisfy," "priority," and "needs," based on local conditions and values. An essential medicines list is a way to operationalize these ideas. The responsible agency compiles a list of medicines—organized by therapeutic category, together with formulations, dosages, and uses for each—that it believes should be available to the population.

WHO argues that an essential medicines list should reflect both the most prevalent diseases and the most cost-effective drugs. It periodically updates a global "Model List" that is intended to serve as a guide for the development of national and institutional lists. An EML can be used in various ways. Governments can use it to determine which medicines to stock in public clinics and hospitals. In countries with a social health insurance system, the list can be used to guide decisions on which medicines the plan will cover. It can also be applied to aspects of the private sector—for example, through decisions on which medicines to register in a country.

Updating the National Essential Medicines List

Five months later, the minister, the PCD chief, a representative from the regional WHO office, and the other members of the Essential Medicines List (EML) Review Committee sat around three sides of a square conference table. On the fourth side, facing the table, were many rows of chairs in which sat about 50 people. At the back of the room were two television cameras and a cluster of newspaper and radio reporters. This was a public hearing on updating the national EML.

The update process had already gone through two phases: First, some technical staff from the PCD and other committee members and consultants had met to review the existing EML by comparing it with the lists of other countries in the same socioeconomic situation and with the WHO Model List. The existing list had not been revised in some years, and the drugs on it were primarily standard, generic forms of single compounds used to treat common infectious diseases. It also included some treatments for chronic diseases, such as insulin, simple statins as anticholesterol drugs, and basic antihypertensives such as diuretics.

The committee had received quite a number of proposals from medical, industrial, and civil society interest groups to add other kinds of medicines to the list. The main options under debate included the following:

- Newer treatments for cardiovascular diseases and diabetes (including advanced antihypertensives such as angiotensin receptor blockers and artificial insulin)

- Chemotherapy for cancers common in Sudamerica

- Antiretrovirals for the treatment of HIV/AIDS and the prevention of vertical transmission from mother to infant

- Second-line treatments for antibiotic-resistant infectious diseases, including tuberculosis

- Fixed-dose artemisinin-based combination antimalarials

- Various injectable and implantable contraceptives, as well as intrauterine devices and barrier methods for family planning, and misoprostol for emergency obstetric care

- Children's formulations of antibiotics and antimalarials

- Psychotherapeutic medicines for major depressive and psychotic disorders

- Antivirals for pandemic flu

- Prolonged-release morphine for palliative care

- Various herbal tonics popular among traditional communities.

An analysis by the ministry's economists indicated that if all of these were approved and provided to all citizens who needed them through the national public health system, public drug costs would triple, and the proportion of the national health budget allocated to pharmaceutical products would increase from 14 percent to more than 40 percent. Obviously, that was not feasible.

The next step in the process had been an outreach campaign to invite public comment. In addition to publishing various proposals on the ministry's website and arranging for public service announcements on the radio, the ministry had reached out to civil society groups representing a cross-section of Sudamerica's population. It had run policy analysis workshops with groups that were less familiar with the issues, so that they could participate effectively in the process. Written responses had been solicited, and now the public was invited to participate in this hearing.

(The minister had faced criticism in the opposition press for the workshop activities, which were described by her detractors as "biased" and "encouraging class divisions." She had defended herself by replying scathingly to a television interviewer that, given the elaborate submissions they had produced, the professional and corporate organizations clearly needed no aid from the government in getting across their views.)

The Public Hearing

The variety of people who had actually come to speak at this hearing reflected the ministry's efforts. They included self-confident medical school professors, representatives of patient groups, and some executives from the pharmaceutical industry. Also present were a cluster of Catholic priests, community organizers in jeans and knit shirts, several people in wheelchairs, and a couple of families wearing pins with the faces of relatives in the center, surrounded by their birth and death dates. Some people were wearing suits, others were in traditional dress, and some looked as if they had just gotten off the bus from the interior and had tried to smooth their wrinkled clothes in the building's restrooms.

Each speaker was given three minutes to make a statement to the committee. The committee would then sort through the proposals to decide on a feasible and affordable EML.

Selected Statements from the Hearing

- Director of a provincial government hospital: "Treatments for the most common conditions that bring people to my hospital are the ones that should be included on the list. Our pediatric ward is full of children with pneumonias, gastrointestinal conditions, and malaria. Our adult wards are mostly populated by people with advanced heart disease and diabetes, as well as complications from malaria. We need safe and effective treatments for these to be available in our pharmacy all the time in order to serve the greatest number of people. They understand when we tell them, 'That is a rare disease; we can do nothing about it.' But when we say, 'You have malaria, but you are resistant to the only drug we can provide—go out and buy a more expensive one,' then they are frustrated. It is getting to the point where people in the community are thinking of the government hospital as a place to go to die."

- Women's association representative: "The entire list of products for family planning and women's reproductive health must be included in the EML. For too long the pervasive gender bias in this country has meant that medicines that are only relevant to women have been left off of the list. But this is not just a problem for women. Poor health prevents women from fully contributing to our country's development. Nearly 75 percent of women between the ages of 18 and 49 are employed in the formal or informal sectors. And women and girls of all ages carry out significant unpaid labor in the home and in the community. Now that we have a woman minister, we ask you to take the lead on this and see that women's rights are recognized and protected by the national health system."

- Father of a child who died of leukemia: "From the time my daughter fell sick, at age 13, until she died two years later, we begged for help. We called on our parliamentary delegate, and though it took months to arrange, he got us in to see some of the country's best doctors here in the capital. 'They are good doctors,' he told us, 'trained in America and Europe. They know the latest in medical science.' Yet when they told us the cost of the only medicines that might help her, there was nothing we could do. A course of treatment would have been more than I, my wife, and both of my brothers could earn in ten years. Now I have lost my daughter Carmella, who was so smart and so beautiful and so motivated. Minister, with all due respect, she used to joke that she hoped you did not become president because she wanted to be the first woman president of our country. I am sorry to get so upset, but my daughter had a right to be treated, to try to live, and she was denied that. We say we are a country that respects human rights. Well, if we do, we need to give priority to treating the Carmellas among us. What is most hard for me is that I know that if I were a rich landowner, she might be with us here today. Sudamerica failed me and I failed her."

- Catholic priest: "This is a Catholic country and our policies should reflect our values, not enable the use of dangerous substances that can be used to destroy holy life. For example, you should not put misoprostol on this EML. There are other ways to save the life of a woman hemorrhaging during childbirth. But this misoprostol is a dangerous drug. It is widely used illegally to induce abortions. Likewise, in many places we know that morphine is used to hasten the deaths of people who are dying. We cannot spend our national budget on something that can be used to kill the unborn or our elders before their appointed times. Our budget should be spent to *save* our citizens—not interfere with God's will by preventing their conception. We should instead focus on prenatal and primary care, medicines for common diseases, and providing spiritual succor to those who suffer."

- Spokeswoman for the National Association of Sudamerica's Poor: "The poorest people in this country suffer the most from bad health and lack of access to medicine. The wealthy can buy what they want, but the EML must cover drugs for conditions that specifically affect poor people, especially treatments for diarrheal diseases, respiratory infections, and tuberculosis, as well as vitamins and dietary supplements. Rich people go to private pharmacies when they are ill, but when we poor people get sick we have to choose between feeding our children their one meal a day and buying some drugs at the public hospital. Even when we are not sick, we cannot afford to feed our children a healthy diet. We live in shacks without running water—who can afford meat or fresh vegetables? How can the ministry of health justify spending money on fancy medicines that make money for international companies when these poor children don't get enough vitamins and minerals to grow properly? And how can you refuse to supply the inexpensive tonics that so many of us rely on, just because doctors look down their noses at the treatments we here have known about and used for a thousand years?"

- CEO of a local generic pharmaceutical company: "This EML is not just a medical issue—it's also an economic one. Only drugs that are proven to be cost-effective and are available in affordable generic formulations should be on the EML. That would promote our national economic well-being. Putting patented, expensive drugs on the EML means that too much of our national budget for medicines would be sent out of the country to multinational pharmaceutical corporations. In contrast, we in the local generics industry employ many people and provide reliable, affordable products that save many lives. We understand that the ministry may want to list a few imported drugs for which there is no alternative. But that should only be done when those compounds would have a significant effect in reducing the burden of disease among the productive members of society."

- Professor of cardiology at the national university: "I am here to speak on behalf of my colleagues in the Department of Medicine at the university. We feel that the whole concept of the essential medicines list needs to be rethought, at least in the context of our institution. Yes, we are a government hospital. But at the same time, we on the faculty are the best trained and most experienced doctors in the nation. You know that yourself, Dr. Medina, from your days there as our student (and a very good student you were, I might add). If we are to keep the best-of-the-best practicing here in Sudamerica they have to be free to use their knowledge and judgment to provide the best care to their patients. The only antihypertensives now on the EML are outdated diuretics. Yes, they are off-patent and very inexpensive; and yes, they show up well in clinical trials. And some say you should only add the so-called statins that are about to come off patent. But trials only capture average effects. What is the point of all my training and experience if I cannot prescribe the most modern treatments like Beta blockers, ACE (angiotensin-converting enzyme) inhibitors, and now angiotensin receptor blockers, when in my clinical judgment they are best for a particular patient? My colleagues in other departments feel the same. Either the teaching hospital should be exempt from the rules, or the rules should be changed."

- Economist from the finance ministry: "These decisions are very difficult, I know. But all of us in government have to consider our country's limited resources. The only responsible way to do this is to do it scientifically: to use cost-effectiveness analysis. You need to set a cut-off level in terms of Quality Adjusted Life Years per unit of money spent, the way they do for the National Institute for Health and Clinical Excellence in the United Kingdom. Then the ministry should only approve treatments that have objective clinical evidence to prove they are above that line. Anything else will open up the process to endless lobbying for special treatment, and charges of favoritism from those who lose out. On the other hand, a clear rule can be explained and defended to everyone in the society exactly because it is based on sound science."

The hearing continued for several hours, and for the most part, the committee was reasonably attentive to the witnesses throughout. The TV crews packed up and left after a few of the early star witnesses had spoken. Print reporters stayed longer, trying to get interviews with civic group representatives after they had made their statements. The next day the committee and its consultants met again in the conference room to review and discuss the views presented and to begin the process of actually deciding on changes to the essential medicines list.

Reference

Heuser, Stephen. 2009. "One Girl's Hope, A Nation's Dilemma." *Boston Globe*, June 14, A1.

Reflections on the Sudamerica Case

As the testimony at the hearing makes clear, setting priorities for medicines spending is a genuinely difficult problem. Because resources are limited, there are typically more plausible claimants and advocates than available funding can accommodate. Moreover, the claimants invoke conflicting philosophical positions. The ministry of finance pushes for the kind of cost-effectiveness favored by objective utilitarians. The Catholic priest speaks for his particular communitarian vision. And some have mixed positions—the advocate for the poor supports using cost-effectiveness criteria but also defends the subjective utilitarian goal of responding to what the people want.

Nor is what everyone says to be taken at face value. Even those with obvious economic interests (the domestic pharmaceutical manufacturers) or organizational interests (the professor) feel it necessary to cloak their self-interest in justifications with more general appeal. That Genzyme is using constitutional rights provisions to advance its sales of a very expensive compound is a similar example. And it would not be unusual in many countries for the professor arguing for "the best"—and newest and most expensive—medicines to be supported in various ways by the manufacturers of those medicines.

The decision is made more difficult by the strong emotions involved. It is very difficult for governments to refuse to fund care for those with fatal diseases—to violate the "rule of rescue." But the minister is aware of the ethical arguments on the other side as well. For example, increasing such "rescue" spending will divert funds from programs that protect other, less obviously identifiable citizens (in this case, bonuses to persuade more staff to work in rural areas).

At the end of the day, the minister (and readers of this book who are involved in such decisions) would be well-advised to try to think through their own philosophic commitments in order to make such decisions coherently and defensibly. At the end of chapter 5, we offered one possible stance: maximizing health status gains (which means using cost-effectiveness analysis) but balancing that against equity considerations. The professor (and the international pharmaceutical companies), the priest, and the father of the dead girl would be the ones most unhappy with such an approach. And given their political resources, the minister had best get the politics of this right if she is to have the needed support. She has done pretty well, so far, in using an approach based on "accountability for reasonableness," but the report of the committee is going to need extensive explanation and justification. And rather than leaving that to chance, the minister would be well-advised to facilitate some expressions of support from key constituency groups along the way.

CASE STUDY B

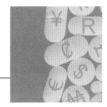

Registering Misoprostol in Sri Lanka

Questions to Consider while Reading This Case

This case relates to issues of ethical analysis for pharmaceutical policy, as presented in chapter 4.

- How would various utilitarians, liberals, and communitarians view this issue? In particular, who would line up for and against the registration of misoprostol?

- Consider the patriotic, nationalistic, and anti-Western rhetoric of the current government in Sri Lanka—where does that fit in the ethical framework we discussed?

- Suppose you wanted to make a human rights argument in Sri Lanka for registering misoprostol. How might you frame such a point of view so that it would have the best chance of public and political acceptance?

Misoprostol is a member of the class of drugs called *prostaglandins*. It was developed by G. D. Searle (now part of Pfizer) and first approved for use in the United States in 1988 under the trade name Cytotec. It was used initially to fight medication-induced gastric ulcers that developed in patients

This case was prepared by Ramya Kumar and Michael R. Reich. It is intended as a basis for class discussion rather than to illustrate either effective or ineffective handling of an administrative situation.

using certain pain medications. The medicine was soon shown to have other properties, and it became widely used globally for evacuation of the uterus after pregnancy failure and for induction of labor. It is also used on its own and in combination with mifepristone (known in the United States as RU-487) to induce abortion.

Misoprostol is also widely used for postpartum hemorrhage (PPH), in countries where emergency obstetric care is not readily accessible, because it is now off patent and inexpensive, stable at room temperature, and easy to administer. In situations where other alternatives (such as oxytocin) are available for treatment of PPH, the World Health Organization (WHO) does not recommend the use of misoprostol (WHO 2009b). In 2005, misoprostol was included in the WHO Essential Medicines List for the induction of labor and in combination with mifepristone for medical abortion (WHO 2006). The listing of the combined preparation includes the addendum, "where permitted by national law and where culturally acceptable." The Expert Committee on the Selection and Use of Essential Medicines at WHO expanded its recommendation for the use of misoprostol to include incomplete abortion in 2009 (WHO 2009a).

Introduction: Sri Lanka

Sri Lanka is a roughly oval-shaped island in the Indian Ocean, off the southeastern coast of India. It is a lower-middle-income country with a population of approximately 20 million. The Sinhalese make up about three-fourths of the population, and a significant proportion of the minorities are Tamils (Lankan and Indian Tamils) and Muslims[1]. The majority of the Sinhalese are Buddhists, and the Tamils Hindu. A relatively small Christian population is made up of both Sinhalese and Tamils and is mostly Roman Catholic (6 percent).

The island was colonized first by the Portuguese in the early 16th century, then by the Dutch in the mid-17th century, and finally by the British in the early 19th century. It became independent in 1948, continuing to use its British name, Ceylon. In the 1960s, under the leadership of Sirimavo Bandaranaike, the world's first woman prime minister, the country became a leader in the nonaligned movement and embarked on an economic strategy based on greater state involvement in the economy, together with the expansion of social welfare. In the late 1970s, the country adopted economic liberalization and a more pro-Western foreign policy. It also took a new name, Sri Lanka, in 1972 and is now officially known as the Democratic Socialist Republic of Sri Lanka. The constitution guarantees the right to equality and the right to freedom from torture but contains no explicit provision guaranteeing a right to life or a right to health.

In May 2009, the government led by President Mahinda Rajapaksa defeated the Liberation Tigers of Tamil Eelam (LTTE), ending the civil war that had ravaged the country for 30 years. The president had come to power five years earlier on a platform of negotiating with the LTTE, but over time his government increasingly pursued a military solution. The conflict arose from the response of the Tamil minority to its marginalization by the Sri Lankan state since the 1950s.

After the war, critics of the government's conduct raised allegations of war crimes, especially in the last phase, when civilians and LTTE rebels were crowded together in an ever-smaller enclave. In June 2010, United Nations Secretary General Ban Ki-Moon appointed a panel of experts to advise him on accountability for alleged violations of international human rights and humanitarian law during the final stages of the conflict.

Those allegations have not been well received by the government and its allies. Interventions by the international community toward the end of the war (directed at aiding civilians in the LTTE enclave) were perceived by many allied with the government as aiding the LTTE. That view of international intervention also grew out of the failure of the peace process facilitated by Norway in 2002. Within Sri Lanka, the international community, including foreign-funded nongovernmental organizations (NGOs), especially those with a human rights (or women's rights) agenda, came to be viewed with suspicion. The government has sought to consolidate its power by promoting Sinhala-Buddhist nationalism. It has also faced allegations that it is using repressive tactics to control the news media and other public institutions. In November 2010, Mahinda Rajapaksa began his second term as president after winning 58 percent of the vote in elections held in January of that year.

Maternal Health in Sri Lanka

Sri Lanka is often cited, along with Costa Rica and the State of Kerala in India, as an example of a poor country that has made remarkable progress in health at low cost. In 2008, 4 percent of gross domestic product was spent on health (WHO 2011), and many national health indicators are very positive.

Sri Lanka has also made impressive achievements in maternal health. The country is on target to achieve the Fifth Millennium Development Goal of improving maternal health by 2015. The maternal mortality ratio (MMR) was 39 per 100,000 live births in 2008, the lowest in the South Asian region

(WHO 2011). The percentage of births attended by skilled health personnel and the proportion of births delivered at a health facility were both exceptionally high, at 98 percent in Demographic and Health Survey for 2006–07 (Sri Lanka 2008), although the survey excluded five districts in the Northern Province that were severely afflicted by the civil war. The figures are national averages, however, and some poor districts did not do as well. For example, in 2003 the proportion of home deliveries in Mannar district in the Northern Province was estimated to be 38 percent, when the national average was 4 percent (Ministry of Healthcare and Nutrition 2007). Similarly in 2005, when the national average was 44, the MMR in Moneragala district in Uva Province was 128 per 100,000 live births (Family Health Bureau and UNICEF 2009).

The advances in maternal health in the first half of the 20th century in Sri Lanka have been attributed to, among other factors, provision of free health services, expansion of health facilities, and the improved social status of women. More recently, the expansion of emergency obstetric care services (including blood transfusion facilities, an effective health referral system, and the establishment of a functioning maternal death surveillance system) has been identified as contributing to further reductions (Family Health Bureau and UNICEF 2009).

Abortion Laws and Abortion in Sri Lanka

Sri Lanka's Penal Code was enacted in 1883 and has undergone little change since. Abortion is only permitted to save a woman's life. An attempt was made to liberalize the law in 1995, when a series of amendments to the Penal Code were proposed. Paragraph 3 of the proposed amendments would have permitted abortion in cases of rape, incest, and gross congenital abnormalities. Parliament passed all the proposed amendments to the Penal Code with the exception of that paragraph.

Opposition to paragraph 3 came in part from members of the parliament (MPs) who questioned the amendment from Catholic and Islamic perspectives (Government of Sri Lanka 1995). One MP stated that "any attempt to legalize abortion or liberalize the existing laws on abortion ... will be strongly opposed by all sections of society" and that doing so would "affect the fundamentals of the social life and the cultural life of the people of this country." The MP added that Christians, Buddhists, Muslims, and Hindus all believe in "the supremacy of life." Other MPs voiced concern that liberalizing the law would result in an increase in "promiscuity" among women. No further attempts to liberalize abortion law have been made since 1995.

The 1995 legal developments occurred even as unsafe abortions were a leading cause of maternal death in the country (following postpartum hemorrhage, pregnancy-induced hypertension, and heart disease). Admittedly, Sri Lanka has achieved a commendable MMR, but unsafe abortion is still responsible for about 15 to 20 such deaths (out of about 150 maternal deaths) every year.

These deaths occur in part because unsafe abortion is in fact quite common in Sri Lanka, where about 500 to 750 abortions are thought to occur every day. A study supported by the United Nations Population Fund (UNFPA) in the late 1990s estimated the abortion rate to be as high as 45 abortions per 1,000 women of reproductive age, and even higher among married women living in rural areas (Rajapaksa 2002). A more recent study of women seeking abortion found that over 50 percent of the study sample desired an abortion to limit or space their family, reflecting the reality that abortion was widely used as a family planning method (Thalagala 2010).

Despite the illegal status of abortion, until recently abortion services were reasonably accessible in Sri Lanka. They were provided through a chain of clinics run by Marie Stopes International, an international NGO specializing in sexual and reproductive health care services. Such procedures were carried out under the heading of "menstrual regulation." Until 2007, the Sri Lanka government turned a blind eye on the clinics, which had operated in the country for more than 20 years. In that year, the government suddenly closed the clinics, making abortion much less accessible. The move was attributed by many to pressure from the Roman Catholic Church, especially from a global antiabortion organization that was thought to have approached the government through the first lady, Shiranthi Rajapaksa, a Roman Catholic. Her meeting with the group was reported in a Roman Catholic periodical published in Sri Lanka (Bastians 2007).

In 2010, the stance of the ministry of health on the problem of unsafe abortion was that Sri Lanka's restrictive laws precluded providing safe abortion services through the health system. Instead, the ministry developed projects focused on improving access to family planning services and post-abortion care.

Advocacy for Abortion Law Reform in Sri Lanka

The website of the Family Planning Association of Sri Lanka (FPASL) states that the association's aim is "to ensure the right of access to safe and legalized abortion and a decreased incidence of unsafe abortion" by raising awareness on unsafe abortion and advocating safe abortion services "under specific circumstances" (FPASL 2011). Its position has been to advocate amending the law to permit abortion in cases of rape, incest, and gross congenital abnormalities. FPASL has not made any public statements on misoprostol.

Other than a media campaign to generate public debate on abortion law reform, which was launched in 1999 by the Sri Lanka Women's NGO Forum, little organizing has taken place among women's groups around the abortion issue since 1995. Misoprostol registration was not on their agenda in 2010.

Physicians appear to be divided on the need for abortion law reform in Sri Lanka, although they agree that unsafe abortion is a public health issue. Policy makers are of the opinion that the support of the medical community would be crucial to advocating for reform.

National Pharmaceutical Policy in Sri Lanka

Sri Lanka has been called a "global pioneer" in progressive pharmaceutical policy (Reich 2005). The first national pharmaceutical policy was developed in 1970 to rationalize the sector by increasing government purchases of low-cost generic medicines, reducing the number of private products on the national market, and reducing the use of brand names. The State Pharmaceutical Corporation (SPC) was established in 1971 and controlled all drug imports by 1973. In 1977, reflecting the economic policy of the new regime, the private sector was allowed to import drugs, although the SPC continued to supply drugs to government hospitals.

Today, only drugs registered in the country may be legally imported. The government controls the registration of drugs through the Sri Lanka National Drug Regulation Authority (NDRA) of the Ministry of Health. The NDRA's activities are guided by the Cosmetics, Devices, and Drugs Act of 1980. Applications for registration are reviewed by the Drugs Evaluation Subcommittee. Its decision is forwarded to a Technical Advisory Committee, which advises the minister of health. The committee makes the final decision on registration and usually concurs with the decision of the subcommittee. Drugs on the WHO Essential Medicines List have generally been registered by the NDRA without controversy.

From a legal perspective, advocates of registering misoprostol believe that the provision in the current law that permits abortion to save the life of a woman could be used to justify such registration, to make it available for women who fall into that narrow category. The registration of misoprostol might also be justified on the basis of providing treatment for PPH in those limited areas of Sri Lanka where oxytocin is not readily available in public health clinics.

Availability of Misoprostol in Sri Lanka

In spite of its unregistered status, misoprostol (as well as mifepristone) is available and used in the private sector (and even in the government sector to a lesser degree). Two distinct supply chains operate.

First, misoprostol is apparently smuggled into Sri Lanka from India and Pakistan, where the drug is registered and easily available at affordable prices. The drug is not accessible over the counter in most pharmacies, but it is available by prescription when the prescriptions are written by doctors who have specific "relationships" with certain pharmacies. Smuggled drugs are also directly available from certain pharmacies, at exorbitant prices, especially in peripheral areas of the country where law enforcement is weak. A recent newspaper article reported that a combination regimen of mifepristone and misoprostol could be purchased in such locations for 10,000 Sri Lankan rupees (about US$100) (Mohamed 2010).

More often, misoprostol and mifepristone are supplied by pharmaceutical company representatives directly to consultant obstetricians and gynecologists who use the drugs in their private practices. In private clinics and hospitals, misoprostol is used to treat a number of conditions (including induced abortion), on its own or in combination with mifepristone. Misoprostol is less frequently used in government hospitals, and where used it is prescribed on patient records as "prostaglandins." In government institutions, misoprostol is typically used only for the treatment of "incomplete" and "missed" spontaneous abortions.

The ministry of health has not made any public statements about the need to register misoprostol in Sri Lanka, except to express concern about its unregistered use (Perera 2010). Given that misoprostol is unregulated in Sri Lanka, it is difficult to assess the safety of the products that are entering the country, and little is known about the quality of the products currently available to women.

Trying to Register Misoprostol

In 2010, an application to register misoprostol was submitted to the NDRA by a pharmaceutical company. The application was reviewed by the Drugs

Evaluation Subcommittee, and a decision was made to seek a recommendation from the Sri Lanka College of Obstetricians and Gynaecologists (SLCOG). Although the practice is not routine, such recommendations are sought when there is a conflict of opinion within the Drugs Evaluation Subcommittee. In November 2010, the SLCOG responded with a recommendation that misoprostol be registered but available only through the public sector.

One month later, in December 2010, the Drugs Evaluation Subcommittee met to review the application. The committee includes physicians with expertise in many different clinical areas, including obstetrics and gynecology, as well as different health professional groups. About half of the committee's members are women.

At the meeting, members disagreed regarding the registration of misoprostol. Some members were vehemently opposed, in spite of the recommendation from the Sri Lanka College of Obstetricians and Gynaecologists. (It is interesting to note that SLCOG supported the recommendation, even though some of its members are likely to lose financially if misoprostol is registered.) Eventually, the committee agreed to keep the decision pending. Such decisions do not progress to the Technical Advisory Committee and are unlikely to be reviewed.

Concerns raised by members of the Drugs Evaluation Subcommittee were focused on the possible side effects and complications of misoprostol use. The potential for widespread use of the drug for induced abortion was not discussed. Anecdotal cases in which misoprostol had been used for labor induction and resulted in two maternal deaths in the recent past appear to have played a large role in the decision. The debate appears to have been confined to the medical community and health ministry bureaucracy. Women's rights advocates and the pharmaceutical industry did not participate. (The pharmaceutical industry is represented at the Technical Advisory Committee but not on the Drugs Evaluation Subcommittee.)

Factors that May Have Influenced the Decision

It is difficult to know exactly what happened in the subcommittee because there is no public record of deliberations by subcommittees of the NDRA. Policy makers involved in the drug registration process, however, have conflicting opinions on why misoprostol was not registered. One possibility is that subcommittee members' focus on the complications of "inappropriate" use allowed them to avoid even considering the issue of abortion. However, other knowledgeable observers are of the opinion that the abortion issue silently influenced the decision.

A number of arguments against registering misoprostol exist in the medical community, and those may be sincerely held or may mask other agendas. Although some believe that the illegal status of abortion does not create a barrier to registration, some in the medical community apparently do believe that registering misoprostol itself would be unlawful. Others question the need to register misoprostol for treating PPH, given the high proportion of institutional births and the widespread availability of oxytocin in hospitals. They argue that the maternal deaths from PPH that occur are mostly the results of delays in receiving appropriate care in a hospital. Others contend that reductions of maternal mortality from unsafe abortion cannot be achieved by registering misoprostol, given that the illegal status of abortion will necessarily restrict its use.

The question also arises of whether the medical community has any real interest in making these drugs available to women on an outpatient basis. Cynics point out that access to such abortion medicines could weaken the monopoly that physicians presently have over providing abortion services, which are even more lucrative because they are illegal.

Why then was induced abortion not even discussed at the meeting of the Drugs Evaluation Subcommittee? Could cultural or social conservatism have influenced the members' decision? The possibility of greater sexual liberation, which these drugs could provide, may have been threatening in a conservative society that places great value on women's role as mothers within traditional family structures.

What Room Is there for Further Advocacy?

If advocates wanted to reopen the issue, how might that be done? Opponents are sure to argue no need exists for misoprostol to treat PPH or for induction of labor. But a demand for misoprostol clearly exists in Sri Lanka. Research has established that the country has high rates of abortion. Experience also shows that there is an active black market for misoprostol that is smuggled into the country or distributed by pharmaceutical representatives. In addition, obstetricians have expressed their limited support, in the form of a recommendation for registration and use in the public sector from the Sri Lanka College of Obstetricians and Gynaecologists.

It is possible that arguments for registering the drug could be framed around reducing harm and providing safer abortion services. But that would mean reopening the whole abortion issue. That might be done from a women's rights perspective. Sri Lanka is a signatory to the International Covenant on Economic, Social, and Cultural Rights and the Convention on the

Elimination of All Forms of Discrimination Against Women. But is there room for such discourse in Sri Lanka today?

The Family Planning Association of Sri Lanka has publicly advocated reintroducing the omitted paragraph 3 that would permit abortion in cases of rape, incest, and the presence of gross congenital abnormalities. But apart from that group's work, activism on the issue is quite limited, and not much public debate about the misoprostol decision has occurred. Indeed, some political observers claim that the climate in Sri Lanka today is not conducive to raising such issues. With the public promotion of patriotism and nationalism by the current regime, human rights (including women's rights) claims are increasingly looked on as "Western" and intrusive. And then there is the first lady's affiliation with the Roman Catholic Church.

Note

1. The 2001 Census was carried out completely in 18 of 25 districts; the remaining districts were partially enumerated or completed excluded from the census owing to the civil war. The people residing in those districts are primarily Tamil and Muslim, and therefore the results of the census are not truly reflective of the ethnic and religious breakdown of the population. Based on 1981 statistics, the ethnic breakdown of the population is as follows: Sinhalese, 74.0 percent; Sri Lankan Tamils, 12.7 percent; Indian Tamils, 5.5 percent; Muslims, 7.1 percent; Burghers, 0.3 percent; Malays (followers of Islam), 0.3 percent; and numerous other small groups, 0.2 percent. The breakdown on religion in the 1981 census was as follows: Buddhist 69.3 percent; Hindu 15.5 percent; Muslims 7.6 percent; Christians (including Roman Catholics) 7.4 percent.

Acknowledgment

This case includes material that was collected in direct interviews with policy makers in Sri Lanka during January 2011. The authors appreciate the cooperation of the people who were interviewed at that time.

References

Bastians, D. 2007. "The Uterus Wars. Inside an Abortionist's Lair." *The Nation* (Colombo), December 2.

Family Health Bureau and UNICEF (United Nations Children's Fund). 2009. *Overview of Maternal Mortality in Sri Lanka 2001–2005*. Colombo: Ministry of Healthcare and Nutrition.

FPASL (Family Planning Association of Sri Lanka). 2011. "Strategic Focus." http://www.fpasrilanka.org/strategic_focus.php. Accessed March 12, 2011.

Government of Sri Lanka. 1995. *Parliamentary Debates (Hansard)*. September 19, 89–128.

Ministry of Healthcare and Nutrition. 2007. *Medium Term Plan on Family Health 2007–2011*. Colombo: Family Health Bureau.

Mohamed, R. 2010. "The World's First Abortion Pill Gains a New Lease on Life in Sri Lanka." *Sunday Leader* (Ratmalana), October 31.

Perera, S. 2010, "Mifepristone and Misoprostol Sold on the Sly." *The Island* (Colombo), October 9.

Rajapaksa, L. C. 2002. "Estimates of Induced Abortions in Urban and Rural Sri Lanka." *Journal of the College of Community Physicians of Sri Lanka* 7: 10–16.

Reich, M. R. 2005. "The Politics of Health Reform in Developing Countries: Three Cases of Pharmaceutical Policy." *Health Policy* 32: 47–77.

Sri Lanka. Department of Census and Statistics and Ministry of Healthcare and Nutrition. 2008. *Demographic and Health Survey 2006/07. Preliminary Report (Draft)*. Department of Census and Statistics, Colombo. http://www.statistics.gov.lk/social/DHS%20Sri%20Lanka%20Preliminary%20Report.pdf. Accessed March 6, 2011.

Thalagala, N. 2010. *Process, Determinants, and Impact of Unsafe Abortions in Sri Lanka*. Colombo: Family Planning Association of Sri Lanka.

WHO (World Health Organization). 2006. "The Selection and Use of Essential Medicines, Report of the WHO Expert Committee, 2005." Geneva: WHO. http://whqlibdoc.who.int/trs/WHO_TRS_933_eng.pdf. Accessed on March 11, 2011.

———. 2009a. "WHO Model List of Essential Medicines 16th List." http://www.who.int/selection_medicines/committees/expert/17/sixteenth_adult_list_en.pdf. Accessed February 27, 2011.

———. 2009b. "WHO Statement Regarding the Use of Misoprostol for Postpartum Haemorrhage Prevention and Treatment." Statement WHO/RHR/09.22.

———. 2011. "Global Health Observatory." http://www.who.int/gho/en/. Accessed February 26, 2011.

Reflections on Sri Lanka

This case illustrates several important points about the ethical analysis of pharmaceutical policy decisions. First, no simple correspondence exists between the basic ethical viewpoints discussed in chapter 4 and policy decisions made in practice. Sometimes different ethical viewpoints can lead to the same policy conclusion. And sometimes people with the same viewpoint can reach different conclusions, based on small variations in interpretation or understanding.

In the case of registering misoprostol in Sri Lanka, most utilitarians and most liberals would support registration. For both objective and subjective utilitarians, the case is almost too obvious to warrant much discussion. Registration would increase satisfaction in a way that would please subjective utilitarians (as indicated by widespread illegal use). It would also improve health status (helping to decrease adverse outcomes), as valued by objective utilitarians.

Rights-based views would also favor registration. Libertarians who focus on negative rights and egalitarian liberals who endorse both negative and positive rights would both support registration. Not allowing individuals access to the drug infringes on the negative right of women to control their own bodies—which is valued by both sorts of liberals. In addition, egalitarian liberals would note that access to abortion services has been especially difficult for rural and poor women. Access to smuggled misoprostol would be similarly difficult for those women, as illegal supplies are typically available directly from physicians at private hospitals or from pharmacies with a prescription written by a physician. Egalitarian liberals would thus support registration because it would improve the well-being of those at the lower levels of the socioeconomic hierarchy, which is the main concern of egalitarian liberals.

The primary opposition comes from various groups of communitarians who see abortion as a moral wrong. Some are universal communitarians who believe that there is one (divinely revealed) correct way for all human beings to live and that they know what that is. Others are relative communitarians who believe that Sri Lanka can and should defend a moral vision based on its own particular history and culture. That vision is not universal, but it does apply to all members of the country's distinct society. The current government, with its connections to Sinhala Buddhist nationalism, fits in that camp.

But even within those groups, disagreements can exist. Some in the medical society appear to accept the objective utilitarian health maximization view. But then they seem to argue that in the particular Sri Lankan context, registering misoprostol is unnecessary and will do more harm than good. That illustrates the point that even among consequentialists who accept the same outcome metric, disagreements can still arise based on varied predictions and projections of the likely consequences of alternative actions.

Similarly, not all communitarians would accept the nonregistration position. Several schools of feminism can be understood as forms of universal communitarianism (not all universal communitarians agree on what constitutes virtue). And those supporters of feminist beliefs would surely favor registration.

Finally, how could misoprostol advocates formulate persuasive arguments in the Sri Lankan context? Trying to convince the most vocal universal communitarian opponents in parliament (including the Christian and Muslim MPs who opposed abortion law reform in 1995) is not likely to be successful. If God has told you the one right way to live, you are unlikely to change your mind in response to a press release from Planned Parenthood. Suggesting to strict religious believers that they should not try to control the behavior of people with different ethical views will only appeal to the more moderate and tolerant believers.

These reflections conclude with a few ideas about how to produce change in the policy for misoprostol in the Sri Lanka context. We do not know if the ideas would make sense in the Sri Lanka context. But we offer them here to illustrate a more general point about argument (which is discussed in chapter 11, on persuasion). It is very difficult to convince people to change their deeply held views simply by telling them that they are mistaken. A more fruitful approach relies on helping them to understand that the view or behavior you are advocating is in fact consistent with their own positions and needs—properly understood.

So, for example, one approach in Sri Lanka would be to argue that it is not abortion rights that are non-Lankan, but rather the prohibition of abortion, which has its roots in Western (originally British) law. A complementary claim would involve suggesting that Western ideas need to be adopted selectively to fit with national culture. Given the high levels of female literacy in Sri Lanka, its outstanding maternal health indicators, and the fact that the country had the world's first woman prime minister, registration advocates might claim that women's rights are more advanced in Sri Lanka than elsewhere. Thus, registration might be framed as a way of respecting local traditions and continuing the nation's long-standing efforts to advance the social status of women.

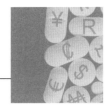

CASE STUDY C

Disentangling Prescribing and Dispensing in the Republic of Korea

Questions to Consider while Reading This Case

This case relates to issues discussed in chapter 6 on managing the politics of reform.

- In responding to the problem posed at the end of the case, first do a stakeholder analysis. Who are the key groups? Identify the power, position, and commitment of each.

- Next, think about a potentially winning coalition. Which opposition groups could be convinced to switch positions or lessen their opposition? How could the power and influence of supporters, or their level of commitment, be increased?

- Finally, what political strategies could the president and his advisers follow to assemble that coalition? Could they offer compromises with the reform plan or trade-offs in other policy areas? Are there any groups who might be convinced to change their position? How should appeals to the public be framed to increase their support for reform?

This case was prepared by Anya Levy Guyer and Michael R. Reich. It is intended as a basis for class discussion rather than as an illustration of either effective or ineffective handling of an administrative situation.

Since the 1960s, the Republic of Korea's health policy makers had discussed the idea of separating the prescribing and dispensing of medicines. But the idea gained little traction over the decades because of a combination of inertia and opposition from both pharmacists and physicians, whose incomes depended on profits from selling medicines. In the late 1980s, however, the issue began to gain increasing policy attention. In 1993 an intense political controversy erupted involving traditional herbal medicines, which returned the issue to the policy agenda (Kim and Ruger 2008).

The 1993 controversy focused on Korea's traditional *Hanbang* medical practice (which originated in China two thousand years ago). In particular, could biomedical pharmacists, not trained in Hanbang, prescribe and dispense herbal products? After several years of vigorous legal, legislative, and political conflict, a civil society organization, the Citizens' Coalition for Economic Justice, helped negotiate a compromise between the traditional practitioners and the biomedical pharmacists. The final agreement, which became law in December 1993, specified that within five years a new system would be put in place that allowed only licensed traditional doctors to prescribe Hanbang remedies. Licensed traditional pharmacists, a new licensure category, would also become the sole dispensers of herbal medicine.

The agreement also included a commitment that by July 1999 the government would pass legislation to establish a standard structure separating the prescribing and the dispensing of *all* medicines in the Korean health system. The prescribing role would belong exclusively to doctors, and the dispensing role only to pharmacists. This mandate set the stage for continued conflict over the prescribing and dispensing of medicines in Korea, which played out during a period of rapid political upheavals and transformations.

Background

After the 1953 armistice that ended the Korean War, the government of the Republic of Korea, eager to recover from the devastation the war had caused, invested heavily in rebuilding infrastructure and promoting economic growth. Health care, which was seen as nonproductive, was left primarily to the private sector. As the country developed, the health sector became dominated by physician-owned clinics and hospitals, pharmacist-owned community pharmacies, and Hanbang practitioners. Korean doctors were accorded respect and deference for their healing work and were generally perceived to be agents of their patients' health. At the same time, health care functioned mostly as a for-profit business.

In 1977, the government established a national health insurance scheme for government and industrial employees, and in 1989 it extended coverage to all citizens through a network of locality- and employer-based insurance societies. Payments to physicians were based on a national fee-for-service schedule. From the beginning, many physicians viewed the fees as insufficient. Leaders of the Korean Medical Association (KMA) stated that the fees covered "less than 80 percent of the cost of the service" (Lee 2004). Meanwhile, the country was experiencing a relative shortage of physicians, so that pharmacists (especially in rural areas) often filled the primary care gap by providing diagnostic services as well as dispensing and selling medicines. They sold products to clients who came either for brief consultations or with requests for specific products (based on personal experience, word-of-mouth recommendations, or manufacturers' advertising).

The insurance system also provided reimbursement for medicines that physicians (and pharmacists) dispensed, and at rates that were higher than the prices that physicians paid for them. This price difference, known as "the drug margin," provided nearly half of the income for physicians who operated private clinics.

Korea's domestic pharmaceutical industry actively supported this model. Primarily made up of small companies, the domestic industry specialized in the production of generic copies of off-patent medicines (in part because Korea did not have a law to protect product patents until 1986). Competing vigorously among themselves, the companies relied on deep discounts and commissions to physicians and pharmacists to expand and maintain their markets (Cho 2001).

The Situation in 1999

Two years before the 1999 deadline for separating prescribing and dispensing, a major political transition occurred. In December 1997, in the midst of the Asian economic crisis, Korea held elections for president. With two candidates splitting the conservative vote, longtime opposition politician Kim Dae-Jung was elected. His inauguration in February 1998 marked the first peaceful transition in postwar Korea from the ruling party to an opposition party (Frängsmyr 2001).

The election also marked a transformation in the civic culture of Korea. Civic organizations, which for many years had focused on working for democracy, strongly supported Kim Dae-Jung (known as "DJ") and his party. (At the time, the party name was the National Congress for New Politics; it later changed its name to the Democratic Party.) Those organizations were led by academics and social progressives who endorsed DJ's emphasis on creating space for civil society to engage in policy and governance (Kwon and Reich 2005). Other associations, including the KMA and the Korean Pharmacists Association (KPA), became connected with political parties when leaders from those organizations engaged in party politics.

President Kim had campaigned on a platform of "One Hundred Reform Policies," including a policy for the separation of prescribing and dispensing, as required by the 1993 law. Apart from the legal mandate to do so by mid-1999, the policy was popular among the leaders of the civil society organizations that had supported DJ in the presidential campaign and who then shifted their attention to promoting the reform policies he had promised.

Shortly after taking office, President Kim called on his supporters to help develop his proposed health reforms. He convened a steering committee of health care policy experts, under the direction of the vice minister of health, to develop a plan for the separation of prescribing and dispensing. The committee had 20 members, including academics, ministry bureaucrats, and two representatives from civil society (from the Citizens' Coalition for Economic Justice and the Korea Consumer Federation), as well as others. It began its work in late May 1998, and at its fourth meeting, on August 24, 1998, a proposed policy was agreed upon (including basic principles and the extent of separation by different health care providers). The implementation date was to be just under a year later, July 1, 1999.

Supporters of reform argued that the then-current system suffered from a number of problems. First, it promoted both misuse and overuse of medicines (contributing to excessive expenditures as well as increased antibiotic resistance). The drug margin and direct sales by physicians and pharmacists created economic incentives for both to dispense large volumes of medicines to patients. Second, with the mixed dispensing and prescribing system, no cross-checking by different professionals of the appropriateness of the medicines provided to patients was taking place. Third, the mixed system encouraged intense competition among pharmaceutical companies, which used deep discounts and rebates to physicians and pharmacists to promote their products. The result was excessive expenditure on promotion, rather than investment in the research and development of new products. Finally, in the mixed system, consumers did not receive adequate information about their medicines. Physicians typically dispensed multiple products without telling patients what the pills were or what side effects might occur. This "polypharmacy" promoted the loyalty of patients who expected to receive multiple drugs from a practitioner and increased practitioners' incomes. This lack of information also served to protect the monopoly of medical knowledge and the status of pharmacists and physicians.

The reformers argued that the new policy would have the following positive effects:

- Promote transparency in pharmaceutical transactions.

- Remove conflicts of interest created by economic incentives.

- Introduce checks on the prescribing of medicines (where pharmacists could review physician choices).

- Improve the quality of information given to consumers.

- Reduce the misuse and overuse of medicines (by removing perverse incentives).

- Contribute to better quality health services.

- Increase satisfaction among patients.

Physicians, on the other hand, opposed the reform because they feared that it would significantly lower their income, especially because the insurance system reimbursed them at low levels for the services they provided. Many believed that they would see more patients if patients could no longer go directly to pharmacies for many drugs. But they doubted that that would compensate for the loss of drug margin revenue. As part of the reform, therefore, they wanted significant increases in their reimbursement fees for services.

The KMA recognized, however, that the general public did not much care about physicians' incomes. So it publicly opposed the reforms on other grounds, namely, patient safety and convenience. Patients, they said, now would have to visit both a physician and a pharmacy to obtain medicines and could no longer obtain medicines from the most trustworthy source, their family doctor. The KMA's position was somewhat complicated, however, by the fact that not all of its members were private-clinic-based general practitioners. It also included subgroups based on medical specialty (pediatrics, internal medicine, psychiatry, and so on) and institutional setting (such as hospitals). Not all of them had the same economic interests as the private general practitioners.

Pharmacists likewise were upset that they would no longer be allowed to provide prescription drugs based on their own judgment. That threatened their autonomy, professional standing, and income because they would no longer be able to serve as primary care providers. Others worried that if pharmacists were no longer care givers, with relationships to their customers, it would undermine small-scale, pharmacist-owned shops in favor of corporate conglomerates (Kwon 2003). The KPA also argued that the policy should require the complete separation of medical institutions from pharmacies, so that physicians could no longer send patients to pharmacies owned by family members. Many pharmacists saw some advantages in the new plan—as physicians would no longer be able to sell drugs. But for many that was not enough to compensate for the change in their role that the new system would impose.

The Challenge

When the reform proposal was publicly announced, many physicians and some pharmacists were deeply opposed and objected to their parliamentarians. In the face of that strong opposition, the expert committee's plan was initially rejected by the National Assembly. But the legal mandate from 1993, to implement the separation of dispensing and prescribing by July 1999, was still in place, and time was running out.

In deciding what to do next, President Kim knew that the proposed reforms could serve as a prime example of the progressive and pro-democracy policies for which he and his party stood. After so many years in opposition, and allowed only one five-year term, Kim was ready to produce comprehensive reform. In particular, he felt that it was time for the government to emphasize a regulatory (rather than market-based) approach to health care. Others in the party, however, with longer political futures ahead, took a different view and hesitated to antagonize the medical professions.

As he considered his options, even beyond the doctors and pharmacists, DJ and his team were faced with a complex political landscape that included a number of significant players:

- *Ministry of health and welfare.* Because none of President Kim's predecessors had taken much interest in health policy, ministry bureaucrats had long dominated a top-down policy process. Despite the role of the vice minister in leading the reform committee, most at the ministry were skeptical about the feasibility of making such a radical change. Over the years, ministry bureaucrats had also developed close relationships with health care providers and with pharmaceutical manufacturers and distributors. They were not eager to disrupt those relationships. Those attitudes help explain why they had never enforced an existing law that set a maximum allowable profit margin of 24 percent in medicine sales by physicians (Kwon 2003).

- *Civic organizations.* The recently established nongovernmental organizations were primarily led by progressive academics, whose expertise gave their groups significant legitimacy. They were generally strongly in favor of the reform, based on their analyses of the existing system's perverse incentives. The civic groups were experienced in advocating for democracy and were savvy about working with the media. However, they lacked a large grassroots base.

- *Pharmaceutical industry.* The existing system of prescribing and dispensing by medical professionals worked well for Korea's domestic pharmaceutical companies. Drugs succeeded less on quality or cost-effectiveness and more on the profits that doctors and pharmacists could earn from them. Because the companies did little research and development, new brand-name drugs came largely in the form of imports by multinational companies. That market was limited, however, because domestic companies offered physicians and pharmacists larger drug margins. The multinationals were therefore likely to benefit from reform because physicians would no longer have that incentive. However, they did not want to arouse opposition by drawing public attention to the likely shift in consumption.

- *General populace.* Many Koreans were frustrated by the high costs of drugs and the tendency of physicians to overprescribe. In addition, many people criticized physicians for their high incomes and their opposition to a policy that was intended to protect the health of the population. However, the population liked the convenience of being able to obtain drugs at any clinic or pharmacy.

Put yourself in the position of an adviser attending a high-level staff meeting with the president, at which the positions of these various groups have just been reviewed. President Kim's secretary interrupts the discussion to tell him that an urgent meeting is being called to discuss security issues with the Democratic People's Republic of Korea. As he leaves the conference room, DJ asks you and the rest of the group to design some strategies to move the reform policy forward.

References

Cho, B.-H. 2001. "Doctors on Strike: Conflict of Interests in Medical Policy Reform." *Korea Journal* 41 (2): 224–43. http://www.ekoreajournal.net/upload/html_20030820.org/HTML4128. Accessed September 1, 2009.

Frängsmyr, T., ed. 2001. "Kim Dae-jung: The Nobel Peace Prize 2000." *Les Prix Nobel. The Nobel Prizes 2000*. Stockholm: Nobel Foundation, 2001. http://nobelprize.org/nobel_prizes/peace/laureates/2000/dae-jung-bio.html. Accessed September 25, 2009.

Kim, H.-J., and J. P. Ruger. 2008. "Pharmaceutical Reform in South Korea and the Lessons It Provides." *Health Affairs* 27 (4): w260–w269.

Kwon, S. 2003. "Pharmaceutical Reform and Physician Strikes in Korea: Separation of Drug Prescribing and Dispensing." *Social Science and Medicine* 57 (3): 529–38.

Kwon, S., and M. R. Reich. 2005. "The Changing Process and Politics of Health Policy in Korea." *Journal of Health Politics, Policy and Law* 30 (6): 1003–25.

Lee, W.-J. 2004. "What Drove Korean Doctors into the Streets?" *Virtual Mentor* 6 (January). http://virtualmentor.ama-assn.org/2004/01/msoc1-0401.html. Accessed September 2, 2009.

Reflections on the Korea Case

This case provides an opportunity to analyze the politics of policy reform. The first step in thinking about how to promote the policy of separating dispensing and prescribing of medicines in Korea is to conduct a stakeholder analysis of opponents and supporters.

The most powerful opposition group was the Korean Medical Association, whose main concern was the income that members feared they would lose if they could no longer make a profit from dispensing medicines. The KMA had substantial organizational resources (money and people), credibility with the public, and access to parliamentarians, making it a major political force. Ultimately it used those resources when it resorted to a series of public strikes in its efforts to stop the policy.

How did the president and his advisers deal with the KMA opposition to the policy? One strategy was to increase reimbursement for medical services under the insurance system to try to compensate physicians for lost income from dispensing medicines.

Another potential opponent was the domestic pharmaceutical industry. A large group of highly competitive small firms, it had a hard time getting itself organized and mobilized to influence the reform process. The fact that the international pharmaceutical companies had different interests helped to diminish the influence of domestic manufacturers.

The pharmacists hoped to see some economic gains from additional business (when physicians could no longer dispense medicines), but they were concerned about lost status and influence and possible competitive turmoil. The pharmacists association was divided and did not strongly take a position on either side of the issue.

The civil society groups connected to the president's party and the reform movement that the party represented were the strongest supporters of the policy. They belonged to a younger generation in Korea, who had protested the military government and fought for democratization. They welcomed the new democracy in Korea that encouraged civil society participation in public policy. They mobilized technical expertise and had direct access to policy making circles, even though they did not have much of a grassroots base. The groups' main policy argument was the need to remove the conflicts of interest that both physicians and pharmacists confronted. They wanted to end a system that combined prescribing and dispensing, so that patients would receive appropriate medicines, not ones based on the size of the margins or rebates that providers might enjoy.

The international pharmaceutical companies maintained a low profile in the policy debate, so that they did not antagonize the physicians, while waiting for the reform to be adopted.

What Happened in Korea

In early 2000, the Korean congress passed a reform law that was slated for implementation in July of that year. The government thought it had a deal with the physicians association (that included a 22 percent increase in medical service fees). But the doctors were not really on board and began a series of strikes—in April, June, August, and October. The strikes shut down between 70 percent and 90 percent of the health care system, and after the second one, in June, the government arrested the leaders of the KMA on charges of violating fair trade and antitrust laws. That radicalized the physicians, even as the public became increasingly unhappy at the disruptions the strikes caused. But many citizens continued to sympathize with the physicians' desires for reasonable incomes.

In October 2000, a compromise was reached that included a 44 percent physician fee increase and took away the pharmacists' ability to substitute generic for brand-name drugs. Injections (which played a large role in Korean medical practice) were also exempted from the new system, allowing physicians to continue to prescribe and dispense injections. The chaos over these reforms significantly changed the political landscape and the feasibility of other health reforms. As a result, the administration was unable to proceed with its plans to change the payment system from fee-for-service to a case-based or admission-based system.

After the separation policy was implemented in Korea, physicians responded by increasing prescriptions of brand-name drugs. That has produced a substantial increase in pharmaceutical expenditures and a significantly increased role of multinational companies in the Korean market. Together with the fee increases to compensate physicians, the reforms have generated significant fiscal burdens on the national insurance system.

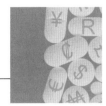

Last Mile Logistics for Essential Drugs: The Case of Zambia

Questions to Consider while Reading This Case

This case relates to issues of organizational change presented in chapter 9.

- Why was Zambia able to keep medicines stocks at the district level but not at the health centers?

- What are the various possible explanations for why the health centers failed to do a better job of reporting stocks and ordering supplies?

- What are the advantages and disadvantages of each of the three options being considered for dealing with the problem?

- What organizational change difficulties are common to all these options, and how could they be overcome?

In Lusaka, Zambia, in early 2007, consultant Prashant Yadav sat in the canteen at the national warehouse run by Medical Stores Limited (MSL) with Tom Brown, the logistics director of MSL, reflecting on the supply chain challenges that were limiting the provision of health services in

This case was prepared by Laura Rock Kopczak, Prashant Yadav, and Marc J. Roberts. It is intended as a basis for class discussion rather than to illustrate either effective or ineffective handling of an administrative situation. The facts and figures presented may be dated.

Zambia. (Although it was a parastatal agency, MSL was operated by a contractor, a United Kingdom–based company called Crown Agents.) Responding to Zambia's health problems required providing a variety of products to more than 1,500 health centers scattered across the large and predominantly rural country. Although some products were being reliably supplied, the figures on health center stock-outs were dismal. In particular, a lack of malaria medicines in public health centers was leading to poor health outcomes or forcing patients to seek substandard treatment in the private sector. Prashant Yadav, a professor of supply chain management at the MIT-Zaragoza International Logistics Program, was part of a team that was working closely with the government of Zambia to help address these problems. The team included Tom Brown from Medical Stores Limited, a team from the World Bank led by Monique Vledder, Michael Borowitz from the U.K. Department for International Development, and colleagues from John Snow Inc.

After spending three weeks mapping out replenishment and delivery processes Yadav observed that although "product" was flowing to the district-level stores, it was not getting the "last mile"[1] to the health centers (see figure D1). The team had generated a number of ideas about how to address that problem, but they knew that any solution they proposed would have to work in the Zambian context and within the limited budget of the ministry of health.

Figure D1   Current Public Health Sector Distribution System

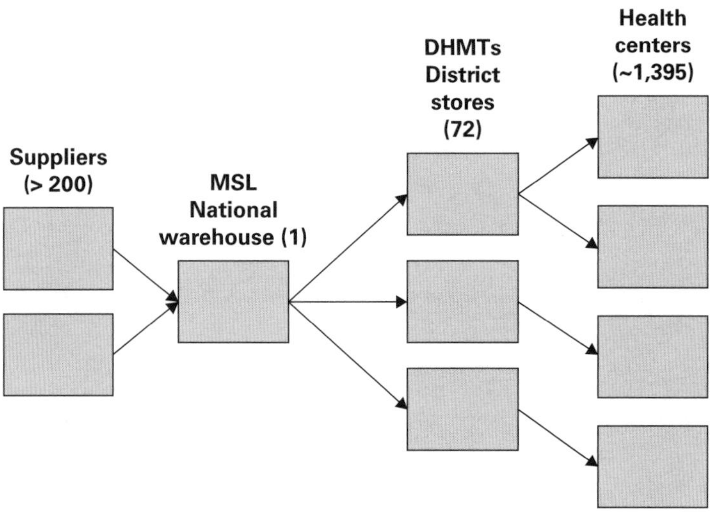

Source: Prashant Yadav.

Note: DHMT = District Health Management Team; MSL = Medical Stores Limited.

Health Care in Zambia

Zambia is a low-income country composed of 72 districts, situated on a large, landlocked plateau. Only 38 percent of its population of 11.6 million people live in urban areas, and 87.4 percent live on less than US$2 per day. Life expectancy at birth for both sexes is approximately 43 years. In 2004, Zambia had 3.5 million malaria cases. Approximately 1.1 million people were living with HIV/AIDS, of whom only 75,000 were on antiretroviral therapy.

The public sector is the largest provider of health care (85 percent of all facilities), followed by the Churches Health Association of Zambia (CHAZ) and hospitals operated by mining companies (see table D1). Although the mining companies originally started their hospitals for their employees, they now have quasi-public status, and many receive drugs from the public sector. The for-profit, private sector is small. Public facilities are located throughout the country. Mission facilities are concentrated in rural areas, and mine hospitals in the Copperbelt province. International nongovernmental organizations (NGOs) operate some health facilities along the borders with the Democratic Republic of Congo and Angola, to cater to the health needs of refugees.

Zambia's public sector consists of modest district hospitals and a general hospital in each provincial center. There are typically at least 20 primary health centers in each district, but the number varies by region. Some areas also have smaller health posts that offer a very limited range of services.

Private, for-profit clinics and hospitals (which also dispense drugs) and retail pharmacies are concentrated in Lusaka and the Copperbelt. Medicines are also sold over-the-counter in drugstores and in informal outlets called "kantembas" in rural areas and the shanty neighborhoods around Lusaka.

Table D1   Health Facilities

Type/level	Public	Mission	Private	Total
Hospitals	53	27	17	97
Health centers	1,052	61	97	1,210
Health posts	19	0	1	20
Total	1,124	88	115	1,327
Percentage of total	85	7	9	100

Source: Republic of Zambia 2006.

MSL provides storage and distribution services for public sector health facilities. CHAZ provides medicine procurement, storage, and distribution for its own members. According to estimates, 20 percent to 30 percent of health care in Zambia is provided through CHAZ, although the proportion is much higher in rural areas.

Public Sector Procurement

Yadav was encouraged by the supply chain improvements that had occurred during the previous seven years. Zambia received funding for drug purchases from many different donors, resulting in fragmented financing and procurement processes. A Procurement Technical Working Group (PTWG) was therefore established in 2002, and it had significantly improved operational coordination between the ministry of health and its funders. In addition, a Drug Supply Budget Line (DBSL) had been created in 2005 to foster centralized, accountable, and efficient procurement.

Within the ministry of health, the Pharmacy Unit carried out demand forecasting in consultation with national program managers for various vertical disease programs. In conjunction with stock-level reports and replenishment requests from MSL, those forecasts were used to create a procurement plan. Tenders were then floated by the Zambia National Tender Board (ZNTB) and the ministry of health. Some donors required Zambia to purchase through an international nonprofit procurement agent, such as the International Dispensary Association (IDA) or United Nations Children's Fund.

Yadav noted that long procurement lead times and the use of annual tenders were limiting Zambia's ability to adjust procurement to actual use. Nevertheless, the PTWG and DSBL initiatives had greatly improved product availability.

In the public sector, the receipt, storage, and initial distribution of drugs and other supplies were managed by MSL. The government budget supported MSL's operating expenses. Capital investments were financed by borrowing against operating revenue; these were periodically evaluated by the MSL board. Such investments had recently resulted in improved physical infrastructure at MSL, including a fleet of 14 ten-ton trucks.

As a parastatal agency, MSL was able to act like a private enterprise in some key areas. It offered performance incentives to its workers, had flexibility in hiring and firing, and was able to make significant investments in technology, such as global positioning system tracking of its fleet. As a result, a study of the availability of 20 essential medicines over a recent one-year period had revealed that only two medicines had faced a stock-out during that time.

Distribution Processes

MSL was responsible for distribution to district-level stores and hospitals. Distribution from a district store to health centers was the responsibility of each District Health Management Team (DHMT). The team provided drugs to health centers through a variety of supply processes:

- *Kit-based push delivery.* Zambia used a primary health care "kit" of 52 items, including 20 basic medicines and products such as sutures, Band-Aids, and oral rehydration salts. A kit was supposed to provide adequate quantities to meet the needs of a typical clinic for two months. Kits were received from the supplier twice a year and stored at the MSL warehouse. The ministry allocated a specific number of kits to each clinic based on its size, service area, and past use. MLS made monthly scheduled deliveries to each district store. Districts in turn made monthly deliveries to the clinics. Consumption data were not collected, so there was no way to know how well the kits matched actual needs.

- *Pull-based supply.* For non-kit products, apart from antiretrovirals (ARVs), districts placed monthly orders and received monthly deliveries from MSL along with the kits. If districts had unmet demand for kit items, they ordered the items as "supplemental drugs." Districts had to place their orders in time to mesh with scheduled deliveries. Districts communicated their orders to MSL via phone or fax, or by giving a requisition slip to the MSL delivery driver.

  Health centers, in turn, were supposed to place orders with the district based on their needs. Delivery or pickup was "as needed," rather than being scheduled. Although the products under the pull-based delivery system were reliably in stock at the district level, health centers were often out of many of them because they had not placed orders.

- *The malaria push-pull system.* The vertical malaria program had started the distribution of the new recommended drug, Coartem®, an artemisinin-based combination therapy (ACT), as well as rapid diagnostics test kits using a push system for moving the products to the district level. The National Malaria Control Program estimated monthly district needs for these and directed MSL to ship that amount to each district. This was followed by a pull system from district stores to health centers. Many health centers, however, did not place product orders on time or for the right quantities, resulting in shortages and delays in adoption of the new treatment regime.

- *Direct HIV/ART supply.* ARVs and other HIV/AIDS commodities were directly supplied to Zambia's 200 antiretroviral therapy (ART) centers by MSL. By a set date each month, ART centers placed their orders with MSL, where a special Logistics Management Unit validated and packed each one. They were then sent either to the ART clinic or its district store. This process was working well, in part because the sites had special donor funding, were well staffed and equipped, and were relatively few in number. The USAID/DELIVER project was instrumental in the design and operation of this system.

- *Prepositioning.* There were times each year when certain health centers could not be reached due to seasonal flooding. For these centers, stocks of medicines had to be "pre-positioned" before the start of the rainy season. The quantities to be pre-positioned were determined on an ad-hoc basis by the relevant DHMT, usually without accurate stock data. Limited storage capacity at a health center often restricted what could be pre-positioned there.

Challenges in Health Center Supply

Getting kits from the district stores to the health centers was not easy. Loads were small, destinations were spread out, and getting through often required using off-road vehicles. At the district level, not enough vehicles were available, and they broke down regularly because of poor roads and inadequate maintenance. Districts lacked adequate transportation budgets, so some sought help from the military or NGOs to distribute needed supplies.

Health center staff traveled to the district store to pick up supplemental items using their own budgets, which were also very limited. About 25 percent of health facilities surveyed reported having debts, many related to transport and fuel costs. Although some health facilities could borrow from their DHMT, their indebtedness restricted their ability to contract for transport, exacerbating stock-out problems.

Communication between districts and health centers was difficult, relying on an old and poorly functioning radio system and staff members' personal cell phones (whose use some health centers subsidized). Although cell phone coverage was high in most parts of the country, some remote health centers were still not covered by a network.

Human resources were also in very short supply, especially at rural health centers. More than half of all posts were unfilled in rural areas, including 90 percent of all slots for doctors and 65 percent of slots for pharmacists (see figure D2). As a result, inventory tracking, re-ordering and other non-critical activities were often neglected. While all districts and health centers had received logistics training that included clear guidelines for ordering and stock management, adherence to these policies was poor and record keeping spotty at best. As a result, there was little information from health centers on which to base decisions.

Options for Improvement

The team had solicited opinions from a wide range of people at all levels of the health system about what might be done (see table D2). After much

Figure D2   Unfilled Posts in the Health Sector

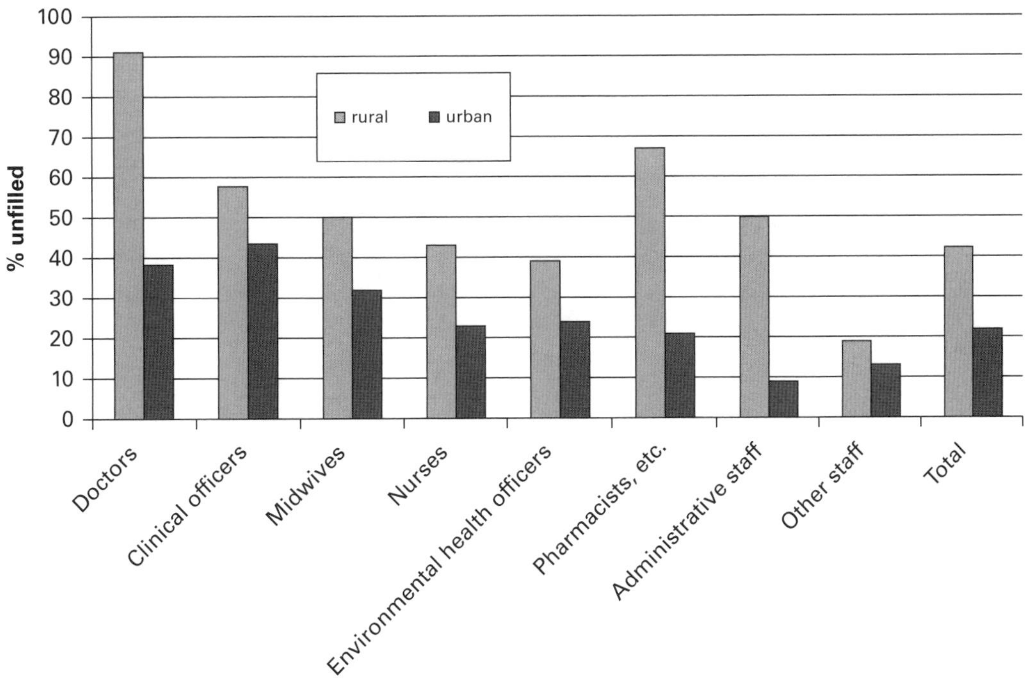

Source: Authors' Compilation.

Table D2 Supply Chain Improvement Alternatives

Suggested solution	Obstacles
Deliver directly from MSL stores to clinics.	The 14 ten-ton trucks owned by the MSL cannot travel on the rural roads. Transport costs would go up drastically.
Outsource delivery to a commercial logistics company.	"We will have insurance trouble. If there is a fire … the insurance is bought by the government."
	"There is no third-party logistics company that can deliver to the rural districts. They only go to the Copperbelt and Livingstone."
Replicate the ARV model.	The other clinics are not nearly as capable as the 200 clinics that handle ARVs.
Increase inventory levels at the clinics.	Clinics lack enough space: "I already put medicines under each bed."
Have district personnel visit the clinics to do stockkeeping and deliver what is needed.	But would this person receive extra pay or exert extra power for doing this additional work?

Source: Authors.

discussion they were considering three options, all of which involved enhancing the role of either the DHMTs or MSL to improve stock levels at health centers.

- *Option 1: Enhance District Capacity.* The first option was to enhance information processing, stock management, and transport capabilities at the district. Districts would be provided with a new staff position, a "commodity planner," and equipped with additional vehicles earmarked for deliveries. Health centers, while continuing to get kits, would report stock levels and usage and place supplemental orders to the commodity planner, using cell phones or radio, at fixed, 15-day intervals. The commodity planner would plan stock levels for the district and place orders with MSL. Delivery from district stores to health clinics would be done using the earmarked vehicles.

  This option would require significant resources for equipping each of the 72 districts. The ministry of health would have to hire and train new staff and procure about 150 vehicles. Another difficulty was figuring out the best organizational situation and reporting relationships for the district commodity planners. The planners would need to work well with both the DHMT and MSL, but to whom should they report?

Being part of MSL would produce better coordination and supervision and the ability to provide performance incentives. The DHMTs, however, would almost surely see this as a loss of power. The role of the provincial pharmacist was also unclear—would he or she have oversight responsibility for the commodity planners in the districts within the province? It would also be necessary to address certain ministry of health guidelines; for example, MSL employees were not allowed to drive ministry vehicles.

- *Option 2: District Crossdock.* The second option was a version of the current ARV system, in which the district would just act as a "crossdock" or transfer point. Decision making on order quantities would be shifted from the district level to MSL. Districts would receive stock from MSL that would already be packaged and earmarked for specific health centers (and also for district hospitals). Those packages would not be shelved but instead immediately loaded onto the new, dedicated vehicles and expeditiously delivered to the intended recipient clinics. As in Option 1, each district would be staffed with a commodity planner to gather stock and use information and relay it to MSL. MSL in turn would need additional stock pickers to assemble the health center orders.

    How the DHMTs would react to the even-more-significant loss of power this would involve was another story. An additional challenge related to how "order picking" would occur at the national store. Individually procuring all 50 items now provided in the kit was likely to overwhelm the ministry's procurement function. The most efficient process therefore might be for MSL to continue to procure kits and then, after they arrived, open them up and redistribute the medicines. However, some worried that sooner or later an "accounting type" from Washington or Geneva, who did not understand why the government would buy a kit and then break it up, would decide that this was some kind of corrupt practice.

- *Option 3: "Vending Machine" Model.* As in the other two options, this third option would also require equipping each district with a commodity planner and usually two earmarked delivery vehicles. The commodity planner would travel along on delivery trips to check stock levels at the health centers. Replenishment would be made instantaneously from the supplies carried in the delivery vehicle. The commodity planner would plan the stock to be held by the district, place orders, and send health center stock data to MSL. To implement this option, delivery vehicles would have to be large enough to carry adequate stocks of a full range of items, adding to the cost of the scheme. The time taken at each clinic would also increase, reducing delivery efficiency.

Some people raised concerns that because the national monitoring and evaluation system was based on assessing a small subset of tracer drugs, the commodity planner might carry too many of those items at the expense of other supplies. Clinic staff might also object because many liked the opportunity to go to the district town periodically, combining drug pickup with shopping and socializing. The "kit breakdown" issue would arise here as well.

Conclusion

Any of the three options would require adequate additional funding, political will to bring the reform about, and sufficient technical and organizational capacity to implement the needed changes. Various sources of resistance would also have to be dealt with, particularly concern from a number of quarters about how the new staff would relate to the existing bureaucratic structures. Another uncertainty nagging at Prashant Yadav and Tom Brown, as they sat sipping tea in the canteen, was exactly how the organization would operate at the level of the frontline workers who actually did the work. Did the capacity and motivation exist, particularly at the district and health center levels, to make any reform function effectively? The fact that the health centers were doing such a poor job of ordering under the current system suggested some unresolved structural issues. Yadav did not know the answers to those questions, he realized, and he was not sure even whom to ask.

Note

1. Although most countries use the metric system, the term the "last mile" is a technical term used in supply chain management.

Reference

Republic of Zambia, Ministry of Health. 2006. *Health Sector Annual Review Report 2005*. Lusaka: Republic of Zambia.

Reflections on the Zambia Case

Reading this case makes it clear just how underresourced public health centers are in rural areas in Zambia; 90 percent of centers lack a physician on staff, and fully half of all posts are unfilled. Is it any wonder that the mission health facilities play such a large role in rural health care? Indeed, the existing drug distribution system—which relies heavily on a "push" kit-based system—would seem to be a response to that situation. It has clearly been designed to deliver basic supplies and medicines to health centers more or less without their involvement. In fact, both the "pull" system for supplemental orders and the separate system for supplying ACTs for malaria appeared to break down because the health centers could not effectively place the needed orders. Inasmuch as the country has reasonable cell phone coverage, the problem could no longer be just a matter of communications, which had been a problem until recently.

All of the ideas put forward by Yadav and his team responded to the situation by enhancing capacity at the district level through some role for a district commodity planner. In the first option, that individual would contact health centers every 15 days to plan and place orders with the central medical supply. Then the districts would package and deliver the order. In the second model, the district commodity planner would still collect and transmit information, but the picking and packaging of all health center supplies would be done at central stores—and be delivered prepackaged to the districts for transshipment. The third model involved actually sending the commodity planner to the health centers with a truck full of supplies, so that health center stores could be directly assessed and replenished.

If the key problem is the inability of the districts to track their own stocks, then only the third option really responds to the problem. In the first two options, the district commodity planner is still at one end of a cell phone call, trying to get the health center personnel to assess and report on stock levels. It is just not clear why they would respond more effectively to such a person than they do now in the existing reporting chain.

The difficulties of implementing the third option are both financial and organizational. With more than 70 districts, a large number of fairly large four wheel drive vehicles will be required to carry the stock for resupplying the centers, and they will be both costly and difficult to maintain. And what happens when a vehicle goes out of commission in a district for days or weeks at a time?

Moreover, for any of these options the existing organizational structure will have to be readjusted. The new commodity planner will suddenly become the most powerful person in the district in terms of controlling pharmaceutical supplies. Will the District Health Management Team—especially the district director and the district pharmacist—be happy with such an arrangement? Resentment (and lack of full cooperation) will be a particular risk if the new position is actually within the organizational structure of the quasi-public central medical stores system, which is run under contract by Crown Agents. And if the new person reports to the team, what is to ensure technically expert (and corruption-free) implementation of the plan?

The case thus makes very clear that technical supply chain issues—like all issues of organizational functioning—come down to the behavior of frontline workers. The question always is how any reform will affect the six keys to organizational performance. In this instance the issues that are especially relevant are the incentives to health center workers, on the one hand, and their skills and values, on the other. For the various organizations involved to accept new arrangements, important change-management tasks would need to be accomplished. New materials-handling systems, new flowcharts, and new reorder schemes are not self-implementing. Yadav was right to worry about the human dimension as he sat in that cafeteria, for that could easily undermine the effectiveness of the vending machine model that he ultimately chose to try in a number of districts.

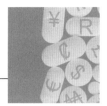

Drug Procurement in East Africania

Questions to Consider while Reading This Case

This case deals with issues of corruption and the organizational and regulatory issues that were discussed in chapters 8, 9, and 10.

- Why did the government of East Africania wind up dealing with this broker, and why then were multiple agencies in the government unwilling to do anything to deal with the situation?

- What factors, apart from corruption, were at work?

- If you were the international consultant who became involved in this case, what, if anything, could you have done differently?

- What would it take for procurement in East Africania to be done more effectively in the future?

East Africania is a fictional low-income country with a history of difficulties in drug supply, a function historically handled by a unit in the ministry of health. In 2004, it had been a long time since the last tender, and drugs were running low. But the country was so short of funds that the ministry of

This case was prepared by Wilbert Bannenberg and Marc J. Roberts. It is intended as a basis for class discussion rather than to illustrate either effective or ineffective handling of an administrative situation.

finance told the ministry of health that there was no money for new drug procurement. After an appeal to international donors, the Department for International Development in the United Kingdom (DFID) agreed to provide US$2.7 million on an emergency basis for acquiring some essential medicines.

Who Actually Supplied the Drugs?

The tender to acquire the medicines was issued by the country's general purchasing authority, the East Africania National Tender Commission. It did so with the normal stipulation that bids were due back in six weeks. For reasons that were never clear, the tender commission took two months after bidding closed to announce its decision. The majority of the contract was awarded to WorldWide Brokerage Ltd., a business in the United Kingdom, with extra payment for air freight delivery because the drug supply situation in public clinics and hospitals in East Africania was now desperate.

After additional delays, products began arriving at the health ministry's central medical stores, although in sea containers and not via air freight. All were labeled as coming from UKPharm. That puzzled two pharmacists attached to central stores because none of the documents that accompanied the shipment listed that name. They consulted three key documents: the bidding documents; the certificate of analysis that is supposed to report laboratory tests of the products supplied; and the certificate of pharmaceutical products, which is issued by the exporting government's drug regulatory authority and attests that the products have been produced according to its regulations. No one in East Africania, and none of the country's international pharmaceutical consultants, had ever heard of UKPharm. (WorldWide had done business in East Africania before, supplying drugs to that country and to some of its neighbors through a number of World Bank procurements.) When WorldWide was queried about what was going on, the company sent a representative to East Africania, whose business cards listed his title as "Senior Director of Quality Assurance." His first act was to inspect the supplies in central stores and re-label all the boxes with the WorldWide name, using labels he had apparently brought with him just for that purpose. After doing that, he began to make the rounds of various offices and agencies involved in drug purchasing and quality control—in order, he said, to establish face-to-face contacts and create communication channels in case any further difficulties arose.

The local pharmacists became increasingly concerned and looked into the documents further. They were totally confused by what they found. For example, one of the major components of the bid was 15 million amoxicillin capsules. The three key documents—the bidding document, the certificate of analysis, and the certificate of pharmaceutical products—bore neither the WorldWide nor the UKPharm name, but rather three other—and different—company names (Pharmgene, Biokem, and Phytokem). A look at the documents for the other compounds produced similar results. There were always at least two different company names in the documents—none of which were WorldWide or UKPharm—even where all the documents were available. (Of the 64 products, certificates of analysis were missing for 16.) Quite a number of different companies, with names that reflected a variety of linguistic origins, appeared at various points in the documents, and several of those were totally unknown to the pharmacists or their consultants.

With the help of their consultants, the pharmacists decided to try to find out who they were dealing with. Their first step was to go to WorldWide's website. It yielded some basic information, such as a telephone number, company officers, business address, and so forth. But as they continued to dig into the situation, the site suddenly became password protected, and they could not access it further.

The information they obtained, however, revealed that the business address of WorldWide was the same as the home address of one of the individuals listed as a WorldWide company director. The Certificate of Good Distribution Practice—which companies had to have as a condition of eligibility to enter the tender process—turned out to have been issued by the chamber of commerce of the smallish English town in which that director lived; it was issued for his home address, as well. Unable to resist further digging, the pharmacists and their consultants pursued the accounting firm that had apparently certified WorldWide's financial statements. No amount of searching on Google and no professional directories in the United Kingdom yielded such an accounting firm. And its telephone number, on the documents it had supposedly prepared, was the same as the WorldWide number.

Quality Problems

As was normal practice, East Africania's National Quality Laboratory, a Division of the East Africania Drug Regulatory Authority, began testing the products that were purchased—choosing 12 of the larger-volume compounds for the initial round of testing. Two of the 12 failed the test, and WorldWide—as required by the contract—agreed to replace them. Saying that he was concerned about the accuracy of the work done by the National Quality Laboratory, the WorldWide representative (who was still in the country six weeks after his first arrival) offered to help resolve any technical problems with the next round of testing. Subsequently, the laboratory reported that all 52 products in the second round of testing had passed their quality checks.

Regulatory Dead Ends

The pharmacists were so puzzled and concerned by all this that they went several steps up their own reporting structure in the ministry of health, only to be turned away. "The drugs are here and have been distributed, and people are getting what they want," they were told. They suggested that the final 10 percent payment to WorldWide be suspended, pending further study of the quality issues. The response was a combination of anger and disbelief. "Why are you causing trouble?" they were asked. "Are you allied with the political opposition? Do you have ties to another supplier?" Aware that they were putting their own positions at risk, they decided to remain in the background of any further efforts.

The international consultants felt less exposed and increasingly uneasy with what was going on. They took their information to several places in the government. Checking with the Drug Regulatory Authority revealed that several of the products supplied were actually not registered at the time they were imported. But the authority seemed totally uninterested in the issue and in the various labeling confusions and document inconsistencies. One of its senior officials hotly rejected any suggestion that any of the drugs should be retested by any other laboratory.

The National Tender Commission likewise expressed no interest. The record of the bidding revealed that several other competitors had been disqualified for technicalities in their documentation. However one commission member contended that the fact that drugs apparently came from sources other than those specified in the bidding documents was "a trivial technicality" and that the documents in question had not been used in the evaluation of the competing bids, so the irregularities in them were irrelevant.

Enter the Department for International Development

At this point, in frustration, the consultants decided to involve the donor who had put up the money. Representatives of DFID reviewed all their documentation and agreed to look into the matter. They went first to the relevant U.K. agency, the Medicines and Healthcare Products Regulatory Agency (MHRA), which confirmed that the Good Distribution Practice certificate was not in keeping with MHRA requirements. Indeed WorldWide had not even applied for a U.K. wholesaler's license until more than a month after the bids had been submitted. The MHRA concluded that the irregularities in the documents would have constituted a violation of the law if the drugs had been exported to a European Union country. But U.K. law did not contain similar prohibitions about exports to other places. The MHRA said it could only proceed further if it received a complaint from the government of East Africania.

The donor representatives then requested a meeting with the ministry of health, at which they reviewed all the facts in detail and asked that the last 10 percent not be paid, pending the outcome of further investigations. The donors saw this as especially urgent because doubts had now been raised about the authenticity of the bank guarantee under which WorldWide had received 90 percent of the funds soon after the contract was executed and before any product was delivered. The ministry representatives agreed to this. In addition, the ministry agreed to transmit the bank guarantee to DFID, agreed to a request that the tender board look into the matter further, and also agreed to a referral to the National Anti-Corruption Commission.

And Now?

Over the next month, DFID discovered the following: (1) WorldWide was paid the last 10 percent, despite the agreed-upon freeze, (2) the National Anti-Corruption Commission ruled that not enough evidence had been presented to justify an investigation and (3) the tender board had ruled that all the relevant rules and regulations had been complied with. In addition, DFID was told that WorldWide's original bank guarantee had apparently been mislaid, and so there was no way to give its representatives the copy of it that they had been promised.

Reflections on East Africania Case

The roots of the situation seem to lie in the joint effect of a number of forces. One undoubtedly is a pervasive pattern of corruption in the government of East Africania. The tender board disqualified several bidders, delayed making the decision, and defended what it had done in a way that refused to take any account of its own rules. Similarly, should anyone really believe the results of the positive tests on the second set of products, in light of the government's adamant refusal to have them retested? Moreover, neither the ministry of health nor the Anti-Corruption Commission was willing to act. That leads one to wonder—just how far up the ladder of authority in East Africania did this web of malfeasance go?

Clearly, the willingness on the part of the broker to circumvent or violate the law was also integral to the situation. Almost nothing about the company's work conformed to appropriate standards—from its U.K. documents and financial statements, to its "missing" bank guarantee, to the certificates of analysis and certificates of pharmaceutical product that it submitted. The company even sent out a representative to change labels and directly supervise the completion of the corrupt transaction—and perhaps provide any last-minute payoffs that might be required.

Brokers of this kind, however, can survive only because of the dysfunctional "organizational ecology" that medicine purchasing practices in some low-income countries help to create. Countries do not appropriate funds on a regular basis. Poor forecasting and leakage mean that politically embarrassing stock-outs intermittently occur in the public sector, creating emergency situations. Donors step in to help, for humanitarian reasons, but are reluctant to take direct control of the purchasing process for fear of provoking an anticolonial backlash. The processes themselves totally lack transparency. Over time, legitimate sellers shy away from even bidding on tender offers from such countries, knowing that they have little chance of being successful unless they offer significant bribes. That leaves the field open to the likes of WorldWide.

Certain manufacturers are also part of this system. Some producers of generic compounds in places such as India and China are quite willing to produce substandard products to order and sell them to brokers like World-Wide at deeply discounted prices. Several Indian state governments (which have the power to issue certificates of pharmaceutical product) are notorious for signing documents without any real quality checks as long as the material is bound for export.

On the buying side, the National Tender Board is harnessed by rigid procedures designed to prevent corruption but that instead merely serve to lock everyone into often pointless formalities. Nor does a body that purchases so many different commodities typically have much in the way of expertise in pharmaceutical purchasing. With many different compounds to acquire, the tender board would be overwhelmed if it tried to manage 30 different tenders. And how are they to know which suppliers of which goods, scattered all over the world, are reliable? It is exactly on this interface between untrustworthy sellers and underequipped and unethical buyers that these kinds of brokerage operations can flourish.

It is a truism of quality management that "every system is perfectly designed to produce the results you observe." And that is so in this case. Given the pervasiveness of corruption in East Africania, the international consultants were unlikely to accomplish very much, no matter whom they went to. After all, as one ministry official says in the case, the procurement did produce drugs in the public sector system, and that dealt with the government's most pressing problem from a political point of view. If the drugs were substandard—with all the health concerns and problems of antimicrobial resistance that that could lead to—who would ever know?

The solution, clearly, is to try to change the system. It needs to be made transparent—perhaps using electronic and web-based technologies. Procedures designed to provide "accountability for reasonableness" (see chapter 4), such as public reporting of deliberations and explicit, written justification of decisions, need to be established. But making such changes will require political pressure. Somehow efforts need to be mobilized to shift the calculation of government leaders from favoring the patronage strategy they now pursue to favoring a strategy of gaining public support through better service. Whether a sufficient coalition can be assembled—from civil society groups, honest manufacturers, and international donors—to do that is very much an open question. And the answer to that question will vary from country to country, depending on the set of stakeholders who can be mobilized and the political skill of those trying to accomplish such a reform.

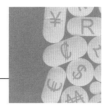

Converting Basic Drug Shops to Accredited Drug Dispensing Outlets in Tanzania

Questions to Consider while Reading This Case

This case relates to issues presented in chapters 9 and 10 on organizing the public sector and using regulation to improve pharmaceutical performance.

- What problem was the Accredited Drug Dispensing Outlet, or ADDO, program intended to overcome?

- How did ADDO differ from most regulatory initiatives?

- What were the differences between the initial demonstration and the national implementation of the program?

- What features of the ADDO program account for the results it has produced?

- To what extent—and why or why not—has ADDO solved the problems it was intended to deal with?

This case was prepared by Tory Ervin and Marc J. Roberts. It is intended as a basis for class discussion rather than as an illustration of either effective or ineffective handling of an administrative situation.

Tanzania is an amalgamation of Tanganyika (a former German colony that the British took over after World War I) and the islands of Zanzibar, formerly a British protectorate. Tanzania is about the size of Nigeria, but with less than a third of the population (about 41 million), and is largely rural and agricultural.

In the early 1960s, Julius Nyerere, a proponent of African Socialism and a prominent figure in the decolonization movement, led Tanzania to independence and into a one-party system. Forced agricultural collectivization produced great economic hardship. Constitutional reforms finally led to the first multiparty elections in 1994. Even today, however, the ruling party remains overwhelmingly popular. In the past 20 years, economic reforms and foreign aid have produced some economic growth (5.8 percent in 2003) (CIA World Factbook 2009). The country has some natural resources, including both minerals and natural gas, and some famous tourist attractions, such as Mount Kilimanjaro and the Serengeti game reserves. But perhaps 85 percent of employment is still in agriculture, and poverty has been a continuing challenge. In 2003, per capita income was only US$630 in purchasing power parity terms (CIA World Factbook 2009).

Because of the government's limited economic capacity, the public health sector run by the Ministry of Health and Social Welfare (MOHSW) has long suffered from deteriorating buildings, a lack of equipment and supplies, and a lack of human resources. At the same time, the system confronts rising levels of HIV/AIDS and high rates of multidrug-resistant malaria. In rural areas, only 27 percent of pregnant women delivered at health facilities, compared to 77 percent in urban areas (United Republic of Tanzania 2006, 17).

The Drug Access Problem

In 2001, Tanzania confronted major drug access problems. An estimated 60 percent of the country's pharmacies were located in the capital city. In rural areas basic medicines were largely supplied by more than 4,000 licensed Cold Drug Shops (Duka La Dawa Baridi, in Swahili, or DLDBs; see figure F1). Unlike urban pharmacies, DLDBs were not supervised by a pharmacist and had a smaller list of approved drugs. In 2001, nearly 70 percent of DLDBs were staffed by nurse assistants or other auxiliaries who had no formal training in drug dispensing (CPM 2003, 30). Yet these shops were often the first point of contact with health services for rural patients. Indeed in 2008 only 620 licensed pharmacists were known to be working in the entire country (FIP 2009, 83).

Figure F1 Tiers of Drug Retailers

Pharmacies

- Able to sell all drugs registered in country

- Do not receive subsidized Coartem

- Are staffed by a pharmacist

Duka La Dawa Muhimu (DLDM/ADDO)

- Expanded drug list by 54 drugs

- Able to sell antibiotics

- Sell subsidized Coartem

- Both shop owner and drug seller receive training
  - Drug seller training: 31 days
  - Owner training: 7 days

- Shop owners and dispensers tend to be clinical officers (2 years training) or nurse or nurse assistant

Duka La Dawa Baridi (DLDB)

- Can sell only limited number of drugs

- Cannot sell antibiotics

- Are staffed by low-level health care workers

Source: Authors' representation.

In addition, the quality of drugs sold by the DLDBs was often problematic: of all the drugs tested for quality in 2000 by the National Quality Control Lab, about 13 percent failed. The stock-out rate for essential medicines in the public sector was 31.5 percent (CPM 2003, 36). Private sector supplies were more available, in part because of the DLDBs, but medicine prices often were not within the economic reach of many citizens. (As in other African countries, street corner vendors and other unlicensed sellers also served these groups.) Moreover, the number of DLDBs was growing, and the country's regulatory agencies were having trouble keeping up. Given their rural location and the country's poor road system, in the 18 months up to July 2001 only 159 DLDBs had been inspected (CPM 2003, 30). With this lack of oversight, the DLDBs often sold unauthorized drugs or even stolen government stock.

Strategies for Enhancing Access to Medicines—SEAM—Enters Tanzania

In 2000, Management Sciences for Health (MSH), a nonprofit international health consulting organization based in the United States, received a US$30 million grant from the Bill and Melinda Gates Foundation to develop ways to improve access to essential medicines using the private sector. With 1,300 employees in more than 60 nations, MSH had long been involved in medicines issues. It publishes the leading reference on how to manage essential medicines in developing countries, *Managing Drug Supply* (MSH and WHO 1997). The program that resulted was Strategies for Enhancing Access to Medicines (SEAM).

More than 40 experts, representing 15 countries, the World Bank, and the World Health Organization, participated in discussions to shape SEAM's approach. Six countries were identified as potential pilot locations, two or three of which were to be selected for long-term projects, depending in part on which governments were committed to the activity and on the available funding.

In the final round of decisions, Tanzania was selected as one of the sites for a long-term project (along with El Salvador and Ghana). It was selected in part because of strong support for the plan from the ministry of health and the Tanzanian Federal Drug Administration (TFDA). Those two organizations took the lead in developing and then piloting the intervention strategy.

The idea was to create a network of private medicine shops that would provide expanded access to safe medicines in rural areas. The new outlets were called "Accredited Drug Dispensing Outlets (or ADDOs)" in English and *Duka La Dawa Muhimu* (DLDMs) in Swahili. They were to be legally able to sell more than 50 additional drugs, including selected antibiotics and birth control products, that the DLDBs had not provided. A diagram of the ADDO program structure appears in figure F2. They were also to be used as a vehicle for public health programs, including Integrated Management of Childhood Illness (IMCI) and family planning. The program began on a pilot basis in one region, Ruvuma, a rural area with a population of 1.2 million in the southwest corner of the country.

Early on, the ADDO process in Tanzania acquired two key champions. The ministry's chief medical officer, Dr. Gabriel Upunda, helped convince some resistant colleagues that with proper oversight the DLDBs could be allowed to sell an expanded list of drugs. The director of the Tanzanian Federal Drug Administration, Margaret Ndomondo, was also an adamant supporter. She argued that because the DLDBs were selling the drugs illegally anyway, it was essential to provide a safer way for them to do so.

Figure F2   Accredited Drug Dispensing Outlet Program Outline

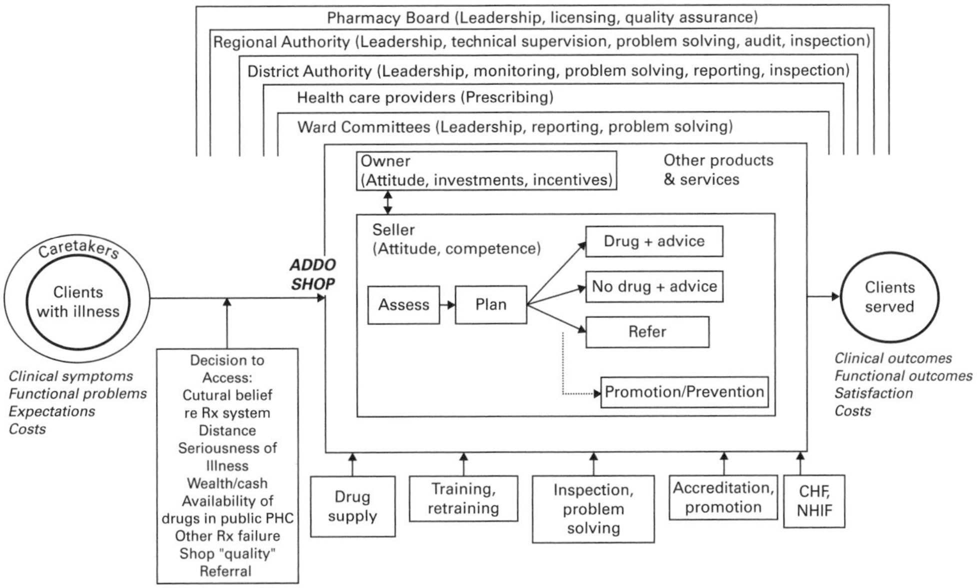

Source: CPM 2003, 74. Reproduced with permission from Management Sciences for Health.

Note: CHF = Community Health Fund; NHIF = National Health Insurance Fund; PHC = primary health care.

MSH provided technical support and funding through SEAM and enlisted other partners, such as the Mennonite Economic Development Associates, for their specific expertise. (After the pilot project was completed in 2005, other donors, including USAID [U.S. Agency for International Development] and the Global Fund, also provided support, as described below.)

With the assistance of SEAM, the Tanzanian Federal Drug Administration developed legally enforceable standards for the ADDOs, including the following:

- Application and approvals procedures

- Building location, design, and layout

- Staffing, training, and continuing education

- Sanitation and hygiene

- Drug list

- Drug quality

- Stock control and handling

- Record keeping

- Inspection and sanctions

- Allowable wholesalers.

By the end of the first year, 150 DLDBs in Ruvuma had been upgraded to ADDOs. In this phase, DLDBs were not required to convert to ADDOs but were highly encouraged to do so. (In fact, more than 90 percent of the DLDBs in Ruvuma did convert, according to program manager Jafary Liana.)

For a DLDB to upgrade to an ADDO, its dispensing staff had to be accredited through a Pharmacy Board–approved course developed by Muhimbili University's School of Pharmacy. Only nurse assistants or above were eligible, and trainees were tested for comprehension at the end of the course. The course provided training on the following:

- Common indications and contraindications for using ADDO-approved drugs

- Dosages and side effects

- When to treat versus when to refer to a health facility

- Collecting and tracking patient information

- Communication skills

- Building layout requirements

- The laws governing dispensing practices

- Management and record keeping

- Practice ethics.

In addition, Mennonite Economic Development Associates provided owners a four-week training course on business skills and management and helped them access loans to upgrade their facilities through local microfinance organizations. After completing their training, the successful candidates received a certificate and ADDO branding materials.

At the end of the pilot in 2004, an evaluation showed that the proportion of unregistered drugs in ADDOs in Ruvuma had fallen from 26 percent to 2 percent. Not all of this was the result of the ADDO initiative however. The Tanzanian Federal Drug Administration had undertaken a variety of quality improvement efforts at the same time, and so, for example, in the neighboring Singida Region, the proportion of unregistered drugs in DLDBs had also declined, from 25 percent to 10 percent. However, the average availability of drugs in Ruvuma was nearly double that in Singida. In addition, in "mystery shopper" tests, just 14 percent of ADDO attendants in Ruvuma inappropriately recommended antibiotics for what were largely viral upper respiratory tract infections, compared to 39 percent of DLDB attendants nationwide in 2001. The percentage of "fever" cases referred to primary care clinics without patients' having first been provided with antimalarials also increased significantly, from 32 percent to 52 percent. This was a practice that had been stressed in ADDO training because overtreatment with those drugs has produced significant increases in drug resistance (CPM 2008).

The Accredited Drug Dispensing Outlet Program Grows and Evolves

Based on the evaluation of the pilot, the decision was made to expand the ADDO program to other regions of Tanzania. By January 2008, rollout was completed in Morogoro, Mtwara, and Rukwa regions, funded in large part by the government of Tanzania. In these four regions, 895 ADDOs were accredited (Rutta et al. 2009, 151). In addition, the decision was made by MOHSW to use the ADDOs as a vehicle for a growing list of other public health programs.

In 2009, the government decided to require all DLDBs to be converted to ADDOs by 2011. All ADDOs within designated regions were given a grace period of three months to convert or cease doing business until they were accredited. In the pilot phase, the costs of training and upgrading had been subsidized with donor funds. In the scale-up, however, DLDB owners and drug sellers had to pay for their own training, at a cost of about US$75.

Decentralization

The Tanzanian Federal Drug Administration was nominally responsible for inspection and enforcement of the ADDO rules, but that was impossible with its limited staff. A key part of the ADDO strategy, therefore, became enlisting and training local government inspectors to provide sensitization, preinspections of shops, accreditation, and enforcement. Local inspectors were to report their findings to a District Drug Technical Advisory Committee composed of the following members:

- The district commissioner, serving as chair

- The district executive director, vice chair

- The district drug inspector or regional drug inspector, secretary

- The district medical officer

- Four other local government officials

- One representative from a local nongovernmental organization

- One consumer representative.

The technical advisory committee, in turn, was asked to report violations to the federal drug administration in the capital, Dar es Salaam. ADDOs that violated standards were to be fined, or in severe cases, shut down. (In practice, few have been sanctioned, and a typical fine has been US$115.) Districts could retain 60 percent of all fees, to help offset the costs of performing inspections.

The decentralization initiative was part of the Tanzanian government's more general efforts in the late 1990s to develop its Local Government Reform Programme. As part of the effort, it decentralized management in a variety of areas to allow local government authorities significantly greater political, administrative, and financial control.

In addition to setting standards, the Tanzanian Federal Drug Administration continued to provide technical assistance and general oversight. The main role of MSH has been technical support. As noted by Keith Johnson, director of program administration for the MSH Center for Pharmaceutical Management, during an interview in September 2009, "MSH's role is primarily now one of helping to scale up [the program] and helping the country facilitate its own program locally." For example, MSH tracks referrals to the local district facilities for integrated management of childhood illness, either dispensaries or district hospitals. That is done through a referral book that is kept at the ADDO and a form that the district facility sends back to the ADDO, once it has seen the patient. This is one of the few formal systems for feedback to the primary intake person in place in Tanzania.

At an ADDO stakeholders' meeting in July 2008, concern was expressed about whether the districts had the money and manpower to carry out all the functions required, especially given the national shortage of individuals with pharmaceutical training (Rutta et al. 2009). Perhaps not surprisingly, the MOHSW wanted the local governments to include ADDO supervision in their plans and budgets. The local governments, in response, wanted the ministry to make more funds available for expenses that they would incur in implementing ADDO. Overall, however, the local governments supported the ADDO idea because it was popular and accepted by the population.

Taking on Malaria

As part of their approved list of medicines, ADDOs can now sell subsidized Coartem®, an artemisinin-based combination therapy (ACT), which is the recommended treatment in Tanzania for malaria. Since 2007 Tanzania, in partnership with the U.S. President's Malaria Initiative, has provided subsidized Coartem, using ADDOs as the private sector distributor in Ruvuma and Morogoro. As of 2009, that was Tanzania's only private sector avenue for distributing subsidized Coartem. Although the unsubsidized market price of Coartem is about US$10 a dose, ADDOs began selling it at about US$1 a dose. ADDOs are required to list the prices for Coartem in a place visible to all customers. The country also received a grant from the Global Fund for AIDS, Tuberculosis and Malaria to subsidize Coartem through ADDOs for all children under five years old.

Future Developments

During the September 2009 stakeholders' meeting, after reviewing the progress of ADDO shops thus far, participants identified several ongoing problems. There was no licensing category either for the ADDO shops or for those who went through the training program. Nor was any mechanism in place for revising the ADDO medicines list. Given the shortage of candidates qualified for training, some participants urged lowering the entry requirements, as well as involving the private sector in providing training (especially because some graduates had left their ADDO shops for better-paying jobs elsewhere).

Enthusiasm was expressed for expanding ADDO in some ways, as was concern about expanding it in others. Problems in access to medicines in poor, periurban areas led to the suggestion that the model should be adapted for those locations, as well as rural areas. But the number of public health functions being added to ADDO was a source of concern to many participants, who urged the government to restrict them to ones deemed truly essential.

References

CPM (Center for Pharmaceutical Management). 2003. *Access to Essential Medicines: Tanzania 2001*. Prepared for the Strategies for Enhancing Access to Medicines Program. Arlington, VA: Management Sciences for Health.

——. 2008. *Accredited Drug Dispensing Outlets in Tanzania Strategies for Enhancing Access to Medicines Program (SEAM)*. Prepared for the SEAM Program. Arlington, VA: Management Sciences for Health.

CIA World Factbook. 2009. "Tanzania 2009." https://www.cia.gov/library/publications/the-world-factbook/index.html. Accessed September 20, 2009.

FIP (International Pharmaceutical Federation). *2009 FIP Global Pharmacy Workforce Report*. The Hague: FIP. http://www.fip.org/files/fip/PharmacyEducation/FIP_workforce_web.pdf. Accessed May 7, 2011.

MSH (Management Sciences for Health) and WHO (World Health Organization). 1997. *Managing Drug Supply: The Selection, Procurement, Distribution and Use of Pharmaceuticals*. 2nd ed. West Hartford, CT: Kumarian Press.

Rutta, E., K. Senauer, K. Johnson, G. Adeya, R. Mbwasi, J. Liana, S Kimatta, M. Sigonda, and E. Alphonce. 2009. "Creating a New Class of Pharmaceutical Services Provider for Underserved Areas: The Tanzania Accredited Drug Dispensing Outlet Experience." *Progress in Community Health Partnerships: Research, Education, and Action* 3 (2): 145–52.

United Republic of Tanzania. 2006. *Millennium Development Goals Progress Report, 2006*. Dar es Salaam: Ministry of Planning, Economy and Empowerment.

Reflections on the Accredited Drug Dispensing Outlet Program

The ADDO case is an interesting example of using the regulation control knob to influence the structure and performance of the private pharmaceutical sector. The underlying problems in Tanzania were typical of those facing many low-income countries. The bulk of drug supply was in the private sector, and yet prices in those shops were often high, and quality was unreliable. That was especially the case in rural areas, where trained manpower was scarce and populations too dispersed to support larger-scale retail enterprises.

What makes this case distinctive is the way in which the initiative evolved. Initially it relied more on "carrots" than "sticks" to elicit participation. It began as a largely voluntary social franchising initiative. In return for following certain guidelines and standards, shop owners were offered training, branding materials, and reliable supplies, and were allowed to sell an expanded range of drugs—including antibiotics. The whole program was supported by an extensive public-private partnership, including funds from the Bill and Melinda Gates Foundation and managerial and technical support from Management Sciences for Health.

Why and how did ADDO evolve into a national regulatory effort? In part the reason was that the evaluation that was done showed real improvement in the pilot region—although the experience in a comparative control group was almost as good on some indicators. (That finding highlights the importance of having a control group in such studies.) Another factor was the strong support it had from some key players in the government, who were very concerned about quality problems in the existing system.

As the program was rolled out nationwide, its regulatory aspect became clearer. Owners had to participate or close their shops, and they had to pay for their own training. In effect, the ADDOs became a whole new class of providers, and the government no longer relied on the notion that increased sales—based on brand identity—would be enough to secure voluntary participation. Those who joined the ADDO system were allowed to sell ACTs at a low price, subsidized by the Global Fund. But that was less for the benefit of the owners than it was a way to use the new infrastructure to distribute the drugs.

Critical to any regulatory initiative is the capacity for inspection and enforcement. And here the ADDO program drew on decentralization ideas (see chapter 9) that were already being followed in Tanzania to transfer responsibilities down to the district level. The usual questions arose of who would pay to support these functions and whether the districts had the necessary technical capacity. But the fundamental approach made much more sense than trying to have a team of specialized inspectors travel over a large and rural country to visit 4,000 relatively small and often-remote locations.

As it evolved, the ADDO initiative found many supporters who wanted to expand its functions and the list of products the shops carried (into family planning, for example). There was also talk of moving the model into periurban slum areas that were also underserved and experienced problems of access to medicines. This is a clear example of a program that was able to achieve *regulatory legitimacy* because of widespread public support for its goals.

But a number of problems also emerged with implementation. It was difficult to find enough qualified personnel to keep the ADDO system going. That was especially so because those who met the qualifications and received the training were sometimes able to move to better-paying jobs elsewhere in the private sector. That risk confronts many efforts to upgrade human resources in the health sectors of low-income countries. Moreover, with the exception of ACTs (and a specific initiative focused on those products), the ADDO scheme did little to bring down prices. As a result, the price and quality difficulties faced by the lowest-income citizens, who often found the ADDOs too expensive and purchased from unlicensed vendors, were not addressed very effectively.

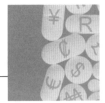

Counterfeit Medicines in Nigeria

Questions to Consider while Reading This Case

This case relates to issues discussed in chapter 10 on the use of regulation to improve pharmaceutical sector performance.

- Why did the government of Nigeria decide to act aggressively on counterfeit medicines at this time?
- What advantages did the new leader of the agency have?
- What particular difficulties did she confront?
- What should her regulatory strategy be? What should she do first and why?
- Where else should she focus her efforts?
- How can she increase the "regulatory legitimacy" of her agency?

Many low- and middle-income countries confront various problems related to the quality of medicines sold in their private sectors (and made available in their public sectors). Key challenges include counterfeit, substandard, and illegal products:

This case was prepared by Eric O. Moore, Michael R. Reich, and Marc J. Roberts. It is intended as a basis for class discussion rather than as an illustration of either effective or ineffective handling of an administrative situation.

- *Counterfeit* products are defined as those whose packaging deliberately misstates what the package contains. This category is commonly called "fake drugs," which are produced to resemble existing products.

- *Substandard* medicines are products that do not meet quality standards because they contain the wrong amount of the active ingredient(s), as a result of poor manufacturing practices or deterioration after manufacturing.

- *Illegal* products are those sold contrary to laws and regulations. They include products imported without a license and ones sold by unlicensed sellers, at illegal prices, or contrary to prescription requirements.

These problems exist to different degrees, and they can intersect. The supply of counterfeit drugs often involves significant criminal activity. Some noncounterfeit supplies are substandard. And many transactions, particularly in the private market, do not conform to legal requirements.

In low-income countries, where many people are poor but are believers in the power of pharmaceuticals, an enormous demand exists for inexpensive medicines. In such situations, there are huge profits to be made from counterfeit medicines. Politicians and even judges may be willing to protect violators for a price. Extensive, uncontrolled borders and widespread skepticism in the population about the capacity of the state to implement policy and enforce laws complicate the issue.

The widespread presence of substandard or counterfeit medicines in the marketplace creates many problems. Medicines with inappropriate or insufficient ingredients will not produce the desired health gains and can contribute to increasing antimicrobial resistance. Illegal retail transactions—especially sales by untrained and unlicensed sellers—can contribute to misuse and poor health outcomes. In addition, consumers who are defrauded (or who suspect that they are being defrauded) are likely to be dissatisfied with the situation and to blame the government for it. Ironically, they may decide to buy higher-priced products to avoid substandard quality, and end up with counterfeit branded products for their trouble.

Such was the situation that Professor Dora Akunyili confronted in Nigeria in 2001, when President Olusegun Obasanjo appointed her to head the Nigerian National Agency for Food and Drug Administration and Control.

Developments in Nigeria

With about 150 million people, Nigeria is the most populous country in Africa and the eighth-largest country in the world. It is also diverse in cultures, languages, and religions, as one might expect in a nation that spans roughly 800 miles east to west and 600 miles north to south. Since gaining independence from England in 1960, Nigeria has been dominated by a series of military governments, mainly controlled by conservative northern Islamic elements. Continuing ethnic tensions and rivalries led in 1967 to a bloody three-year civil war (in which perhaps a million Nigerians died). In response to these fractionalizing forces, much authority has been delegated over the years to the subnational level, and the country now consists of more than 35 states, all with significant governing authority.

The military ruler from 1976 to 1979 was a British-trained general named Olusegun Obasanjo. A commander in the civil war and deputy to the dictator, General Murtala Mohammed, Obasanjo took over when Mohammed was assassinated. Mohammed had announced a timetable for transition to civilian control, and Obasanjo kept to the timetable. The civilian president who was subsequently elected was widely perceived as incompetent and corrupt and was ousted in another military coup in 1985.

Successive military administrations squandered, stole, and mismanaged the country's resources, especially its significant oil revenues. As the world's seventh-largest oil producer, perhaps 40 percent of Nigeria's economy and the bulk of its government revenue come from oil. Nigeria is widely viewed as deeply troubled by corruption, and it has continued to experience internal turmoil stemming from regional, political, and religious differences.

In June 1998, Obasanjo was released from prison on the death of the dictator General Sani Abacha, who had been in power since 1993. Obasanjo had been imprisoned by Abacha after speaking out against human rights violations. Abacha's successors kept his promise to hold elections, and Obasanjo won 63 percent of the vote, carrying both the north and the southeast but doing poorly in the southwest.

Obasanjo began his term by visiting a number of Western countries. He recognized that he needed to improve Nigeria's international image to restore the country's standing in the global community. Focusing on reforms in a number of social and economic sectors, President Obasanjo recognized that it was critical to address the counterfeit medicines problem. Fake and substandard medicines, mainly imported from India and China but also locally produced, were flooding the Nigerian market.

To do that, Obasanjo had to deal with major challenges in the operation of the National Agency for Food and Drug Administration and Control (NAFDAC). NAFDAC was a relatively new, small agency that was widely considered corrupt, with a poorly motivated workforce that functioned without adequate supervision or incentives. Obasanjo knew that he needed an honest and dynamic leader to head NAFDAC if he was to make any progress on this problem. According to some, he also preferred to appoint a woman (Obioha 2009).

Obasanjo Chooses Akunyili

In early 2001, President Obasanjo approached Akunyili about heading NAFDAC. She had been recommended as someone with a reputation for honesty and transparency, who could clean up NAFDAC and the national pharmaceutical market. Akunyili was a pharmacy lecturer at the University of Nigeria, Nsukka, and had also worked for Nigeria's Petroleum Trust Fund, which distributed government oil revenue for infrastructure projects. While serving in the latter position, Akunyili had received US$23,000 from her employer for surgery out of the country. When she discovered that the surgery was not needed, she returned the funds (despite the willingness of her European doctor to write off the amount as spent). It was an act that many Nigerians viewed as extraordinary.

Akunyili's family had also directly experienced the damaging effects of counterfeit medicines: her younger sister, who was diabetic, died in 1988 after receiving fake insulin.

In early 2001, Akunyili received a phone call one Sunday evening from President Obasanjo (Okoro 2005). She went to meet the president the following Tuesday and was subsequently offered the job of director-general of NAFDAC. The president said he wanted her to clean up the counterfeit medicines in the Nigerian market, make the regulatory agency work effectively, and bring Nigeria's food and drug industries up to international standards.

The Problems Akunyili Faced

NAFDAC had been established by Decree No. 15 of 1993 and was expected to perform a wide range of functions (Erhun, Babalola, and Erhun 2001):

- Regulate and control the importation, exportation, manufacture, advertisement, distribution, sale, and use of food, drugs, cosmetics, medical devices, bottled water, and chemicals.

- Conduct appropriate tests and ensure compliance with quality standards for foods, drugs, and so forth, as well as their raw materials.

- Undertake appropriate investigations into the premises producing foods and drugs and establish relevant quality assurance systems, including certification of the production sites.

To carry out those functions, NAFDAC was empowered to compile a wide range of standards, specifications, regulations, and guidelines. It was supposed to undertake the registration and inspection of food and drugs and was also empowered to establish and maintain laboratories and other needed institutions.

In 2001, the agency confronted a very difficult situation. Because of unfair competition and rampant corruption, many multinational companies had left Nigeria in frustration, despite the attractiveness of the large national market. Most genuine drugs were very expensive, driving people to cheaper options, which included counterfeit products. High prices and high demand created great incentives for criminal elements to produce and import counterfeit products. Estimates of the extent of counterfeit medicines in circulation in Nigeria ranged from 48 percent to 80 percent in various studies before 2001.

Nigeria's chaotic medicine production and distribution system made it particularly difficult for regulatory authorities to carry out their responsibilities. The retail system included not only licensed pharmacies, but also nonpharmacists who held licenses as patent and proprietary medicine vendors. Those vendors were involved in the sale of virtually all categories of drugs. Moreover, six or eight of the larger cities had thriving drug markets, chaotic collections of stalls and sellers, often dependent on a small number of wholesalers (some of whom had criminal connections). These drug markets were patronized not only by individual consumers but also by physicians, hospitals, and pharmacies to purchase their pharmaceutical and medical supplies. The total volume of product flowing through them ran into the tens of millions of dollars. Commonly prescribed medicines, such as analgesics and some antibiotics, were openly hawked and sold by petty traders in kiosks, in motor parks, and by the roadside. Drugs were also sold by any number of private and public clinics and hospitals.

Above the retail level were a wide variety of importers, wholesalers, and local pharmaceutical manufacturers. Because of quality concerns, Nigerian drugs were often unwelcome in other African countries. Despite growth in the global pharmaceutical industry, no company had set up a plant to manufacture active pharmaceutical ingredients in Nigeria (NAFDAC Nigeria 2002-5). All raw materials were imported from abroad (mainly from India and China), so that the production taking place in Nigeria was only formulation.

But products imported into Nigeria were not necessarily reliable, and imports accounted for about 70 percent of the country's medicines consumption. Some products being imported were marked "For Export Only." Those labels raised questions about lower quality standards for exports in the exporting country. Moreover, import control was very difficult because of Nigeria's long borders and many small ports. In major transit locations, creative concealment methods were routinely employed by the importers of counterfeit medicines.

The penalties for importing, producing, or distributing counterfeit medicines in Nigeria were too light to be much of a deterrent—imprisonment for between three months and five years or a fine of up to US$3,600. Moreover, enforcement was lax. Government employees were poorly paid and supervised, and drug counterfeiters regularly resorted to bribery, intimidation, harassment, blackmail, threats, and physical attacks on regulators. Growing sophistication by counterfeiters in copying packaging made it increasingly difficult for everyone—customers, enforcers, and pharmacists—to tell the difference between real and counterfeit merchandise.

Imagine that you are a friend of Akunyili. What would you advise her about where to start and where to focus her efforts as the new director of NAFDAC? How can she make a difference in controlling counterfeit medicines in Nigeria? What strategies should she follow? What assets does she have, and how could she take advantage of them?

References

Erhun, W. O., O. O. Babalola, and M. O. Erhun. 2001. "Drug Regulation and Control in Nigeria: The Challenge of Counterfeit Drugs." *Journal of Health and Population in Developing Countries* 4: 23–34.

NAFDAC Nigeria. 2002–05. "The Evolution of Drug Production in Nigeria." http://www.nafdacnigeria.org/drugproduction.html. Accessed July 16, 2009.

Obioha, R. 2009. "Akunyili and Her Critics." *Sun Newspaper* (Lagos), January 23. http://www.sunnewsonline.com/webpages/columnists/obioha/obioha-jan-23-2009.htm. Accessed August 13, 2009.

Okoro, N. 2005. "Nigeria—A One Woman Army." *Probe News Magazine* (Dhaka), September 2–8. http://www.probenewsmagazine.com/index.php?index=2&contentId=269. Accessed August 13, 2009.

Reflections on the Case of Counterfeit Medicines in Nigeria

Professor Akunyili's most important asset in taking on this difficult job was her support from and access to the president. He was a newly elected ex-general trying to establish his credibility with the population. Making progress on an important issue such as fake drugs was one way for him to do that. In addition, Akunyili's technical expertise and well-deserved reputation for integrity served her well when she approached reorganizing NAFDAC, enabling her to attract staff interested in working in a high-profile and non-corrupt environment. She also had a talent for public relations and was comfortable using the media to advance her program (and herself).

NAFDAC needed to make many internal changes to meet its broad range of responsibilities: to simplify rules, develop better testing capacity, and strengthen inspection and enforcement efforts. Moreover, to complement increased enforcement activities, "Professor Dora," as she was widely known, needed to rally public support. The police, the judiciary, and local political elites were not reliable allies. An aroused public was a potentially critical source of pressure to get them to cooperate. Legitimate drug manufacturers and sellers (such as firms whose products were being counterfeited) might also become a source of some support.

Engaging in high-profile actions that attracted media attention was one possible approach. But any grandstanding had to go hand-in-hand with real improvements if gains were to be sustained. Moreover, both the retail sellers of counterfeit medicines and the criminal gangs that controlled much of the business could be expected to use whatever resources they possessed (from political pressure to bribery to violence) to oppose NAFDAC's efforts.

Because this case occurred some years ago, we are able to review what NAFDAC did under Akunyili's leadership.

NAFDAC Initiatives against Counterfeit Medicines

While Professor Akunyili headed NAFDAC, the agency implemented a number of initiatives (Akunyili 2006):

- *A national public awareness campaign.* The agency explained the counterfeit medicines problem in numerous newspaper and radio advertisements. An intensive media campaign communicated the message that all legitimate products (domestic and imported) had to have a NAFDAC registration number on the packaging.

- *Seizure and destruction of counterfeit goods.* From 2001 to July 2005, over 1,000 raids were carried out on drug hawkers, distributers, and transporters. Efforts were made to trace the counterfeit supply chain by pressuring hawkers for information on suppliers and warehouse owners who were their sources. Every few weeks, NAFDAC made a widely publicized show of burning large stocks of confiscated fake medicines, destroying hundreds of millions of dollars in counterfeit supplies.

- *Closure of major drug markets.* The three largest retail drug markets—the source of much of the fake drug supply—were closed for periods of three to six months (including the nation's largest, Onitsha drug market in Anambra state). Associated clinics that provided fraudulent treatment and warehouses used to store the material were also closed.

- *Import controls at the source.* NAFDAC employees inspected factories in India, China, and Egypt to ensure good manufacturing practice (GMP) compliance and to recertify drugs before they were exported to Nigeria. Nigerian banks cooperated by insisting on NAFDAC clearance before processing financial documents for medicine importers.

- *Increased surveillance at ports of entry.* The government restricted medicines imports to two designated airports and two seaports, facilitating increased surveillance of imports. To foster compliance, NAFDAC guidelines specified that aircraft carrying medicines into Nigeria without NAFDAC authorization could be impounded.

- *Streamlining and enforcing registration guidelines.* The requirement that medicines comply with laboratory standards and inspection requirements before being registered was more consistently enforced. Sanctions on noncompliant manufacturers and importers increased steadily, from 2,226 such actions in 2002, to 4,132 in 2005.

- *Increasing international awareness.* To help mobilize cooperation by foreign governments, including exporting countries, Akunyili spoke at many international conferences to promote awareness about Nigeria's efforts to control counterfeit medicines.

Restructuring NAFDAC

- *Staff reorientation and motivation.* A major effort was made to identify and remove corrupt and ineffective staff. Promotion practices were changed and opportunities for foreign training were introduced to motivate workers and reward good performance.

- *Restructuring.* Two new directorates, Ports Inspection and Enforcement, were created to focus those efforts. Procedures and practices were changed to foster delegation and eliminate bureaucratic bottlenecks.

- *Increased capacity.* Ten new state offices were established, and the existing 27 offices were strengthened to cover Nigeria's 36 states and Federal Capital Territory. Three special inspectorate offices were established in the three towns with the biggest medicine markets.

- *Laboratory modernization.* Laboratories were refurbished and two additional ones were built. Standard operating procedures and guidelines were developed, and processes were automated.

Challenges

Despite these changes and initiatives, many challenges remained for NAFDAC:

- *Staffing.* NAFDAC continued to have difficulty obtaining the money and manpower it needed to carry out its many responsibilities.

- *Bureaucratic rivalry.* Nigerian Customs was not receptive to the newly created Directorate of Ports Inspection, which it viewed as intruding into its sphere of operations.

- *Corruption.* Drug counterfeiters continued to bribe customs officials, police, and members of the judiciary to escape prosecution. As of 2010, only about 50 cases had been brought under the anticounterfeit legislation that was passed in 1999.

- *Violent resistance.* NAFDAC's laboratory in Lagos was vandalized, and in March 2004, NAFDAC facilities across the country were burned. Several attempts (including one very close call) were made on Akunyili's life.

- *Smuggling.* With NAFDAC unable to cover all the small ports and overland routes into Nigeria, smuggling became an ever-increasing problem.

- *Quality problems.* As of 2005, NAFDAC claimed that the incidence of counterfeit medicines had been reduced by over 80 percent compared to the situation in 2001. However, in a 2008 study of 144 samples of essential medicines purchased in Lagos-area private pharmacies 18 percent failed basic drug quality tests. Although the sample size is small (and biased toward more reliable sellers), the study suggests that quality problems remain in the Nigerian medicine market (Bate et al. 2009).

- *Consumer attitudes.* Nigerians continued to be concerned about medicines quality. Some questioned whether the highly public burning of fake drugs really solved the problem and whether the progress made by NAFDAC could be sustained.

- *Reopening of urban drug markets.* The major urban drug markets all reopened with only limited regulation and remained a focus for the supply of counterfeit medicines.

Recent Developments

- The sales ban on drugs made in Nigeria has been lifted by neighboring West African countries, and drugs made in or imported through Nigeria are now common throughout the region. Sixteen new drug manufacturing companies were established between 2002 and 2005.

- In 2008–09, contaminated medicine killed more than 84 children in Nigeria between the ages of four months and two years. A "teething mixture" called My Pikin (Oghenerhaboke 2008) was contaminated by diethylene glycol that was sold by an unlicensed chemical dealer in Lagos to the manufacturer (Polgreen 2009).

- In late 2008, Akunyili completed her tenure as the director-general of NAFDAC and began serving as minister for information in the cabinet of President Umar Yar'Adua.

- Dr. Paul B. Orhii was appointed the new director-general of NAFDAC in January 2009. A United States–based lawyer, physician, and pharmacologist, Orhii was a specialist in pharmaceutical litigation.

- In May 2009, NAFDAC confiscated a large shipment of counterfeit antimalarials from China with "Made in India" labels. The packaging was very sophisticated, but laboratory analysis showed no active ingredients (Sen 2009).

- In August 2009, NAFDAC announced that it would open offices in Indian cities that are prominent centers for pharmaceutical production to enhance surveillance and regulation of medicine imports (ET Bureau 2009).

Final Reflections

Professor Akunyili proved herself an adept bureaucratic strategist. Her highly publicized efforts in closing the big drug markets and burning huge volumes of confiscated products brought NAFDAC a great deal of positive attention. The idea that products had to have a NAFDAC registration number was effectively communicated to the public, and legitimate participants in the medicines supply chain became mobilized to support NAFDAC's efforts.

But Akunyili's efforts were more complex than just those public activities, reflecting an awareness of the need for a multifaceted approach. It was sensible to work to control the importation of fake drugs by limiting the number of access points and increasing enforcement capacity. Implementing the registration numbers program also required the creation of more laboratory testing capacity to support the registration process. Local observers agree that real improvements have been made in NAFDAC's levels of competence and professionalism.

The work has not always proceeded smoothly. Smuggling has remained a significant problem. Other police and enforcement agencies (especially customs) have not cooperated in aggressively pursuing cases that NAFDAC has developed. Moreover, under local political pressure, the major drug markets have all reopened, and although the presence of counterfeit drugs in the country has been reduced, it is unclear by how much. Consumers are still worried about medicines quality in a nation with thousands of miles of borders that cannot be policed effectively.

On the plus side, products made in Nigeria are now more widely accepted in nearby West African countries, as NAFDAC has done a better job policing the country's domestic manufacturers. And ironically, the assaults on Akunyili and on some NAFDAC locations suggest that the agency's enforcement efforts were making some criminals very uncomfortable. Akunyili is now well known in Nigeria (and in drug policy circles internationally) and has gone on to a different ministerial job. But until even greater resources and political support are devoted to the problem, no one will be able to declare victory in this particular war.

References

Akunyili, D. 2006. "Women Leadership in Emerging Democracy—My NAFDAC Experience." Speech delivered at the Woodrow Wilson International Center for Scholars, Washington, DC, May 1. http://www.wilsoncenter.org/events/docs/Akunyili_speech.pdf. Accessed July 16, 2009.

Bate, R., T. Ayodele, R. Tren, K. Hess, and O. Sotola. 2009. "Drug Use in Nigeria: An Informal Survey of Doctors, Pharmacists, and Healthcare Workers in Lagos, Ondo, and Ogun, and a Pilot Quality Assessment of Essential Drugs from Lagos Pharmacies." Working Paper, Africa Fighting Malaria, American Enterprise Institute, and the Initiative for Public Policy Analysis, Washington, DC.

ET Bureau. 2009. "Nigerian Drug Regulator to Open Indian Offices." *Economic Times* (India), August 5. http://economictimes.indiatimes.com/News/Economy/Nigerian-drug-regulator-to-open-Indian-offices/articleshow/4860464.cms. Accessed August 5, 2009.

Oghenerhaboke, A. 2008. "My Pikin, the Killer." *Newswatch Magazine*. December 8. http://www.newswatchngr.com/index.php?option=com_content&task=view&id=338&Itemid=48. Accessed September 13, 2009.

Polgreen, L. 2009. "84 Children Are Killed by Medicine in Nigeria." *New York Times*, February 7.

Sen, A. 2009. "China Owns up Nigeria Fake Drugs Cargo." *Economic Times* (India), August 4. http://economictimes.indiatimes.com/News/Economy/Foreign-Trade/China-owns-up-Nigerian-fake-drugs-cargo/articleshow/4854410.cms. Accessed August 5, 2009.

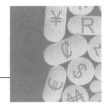

Changing the Use of Antibiotics in Peru

Questions to Consider while Reading This Case

This case relates to issues presented in chapter 11 on using persuasion to influence pharmaceutical use.

- The case sets the stage for the task of developing a social marketing campaign designed to promote the "rational use" of antibiotics in Peru.

- As you read the case, reflect on the extent to which the behavior of key players is or is not "irrational."

- If you were going to persuade these key players to change their behavior, how could you make that new behavior fit with their underlying motivation?

- What specific messages would you formulate? Where and how would you convey them to your target audiences?

Drug resistance is the ability of a microorganism to survive an encounter with antimicrobial drugs. As explained in one World Health Organization (WHO) report, "The use of an antimicrobial . . . in any dose and over any

---

This case was prepared by Anya Levy Guyer and Michael R. Reich. It is intended as a basis for class discussion rather than to illustrate either effective or ineffective handling of an administrative situation.

time period, forces microbes to either adapt or die in a phenomenon known as 'selective pressure.' The microbes that adapt and survive carry genes for resistance, which can be passed on" (WHO 2002). WHO frames campaigns to promote appropriate regulation, prescribing, and use of antibiotics as promoting the "rational use" of medicines (WHO 2009). A key part of the problem of medicine use that promotes drug resistance is that "patients experienced with the benefits of antimicrobials tend to self-medicate, even when they may have access to formal health care services" (Yeager et al. 2006).

In 2003, Peru's ministry of health became very concerned with the problem of growing drug resistance. One report on Peru from the Pan American Health Organization (PAHO) highlighted the problem. "No matter how much we spend on care . . . everything can be wasted if we cannot ensure the antimicrobials that are marketed are of good quality and can produce the therapeutic effect expected" (PAHO/SAIDI 2009, 174). To assess the situation, the ministry collected biological samples from children under five with various bacterial infections, including pneumonia, shingles, and urinary tract infections (INS 2003). Depending on the bug, between 30 percent and 80 percent of the samples were resistant to treatment by standard, first-line antibiotics.

The Peru Context

A lower-middle-income country of more than 27 million people, Peru was racked in the 1980s by a fierce armed struggle against a Maoist insurgency (the so-called Shining Path). During the early 1990s, under President Alberto Fujimori, the insurgency was brought under control and the economy began growing. By the end of the decade, however, an internal political and economic crisis was building, triggered in part by international economic disruptions. In 2001, it finally led to the removal of President Fujimori and his administration. A transitional government was put in place to prepare for new elections in 2002. The two subsequent elected administrations had "heralded transparency and the fight against corruption as key aspects of their political stance" (Ramis 2007).

Peru's public health establishment provides the bulk of its health services. The country has three government-run systems: a system run by the ministry of health, a social security system for formal sector employees, and separate health services for the armed forces and police. These three systems account for over half of the country's hospitals and more than two-thirds of the health centers. In 2004, Peru spent 4 percent of its gross domestic product on health expenditures, a figure that had remained steady for a decade.

In 2004, the ministry of health spent about 10 percent of its budget—nearly US$50 million—on pharmaceutical products, a bit under US$2 per capita. A cost recovery policy for medicines, introduced in the public sector in 1994, had created financial barriers to access for many people. According to a 2004–05 study of 600 outpatients in 20 ministry facilities (including hospitals, health centers, and health posts), 33 percent of patients paid for their medicines directly. The costs of medicines for other patients were covered by various subsidy programs. However, 15 percent of patients did not obtain medicines because they had no money. Meanwhile, Peru was estimated to have more than 11,000 private pharmacies and drugstores, with private drug sales in 2004 averaging US$13.23 per capita, or about 85 percent of all drug spending (Ministry of Health 2006).

In the decades before 2005, Peru had made several efforts to address appropriate drug use. Throughout the 1990s, occasional mass media campaigns focused on the use of antidiarrheal drugs and promoted the use of oral rehydration solutions (Homedes and Ugalde 2001). Other programs were designed to encourage pharmacists and community health workers to promote cost containment and prevent the misuse of antibiotics. In the mid-1990s, efforts were focused on providers to try to stem the rise of drug-resistant tuberculosis in poor urban communities (Mitnick et al. 2003).

In the 1990s, Peru also implemented activities to address antibiotic use in hospitals. The country built laboratory capacity to ensure the quality of available medicines and to help monitor disease-causing organisms for the development of resistance. It put in place administrative efforts to change the use of medicines in hospitals, to prevent the development and transmission of drug-resistant infections in clinical settings.

In 2001, the ministry had begun tightening the regulations governing prescribing. Most prescribing was restricted to physicians. Dentists and midwives were restricted to prescribing only those drugs used in their particular practices. All drugs, whether prescription or over-the-counter, were to be sold only at accredited outlets and not through the informal sector (according to Decreto Supremo No. 021-2001-SA).

To improve use, both prescribers and pharmacists were required to provide patients with a variety of information. This included appropriate doses, period of administration, any adverse reactions and interactions that the drug could produce, and any precautions that were recommended to ensure correct and safe use (Ministry of Health 2006).

Continuing Challenges

The misuse of medicines that led to drug resistance in Peru reflected both supply-side and demand-side factors, that is, the behavior of both patients and health professionals. A ministry study identified multiple behavior patterns and situations in the pharmaceutical sector that contributed to the rise of drug resistance in Peru, including the following:

- Incorrect prescribing (wrong drug or wrong dosage)

- Easy access to antibiotics in pharmacies and markets

- Improper self-medication by patients

- Bacterial contact with pharmaceuticals in the hospital environment

- General overuse of antibiotics for viruses or other diseases (INS 2003).

A ministry publication of 2006 identified several causes of these patterns. First were the economic incentives for doctors to overprescribe and for pharmacists to overlook restrictions on dispensing. At the same time, high prices gave poor patients an incentive to purchase only partial prescriptions. Further, the population-wide effects of inappropriate antibiotic use were rarely immediately evident to the individual users. The ministry also identified a lack of information and education among both prescribers and the general public about the risks of misuse. The use of medicines, wrote the ministry, was influenced by cultural attitudes all along the "chain of health care" (Ministry of Health 2006).

Callao, a coastal area near the capital, Lima, was selected as a pilot site, and several studies of prescribing practices were carried out there. Among the findings were the following:

(1) The proportion of consultations that resulted in a prescription for antibiotics was 64 percent, with an average of 2.38 medicines per consultation; 53 percent of the consultations were for children under five years of age.

(2) Among patients diagnosed as having upper respiratory infection, 71 percent received prescriptions for antibiotics.

(3) The proportion of establishments that sold antimicrobials without asking for a prescription was 79 percent; among private establishments, 92 percent sold antimicrobials without a prescription.

(4) In a representative sample of adults in Callao, 75 percent reported self-medication, and 49.8 percent of those reported that they would purchase only a partial treatment.

(5) Dispensers in both the public and private sectors lacked access to independent sources of information on medicines (PAHO/SAIDI 2009:63).

Based on those results, Peru's government and nongovernmental organization partners, with support from partners in the South American Infectious Disease Initiative (the U.S. Agency for International Development, PAHO, and neighboring countries), began to design a pilot intervention to persuade community members to change the way they used medicines to treat respiratory and diarrheal diseases among children under age five.

- Imagine that you were part of the task force. Identify the main target audiences for changing antibiotic use in these children and the behaviors that each target audience should adopt.

- Assess the underlying determinants of the behaviors that contribute to the development of antimicrobial resistance.

- Propose how you would persuade the target audiences to adopt the new behaviors.

- Identify the four Ps (product, place, price, and promotion) that you think the steering committee should recommend as the main components of the campaign.

References

Homedes, N., and A. Ugalde. 2001. "Improving the Use of Pharmaceuticals through Patient and Community Level Interventions." *Social Science and Medicine* 52: 99–134.

INS (Instituto Nacional de Salud). 2003. *Vigilancia de la Resistencia Antimicrobiana en el Perú*. Informe Perú. Lima: INS.

Ministry of Health (Peru). 2006. "Evaluación de la Situación de los Medicamentos en el Perú." Ministry of Health, Department of Medicines, Consumables, and Drugs (MINSA/DIGEMID), Lima. http://www.digemid.minsa.gob.pe/daum/urm/evasitmedicamentos.pdf.

Mitnick, C., J. Bayona, E. Palacios, S. Shin, J. Furin, F. Alcantara, E. Sanchez, M. Sarria, M. Becerra, M. C. Smith, S. Fawzi, D. Kapiga, D. Neuberg, J. H. Maguire, J. Y. Kim, and P. Farmer. 2003. "Community-Based Therapy for Multidrug-Resistant Tuberculosis in Lima, Peru." *New England Journal of Medicine* 348 (2): 119–28.

PAHO/SAIDI (Pan American Health Organization and South American Infectious Disease Initiative). 2009. *Perfil de País Perú—Resistencia Antimicrobiana*. Washington, DC: PAHO.

Ramis, O. 2007. "Medicines Transparency Alliance—Peru Scoping Study." DFID Health Resource Centre, London.

WHO (World Health Organization). 2002. "Antimicrobial Resistance." Fact sheet N·194, WHO, Geneva. http://www.who.int/mediacentre/factsheets/fs194/en/.

——. 2009. "Rational Use of Medicines." http://www.who.int/medicines/areas/rational_use/en/. Accessed September 24, 2009.

Yeager, B., E. Barillas, A. Sosa, and A. Barojas. 2006. "Workshop with SAIDI National and International Partners to Prioritize the Objectives and Activities of a Plan to Contain and Prevent Antimicrobial Resistance in Paraguay" and SAIDI Steering Committee Meeting, June 20–30. Submitted to United States Agency for International Development by the Rational Pharmaceutical Management Plus Program. Management Sciences for Health, Arlington, VA. http://pdf.usaid.gov/pdf_docs/PDACI133.pdf.

Reflections on the Use of Antibiotics in Peru

The group that developed the campaign in Callao identified mothers of young children as the most important target audience because they were the ones purchasing the medicines and supervising their use. The mothers were busy and not easy to reach. Clearly, they were concerned with the health of their children, but they also had both economic and time constraints to manage. And in communicating to those mothers, the intervention's planners did not want to simply come out against the use of antibiotics. Instead the public health community needed those mothers to continue to use antibiotics but to use them in a more restrained and appropriate fashion.

The second-most-important actors were doctors and pharmacists. As noted in the case, they had obvious economic motives for collaborating in the pervasive polypharmacy. Doctors also desired both to please patients and, in public clinic settings, to move them through quickly. In such situations they had every reason to promptly provide patients with the prescriptions they expected. But neither health professionals nor most mothers wanted to contribute to a rise in antimicrobial resistance that would cause them all significant problems in the years ahead.

After considering these factors, the committee decided that an intensive, one-week campaign was needed to get the attention of the public and to shift the community toward a "healthy culture" focused on the rational use of antibiotics. The campaign was designed in response to the considerations reviewed above: *"Los Antimicrobianos son necesarios . . . debemos usarlos con responsabilidad"* (Antimicrobial drugs are necessary—we must use them responsibly).

The week began with a press conference, and the campaign was announced with huge posters all over the city. During the week, marches, festivals, and other public events were held, all with press coverage. Campaign materials were distributed in schools, in pharmacies, and on the street. Materials with the campaign logo and slogan were produced and distributed:

- 10,000 pens

- 5,500 spiral notebooks

- 10,000 magnetic mini phone books

- 15,000 posters

- 50,000 bifold brochures

- 5,000 plastic bags

- 5,000 folders.

The campaign organizers hoped that a saturation effort would expose most of the target audience repeatedly to the message about "responsible use" as they traversed their life-path points during the week.

The more detailed messages for consumers attempted to spell out the implications of the general slogan and appealed to mothers' sense of responsibility. They included a number of themes designed to move the community toward rational use and away from both self-medication and purchasing medicines from the informal sector:

- Using antimicrobials without a doctor's prescription is harmful to your health and that of your family.

- Antimicrobials from the black market put your life at risk.

- Caring for your health is your responsibility. If you feel ill, go to a health facility.

- Buy antimicrobials in pharmacies and drugstores registered with the ministry of health.

- When you are prescribed medications, complete the entire treatment.

- Taking antimicrobials when you have a virus will not cure your infection.

A complementary set of messages was produced for doctors and other health workers. Miniconferences were held at hospitals and at the local university to convince these professionals that they had a responsibility to improve the use of antibiotics. To appeal to this target audience's intrinsic motivation, the emphasis was on being sophisticated and expert in exercising one's professional responsibility:

- Appropriate use of antimicrobials allows us to treat serious infections.

- An irresponsible attitude toward the use of antimicrobials has a negative impact on the public health of our population.

- Prescribe antimicrobial using internationally recognized terminology, not a brand name.

- Base your antimicrobial prescriptions on independent, evidence-based information, therapeutic guidelines, and treatment protocols.

- Do not be influenced by promotion and advertising of antimicrobials—each patient requires individualized treatment.

The experience with this campaign on rational use of antibiotics in Peru shows that behavior change is not easy to produce. Aggressive and sophisticated efforts are required, and even then, success is hardly guaranteed. Unfortunately, we have not been able to uncover any detailed evaluation of the impact of the efforts in Callao.

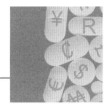

CASE STUDY I

Preparing for Microbicide Introduction in South Africa

Questions to Consider while Reading This Case

This case relates to chapter 11, on using persuasion to influence pharmaceutical use. At the end of the case, you are asked to develop a social marketing plan for the introduction of micro-bicides. As you read the case consider the following:

- What are the alternative target audiences for such a campaign, and what specific behaviors would you want them to adopt?

- Considering those various groups, what motivations would you seek to harness to influence them to choose the behavior in question?

- What, in the beliefs or circumstances of various target audiences, might lead them not to adopt that behavior?

- How do your answers to these questions influence your choice of target audience and your specific marketing plan (product, place, price, and promotion)?

- What additional research would help you do a better job in plan development?

This case was prepared by Anya Levy Guyer, Michael R. Reich, and Marc J. Roberts, with an update on recent events by Pamela Norick. Portions of this case are based on J. Becker et al., *Paving the Path: Preparing for Microbicide Introduction, Report of a Qualitative Study in South Africa* (New York: EngenderHealth, International Partnership for Microbicides, University of Cape Town and Population Council, 2004). This case study is intended as a basis for class discussion rather than as an illustration of either effective or ineffective handling of an administrative situation.

South Africa is one of the most economically and culturally diverse countries in the world. Its approximately 50 million citizens are divided in many ways, in what the country itself calls "the Rainbow Nation." The 80 percent of the population that is of African origin speaks nine officially recognized languages. The 10 percent of the population that is white is of British and Dutch background and is culturally quite divided. Substantial mixed-race communities are also present, as well as Indian and other Asian minority groups.

Economic and social conditions are as varied as the demographics. The average income of the African population is roughly 15 percent of the income of whites, and the income of Indians is 60 percent. The top 10 percent of the income distribution gathers nearly 60 percent of the national income, and essentially all the poor are either black or mixed race, many living in urban areas (Liebbrandt et al. 2010). The unemployment rate among young, urban African men was estimated at 40 percent to 50 percent in 2001 (Kingdon and Knight 2001).

In the low-income, periurban townships, social conditions reflect those economic difficulties. Housing stock is of low quality, and access to utilities uneven. Levels of crime and violence—especially sexual violence—are high. Some analysts believe that the rate of rape is the highest in the world, with up to 30 percent of women reporting such experiences. In one survey in a mixed-race and black community, 25 percent of the men responded that they had committed sexual violence (Jewkes et al. 2009).

Those patterns contribute to rates of HIV in South Africa that are among the world's highest, and HIV is primarily transmitted by heterosexual activity. The problems posed by these high rates have been exacerbated by years of government policy neglect of the issue. In the absence of effective public education, many myths spread in the community—including the idea that sex with a virgin cures AIDS, an idea that has contributed to extensive sexual violence against young girls. Estimates are that about 30 percent of all women attending antenatal clinics in South African are HIV positive, but among women 25 to 35 years old the number is closer to 40 percent. The prevalence among men is somewhat lower, at 15 percent to 25 percent depending on age (www.avert.org/safricastats). (HIV prevalence rates among provinces, however, vary greatly.)

The Potential Role of Microbicides

In the context of this discussion, "microbicide" does not refer to a compound that kills microbes. Rather, it refers to topical products being developed to prevent the transmission of HIV. Microbicides could take many forms, including daily vaginal gels, films, or tablets, or contained in a vaginal ring that releases the active ingredient gradually and provides protection against HIV for up to a month. A microbicide would be a significant complement to other HIV prevention measures, such as condoms, treatment of sexually transmitted infections, safe blood supplies, and other existing approaches. It is also possible that microbicides will be developed that could be used rectally.

Because of the urgency of the global AIDS epidemic, major efforts are now under way to support the accelerated development of microbicides to prevent HIV transmission. In 2002 and during the years since, various groups involved in microbicide development have come together to identify strategies for introducing a microbicide, once a product is developed that is proven safe and effective and is approved for use. Their work has been informed by the realization that historically, technological innovations have sometimes encountered significant obstacles that might have been avoided with more careful preparation. In the case of microbicides, it is obviously important to understand the gender-related, social, economic, cultural, and structural contexts in preparation for introducing these new products.

Conducting a Study

To better understand the issues and problems involved, a consortium of local and international nongovernmental organizations and local researchers conducted a study that included both individual interviews and focus group discussions in Langa, a periurban site in the Western Cape Province of South Africa, and at national and provincial levels. The study took place between September 2002 and September 2003. Those surveyed included community members, health care providers and managers, provincial and national government officials, and representatives from national and provincial nongovernmental organizations and health professional bodies. A local advisory group, which included stakeholders drawn from the community, public health practitioners, and policy makers, supported and informed the research design and implementation.

Apart from its high HIV rates, South Africa was selected for the study because it was the site of a number of clinical trials and acceptability studies of microbicides and had a potentially sizable market for them. Given the country's relatively extensive clinical experience with microbicides, and the urgency of the epidemic, it is likely that South Africa will be one of the first countries to introduce a microbicide once safety and effectiveness are established in the future.

Findings of the Study

The most powerful arguments for microbicides that emerged from the data were the severe effect of the AIDS epidemic on people's everyday lives and the desperate need for new approaches to help curtail the spread of the disease. Respondents clearly understood women's social vulnerability to HIV infection and their limited ability to protect themselves. Many spoke openly—and spontaneously—about the underlying social, economic, and political factors that contribute to women's lack of control over sexual relations. Because microbicides were expected to be mostly female initiated and controlled, participants felt that the products could provide an important way for women to protect themselves, particularly given widespread male resistance to condom use.

Many respondents felt real frustration at the relatively long time before an effective microbicide could potentially be made available. Because of the devastating impact of the HIV/AIDS epidemic in South Africa, a sense of desperation was evident among community participants, providers, and policy makers for something that could help prevent HIV infection. (Since the time of the consultation, a study released in 2010 showed that a particular microbicide gel is effective in decreasing HIV infection rates in women. Confirmatory studies of the gel are ongoing, and a product could be available for introduction in 2013.)

Implications of Introducing a Partially Effective Product

Respondents were concerned about the partial effectiveness of the first generation of microbicides, presented as ranging from 40 percent to 70 percent. Despite apprehensions among a few providers and policy makers about promoting a partially effective method, most saw it as a trade-off, pointing out that no method is 100 percent effective, including condoms with typical use. The severity of the situation led many women to feel that it was preferable to take some action, rather than do nothing, even if microbicides were not 100 percent effective.

Initially, all groups of respondents expressed some unease about the implications of introducing microbicides as stand-alone products, given that they will be less effective than condoms. Many were more comfortable with microbicides as a complement or addition to existing prevention options, as part of a mix of methods that people would be able to choose from. In particular, some felt that microbicides should be positioned alongside male and female condoms as a dual method—and only used as stand-alone products where other, more effective prevention options were not feasible.

Policy makers and providers reflexively positioned condoms as the "gold standard," and expressed some concern that introducing microbicides might lead people to switch from condoms to microbicides, undermining condom use. Some community members confirmed this possibility, indicating that the primary appeal of microbicides was as an alternative to condoms. On further reflection most respondents acknowledged the condom's limitations, particularly because actual use is quite low among many vulnerable groups. That suggests the importance of developing approaches and messages for introducing microbicides that reflect their potential for HIV risk reduction in the situation as it actually exists, rather than in the context of a theoretical ideal.

The discussion illustrated the challenges of accurately conveying complex messages about risk reduction and the options presented by a partially effective product. A striking element of the interviews was the evolution of providers' and policy makers' concerns about microbicides' partial effectiveness. While many began by expressing some apprehension about practical and ethical implications, they often came to a more positive view as the interviews proceeded. That suggests that some initial concerns and assumptions in the general population may also be amenable to change by a carefully designed social marketing campaign.

Covert or Overt Use

Women's lack of power in sexual relationships was cited as both a barrier and an incentive to microbicide use. Some participants, both women and men, strongly recommended partner involvement and open communication about microbicide use, and many believed that such communication would be feasible. Other participants, however, felt that in the context of some relationships, where trust between partners was lacking, covert use would be a necessary alternative. They cited situations where women lacked the power to negotiate the method's use, or where they feared repercussions, including violence. Community members, service providers, and policy makers alike questioned women's ability to negotiate microbicide use in such situations and said that even covert use might be difficult or could result in negative repercussions if discovered.

One of the primary unexpected findings was the degree to which respondents—especially community members—assumed that an important application for microbicides would be for women to protect themselves in case of rape. Women also discussed the utility of microbicides in the case of unplanned consensual sex. Both of these uses assume that women would be able to apply a microbicide as part of a daily routine. That would require that a microbicide have a relatively long duration of action and that it be both affordable and convenient enough to be used daily. That has important implications for microbicide development and for how microbicides are introduced or marketed.

Wetness, Lubrication, and Acceptability

Respondents across categories had different perceptions about how important added lubrication might be in enhancing or hampering microbicide acceptability and use. Consistent with recent reviews of that issue, the extensive discussions and widely varying views of lubrication underscore the need to examine the actual meanings associated with wetness and lubrication in different social groups, rather than rely on assumptions about practices and preferences. Similarly, the different perceptions of policy makers and community members with regard to women's comfort with use of a vaginal product point to the importance of examining actual experience rather than making assumptions. Beliefs and assertions by policy makers or providers that "women won't use them [microbicides]" because they are inserted vaginally could erroneously inhibit support for microbicides, even in settings where women regularly use vaginal products.

Distribution, Marketing, Supply, and Cost

Almost all participants felt that microbicides should be distributed widely. That meant moving beyond obvious locations such as health clinics devoted to family planning or maternal and child health. Instead, the participants recommended focusing on places where women congregated and locations that were easily accessible in the community, such as chemists, supermarkets, and shops where herbal medicines are obtained; local informal shops and bars; and community-based organizations. However, despite a desire for widespread access, many respondents at all levels hesitated to endorse distribution of the products in venues where personal counseling was not available or quality control would be difficult to ensure.

In community focus groups, men and women of all ages and socioeconomic groups stressed the need for media campaigns and for sources of information to be available at such places as churches, schools, libraries, and other community organizations. At the same time, several policy-level respondents warned about problems if demand for the product is created at the community level before supplies are sustainable. Citing some experience with the female condom, they underscored that a reliable and affordable supply needed to be in place before widespread marketing of microbicides began. To address those concerns, and to allow users to become familiar with the products, some suggested a gradual introduction strategy.

National and provincial policy makers, key policy informants, and providers all stressed that microbicides should be accessible to clients and should be provided at low cost or free. Some community and policy-level respondents supported the assertion of social marketers that products distributed in the public sector, or free of charge, are seen as inferior to other products. Finally, a number of policy makers expressed concern about the cost to the health system, the lack of resources throughout all levels of the health system, and the difficult decisions that must be made among competing priorities.

Positioning and Distribution Strategies

Findings from the study suggest that microbicides could be positioned for a wide range of potential users. Although in other settings people often assume that "high-risk groups," particularly sex workers, would be the most likely and appropriate users, respondents in this study suggested a much wider range, including children (in the case of rape) and "older" married women. Providers and community members assumed that younger, unmarried women, including youth, would be important users of microbicides. However, some policy makers were less supportive of targeting youth because of the potential to undermine recent gains in condom use. Strikingly little stigma was associated with microbicides or the people who might use them, and a real sense prevailed that microbicides would be "mainstream" products.

Need for Information

Policy makers, providers, and community participants all stated that they would need information about effectiveness, efficacy, safety, side effects, and contraindications before they would recommend microbicides to clients or support their introduction. Because the first microbicides will not provide complete protection, both national and provincial-level policy makers pointed out that clients must be fully aware of the implications of partial effectiveness. They emphasized a desire for evidence from both animal and human clinical studies to determine whether microbicides were in fact safe and effective. The conversation also revealed that many participants did not fully understand such basic concepts as safety, efficacy, and partial effectiveness. In response some policy makers highlighted the need to grasp how to convey these concepts to potential users, stressing the need for simple yet comprehensive information to facilitate informed choice.

Because understanding is growing concerning how relationships and other circumstances influence condom use, it would be useful to explore explicitly how those forces are likely to play out with respect to microbicides. Concerns about condom substitution will likely shift with any changes in condom use that may occur: if condom use increases before microbicides are introduced, condom substitution may become more of a concern. Because of the long time required for microbicide development and introduction, that issue will need to be continually revisited to take account of any changes in patterns of condom use.

The Situation in 2010

In 2010, ongoing, studies finally produced proof that a topical microbicide could prevent heterosexual transmission of HIV. Data from a study known as the "CAPRISA 004" trial, announced in July 2010, provided "proof of concept" for a particular vaginal microbicide—1 percent tenofovir gel. Tenofovir is an antiretroviral (ARV) that has been used successfully to prevent mother-to-child transmission of HIV. The new trial showed that topically applied to the vaginal mucosa, it could protect against HIV and herpes simplex virus (HSV-2).

The study followed 889 women in South Africa. Overall, it found a statistically significant 39 percent lower HIV infection rate in women after 30 months of tenofovir use, compared with women using a placebo gel, and a 51 percent protective effect against HSV-2. Tenofovir gel was shown to be safe as tested when used up to 12 hours before sex and again within 12 hours after sex, for a maximum of two doses in 24 hours. It was the 12th microbicide efficacy study and the first to demonstrate a statistically significant reduction in HIV transmission. It was also the first study to test a vaginally applied ARV for efficacy. Previously tested products, known as "early generation microbicides," did not act specifically against HIV, and none was proven effective in reducing the risk of HIV infection.

In August 2010, the joint United Nations Programme on HIV/AIDS, the World Health Organization, and the South African government convened a meeting in Johannesburg with more than 80 researchers, regulators, funders, civil society representatives, and policy makers to discuss next steps with the tenofovir gel microbicide. Most of the discussion focused on what additional testing of safety and efficacy should be conducted and what data would be necessary to convince various regulatory authorities (including the U.S. Food and Drug Administration) to accept the product.

Imagine that this meeting, in addition, included a social marketing working group. That group was charged with beginning to think about a plan for introducing the new microbicide, using the information collected in the 2002–03 survey. Because a potential product now existed, the group was asked to think about what the product would be, that is, what pattern of use it would recommend. Who would the target market be? What should be the main messages (promotion)? Where and how should they be communicated (place)? Finally, where should the product be available and at what price? To be convincing, any such plan would have to address the potential motivations of the target group and the difficulties it might face in adopting the promoted behavior and should contain an explanation of why that group was selected.

References

Becker, J., R. Dabash, D. Cooper, J. Harries, M. Hoffman, P. Orner, J. Moodley, E. McGrory, and H. Bracken. 2004. *Paving the Path: Preparing for Microbicide Introduction, Report of a Qualitative Study in South Africa*. New York: EngenderHealth, International Partnership for Microbicides, University of Cape Town, and Population Council.

Jewkes, R., Y. Sikweyiya, R. Morrell, and K. Dunkle. 2009. "Understanding Men's Health and Use of Violence: Interface of Rape and HIV in South Africa." MRC Policy Brief, Medical Research Council, Pretoria.

Kingdon, G., and J. Knight. 2001. "Race and the Incidence of Unemployment in South Africa." Working Paper for the Center for the Study of African Economies, Department of Economics, University of Oxford, United Kingdom.

Leibbrandt, M., I. Woolard, A. Finn, and J. Argent. 2010. "Trends in South African Income Distribution and Poverty since the Fall of Apartheid." Social, Employment and Migration Working Papers 101, Organisation for Economic Co-operation and Development, Paris.

Reflections on Introducing Microbicides in South Africa

This case involves the challenges of persuading women to adopt a new technology that has not previously existed but that has the potential to prevent a life-threatening infection, HIV. That means that they cannot use an existing model to understand what a microbicide is, what it does, and how it is to be used. Indeed, the word "microbicide" may not be immediately understood because in this instance, it does *not* refer to something that kills microbes or germs. Microbicides are designed specifically to kill or inactivate HIV and may also prevent other viruses, such as HSV-2 or herpes. They are a topical product to be used to *reduce* the risk of HIV transmission during sexual relations. The fact that the compounds being tested come in different forms (gels, rings, and films) means that they will vary in method of application, frequency of use, and duration of protection. All of those characteristics of the product (still to be finalized) will have profound implications for user adoption and for social marketing efforts.

As the case indicates, there are important questions about what the "product" will be—and particularly how it should relate to condom use. Most policy makers and providers clearly would prefer that microbicides be used as a complement to, rather than a substitute for, condoms to get full protection. And they are reluctant to do anything that will undermine the modest and hard-to-achieve gains they have made in condom use. But given women's high level of vulnerability and the prevalence of sexual violence in South Africa and elsewhere, as well as the possibility that consensual male partners may object to condom use, it is clear that a great deal of discreet microbicide use will likely occur. Campaigns to promote microbicide use thus will need to be designed in ways to support campaigns for continued male condom use, especially for groups such as couples in longer-term relationships.

Other choices also must be made concerning this product. Will users have to obtain a prescription for it? Will they be required to obtain, or will they have to be offered, counseling on HIV infection before a microbicide is provided? Will they have to have an HIV test, and if so, how often? The point is that, properly understood, the "product" is a complex combination of a technology, the terms of access to that technology, and its pattern of use. It is not just something that comes in a box.

The next question is, Who is the target audience? Is it all women who are HIV-negative? Or should the target be particular groups of HIV-negative women, depending on their level of risk and sexual activities? If one were to select the highest-risk subgroups, that might imply commercial sex workers. Or it might be sexually active younger women who were likely to have multiple partners or little power over their sexual lives. In light of the concerns expressed in the case, one might ask whether any way exists to identify and target those women considered vulnerable to forced sex. Again, the choice intersects with the issue of condom use, as different target audiences will be subject to different risks of otherwise unprotected sex.

The message will depend in part on the target group. The selection of the target group will also affect how the message relates to fears, emotions, and empowerment desires. The admonition to "protect your future children" may work for some and not others. Appeals to female empowerment (such as "woman-controlled risk reduction" or "control your own body and your own future") may be more effective in urban than rural areas. Protecting children will again mean a different kind of campaign.

Cost is also an issue. Almost everyone believes that the first microbicide will need to be highly subsidized in Africa. It will probably have to be offered at very low cost or free to end users. The concerns that community members expressed for ease of access and wide availability imply and assume that the method will be inexpensive and low-risk—and available for general use. But that is not the only conceivable scenario. A microbicide could be free, for example, to young women and to commercial sex workers who agree to an HIV test. All of those decisions will affect the design of a social marketing campaign around product, place, price, and promotion.

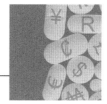

Drug Coverage in Ghana's National Health Insurance Scheme

Questions to Consider while Reading This Case

This case relates to the issues of financing and paying for medicines presented in chapters 7 and 8. The case illustrates the pharmaceutical financing choices facing low- and middle-income countries.

- If Ghana wanted to provide expanded access to medicines, what other choices did it have besides creating something like the NHIS?

- What were the particular problems that the NHIS drug benefit was intended to overcome?

- To what extent, as of 2008, had it accomplished its goal?

- Who ended up actually paying for the benefit?

- What role did decentralization play in the scheme's emerging problems?

- If you were to advise the government, what changes in the scheme would you suggest? How can it make revenues match expenses?

This case was prepared by Nathan J. Blanchet, Marc J. Roberts, and Michael R. Reich. It is intended as a basis for class discussion rather than as an illustration of either effective or ineffective handling of an administrative situation.

In January 2009, Ghana's former vice president, John Atta Mills, of the National Democratic Congress, won a runoff election for president by a very narrow margin—about one half of one percent—and with the narrowest of parliamentary majorities. It was a major victory for a man who had lost the previous two elections in 2000 and 2004. A big decision facing the incoming administration was what to do about the financial crisis that was then developing in the country's recently introduced National Health Insurance Scheme (NHIS), especially with respect to its drug benefits. The scheme had been the centerpiece of the rival New Patriotic Party's program at the beginning of the decade. But by 2008, medicine spending accounted for nearly half of annual NHIS expenditures (46 percent), and funding to support the system was becoming insufficient.

As of 2008, Ghana's health system functioned relatively well compared to those in similar African countries. After two decades of reform, 60 percent of the population lived within an hour's travel time (by foot) of a health facility. With two doctors and nine nurses or midwives per 10,000 people, Ghana's human resource levels were about twice those of its neighbors. About 70 percent of all children received BCG (bacille Calmette-Guerin, a vaccine for tuberculosis [TB]); measles; diphtheria, pertussis, tetanus (DPT); and polio immunization by 12 months. In addition, rates for several individual vaccinations were in the mid-90 percent range. The total fertility rate had also decreased markedly from 6.4 births per woman in 1998 to 4.0 births per woman in 2008 (GSS 2009). Life expectancy at birth was 60 years, and World Health Organization (WHO) data put under-five mortality at 115 per 1,000 live births.

All this had been accomplished with a per capita income of about US$590 and with 29 percent of the population living below the poverty line (World Bank 2009). Ghana had attained the Abuja Declaration target of allocating 15 percent of public spending to health, although total health expenditures remained low (at US$33 per capita, compared to an average of US$75 in lower-middle-income countries) (World Bank 2009). The country was rapidly urbanizing, though about 60 percent of the population still resided in rural areas and agriculture accounted for about one-third of the national economy.

Ghana's health care delivery system included both public and private sector facilities (48 percent and 9 percent of all facilities, respectively) (Segre and Tran 2008). Nonprofit facilities, most notably those run by the Christian Health Association of Ghana, received substantial financial support from the government and were often viewed as an "implementer" alongside the (larger) public Ghana Health Service. However, frequent stock-outs at all these facilities, even of essential medicines, regularly drove patients to the private sector. Because 90 percent of private pharmacies were located in urban areas, in rural areas licensed "chemical sellers" played a prominent role in supplying medicines to the population and were often the first point of contact for patients seeking care.

The disease burden confronting the system had been steadily changing. Infectious diseases still accounted for a large share of outpatient visits, with malaria alone recently accounting for 40 percent. Directly Observed Treatment Short-course coverage for TB had technically reached 100 percent, but the quality of that coverage remained low in many places (USAID 2009). The country's HIV prevalence (between 2.2 percent and 3.6 percent) was below prevalence rates in many other countries in the region (Ballou-Aares et al. 2008). Recent economic growth had led to an increase in noncommunicable diseases. WHO reported rises in hypertension, diabetes, chronic renal disease and cancer, as well as in alcohol and tobacco use and substance abuse (WHO 2006).

The National Health Insurance Scheme

In 2000, the opposition New Patriotic Party (NPP) was voted into power, in part based on its campaign promise to abolish the cash-and-carry drug policy and fees for outpatient services that had been introduced during the severe economic turmoil in the 1980s. (The only two previous elections, in 1992 and 1996, had been won by the ruling National Democratic Congress [NDC]. That party was established by Flight Lieutenant Jerry Rawlings, who originally came to power in a military coup in 1981.) In 2003, the NPP fulfilled its campaign promises by passing the National Health Insurance Act. It did so over the vehement opposition of the NDC, which cooperated with allied unions to organize strikes in protest and even walked out of the legislature in an unsuccessful effort to block passage of the reform.

In this highly charged climate, influential leaders in the NPP decided that the new initiative had to meet three criteria:

- The policy had to result in establishment of a national system that could quickly be scaled up to cover the majority of the population.

- The policy had to be publicly perceived as an NPP initiative, not a continuation of the previous government's efforts.

- The policy had to be formulated and passed through Parliament before the elections in 2004.

The creation of the NHIS followed in 2004, and actual benefits began to be provided in late 2005 (Witter and Garshong 2009). (The NPP was returned to power in the 2004 elections.) The NHIS was intended to be a universal, mandatory system implemented through district-level health insurance schemes. As discussed further below, the commitment to universality in a country with so many low-income families led to a scheme that included low premiums, and a generous exemption policy even from those obligations, as well as an extensive benefit package.

The benefit package, established centrally, was intended to cover 95 percent of the disease burden in Ghana. It covered outpatient services, including diagnostic testing; most inpatient services, including specialist care and most surgeries; dentistry; maternity care including cesarean deliveries; emergency care; and finally, all drugs on the centrally established National Health Insurance Authority (NHIA) Medicines List (NHIS 2009). In sum, the NHIS essentially covered all services except very expensive procedures: certain surgeries, cancer treatments, organ transplants, nonvital services such as cosmetic surgery, and some high-profile items covered under other programs.

The NHIS benefit package was apparently agreed upon over the objections of the technical experts on the steering committee, who thought it too generous. The provisions setting reimbursement rates for medicines were reported to have been heavily influenced by pharmaceutical companies (Rajkotia 2007).

The Structure of the National Health Insurance Scheme

The National Health Insurance Fund (NHIF) subsidizes district-level schemes, which in turn reimburse providers based on claims submitted. Since 1992 Ghana had been experimenting with district-level community financing schemes, which were supported by church groups, United Nations Children's Fund (UNICEF), and the previous government. Politically popular, those schemes were not always well administered and only covered a small percentage of the population. Allowing many of them to be converted into district-level NHIS schemes was politically expedient, and it facilitated the rollout of the new system.

The NHIF is financed from several sources:

- The National Health Insurance Levy (NHIL), a dedicated 2.5 percent value added tax (VAT) on goods and services, which was added on top of the pre-existing VAT.

- Involuntary payroll deductions from formal sector employees (2.5 percent, diverted from a 17.5 percent social security tax)

- Premiums paid by informal sector workers, set at about US$8 per adult by the NHIA

- Other funds voted by Parliament from general revenue and designated to cover the costs of exempt populations

- Additional income from investments, loans, and donations.

The dedicated VAT is the most important funding stream, accounting for 70 percent to 75 percent of revenue. Formal sector social security contributions are next, making up 20 percent to 25 percent, and informal sector premiums represent the smallest share, at 5 percent. However, large parts of the population are exempt from any payment, including all minors under 18, all adults over 70, pensioners, and the indigent. The ministry of health has calculated that the exempt groups may account for as much as 70 percent of the population (Back and Graymore 2007).

By 2008, 48 percent of Ghana's population held an NHIS membership card, according to the NHIA. An additional 10 percent had enrolled in NHIS but not yet received a membership card. Coverage rates varied substantially by region, ranging from 13 percent to 70 percent. As of 2007, roughly 40 percent of the lowest income quintile was enrolled, compared to 70 percent of the highest income quintile (Ballou-Aares et al. 2008).

The National Health Insurance Drug Benefit

The drug benefit was not financed with a separate flow of funds but through the general funding mechanisms described above. Separate financing from various donors covers some specific drugs, such as those for HIV/AIDS and TB and psychiatric medicines. The systems for supplying these medicines operate outside the NHIS drug coverage scheme. For example, antiretrovirals are provided separately under Ghana's National AIDS Control Program.

The NHIS benefit package covered all drugs on the NHIA Medicines List (which is more extensive than the separate essential medicines list established by the Ghana National Drugs Program). District-level schemes must adhere to the benefit package by covering 28 therapeutic classes and hundreds of different drugs and formulations (Ghana NHIA 2009). The NHIA Medicines List is supposed to set a maximum reimbursement price for each drug, based on the median price in the market (Seiter and Gyansa-Lutterodt 2009). Some reports suggest, however, that pharmaceutical companies greatly influenced the prices that were initially specified (Rajkotia, 2007). For an overview of the general pharmaceutical market in Ghana, see annex J1.

To receive the NHIS drug benefit, a card-holding NHIS member (patient) has to obtain a prescription from a physician and fill it at an NHIS participating chemical seller, pharmacy, clinic, or hospital. No co-payment is required. The providers then submit claims to that patient's district insurance scheme, which reviews the claim against Standard Treatment Guidelines, and if it is approved, reimburses the provider according to the prices set by the NHIA Medicines List. This process also applies to any medicines used in inpatient settings.

Some providers have tried to evade the rule against co-payments, for example, by requiring patients to pay for brand-name drugs not on the NHIA list when the listed generics were not available. Other forms of fraud and noncompliance were also reported to occur at times, leading to costs borne by patients (Seiter and Gyansa-Lutterodt 2009).

The NHIS has apparently increased access to health care and to medicines. Outpatient visits per capita increased from 0.55 in 2005, to 0.75 in 2008. Drug utilization also increased. One report found that the number of medicines per prescription rose from 4.5 in 2004 to 6.0 in 2008 (Ballou-Aares et al. 2008). An increase in access to formal care and a decrease in out-of-pocket payments have been documented in at least one district (Witter and Garshong 2009). Some have suggested that the new drugs benefit was driving a shift in Ghanaians' preferences for self-treatment through informal (but very accessible) chemical sellers, toward a preference for formal care and prescriptions. Indeed, some observers worried that the increases in health service use might be pushing demand "beyond what is medically necessary" (Witter and Garshong 2009). However, a preliminary analysis of the top 100 drugs by cost and utilization in the NHIS (based on 10 percent of claims data) shows a pattern of use not inconsistent with the country's disease burden (see table J1). Key health status indicators had

Table J1 Top 100 Drugs in the National Health Insurance Scheme by Cost and Utilization

Drug category	% of Cost	% of Utilization
Antimalaria	21.4	14.80
Anti-infectives (excluding antimalarials)	18.4	20.30
Cardiovascular	13.3	3.40
Diabetes	10.3	0.59
Analgesic (pain management)	7.9	23.40
Antacids and antiulcer	7.7	1.30
Vitamins and minerals	6.6	19.60

Source: Mensah and Acheampong 2009a.

mostly been stable since 2005, although 2008 was too early to expect to see much impact from the program.

Given all these forces, the drug benefit grew to account for nearly half of annual NHIS expenditures (see figure J1). The increase was also reflected in increased turnover in revolving drug funds at the periphery level (Seiter and Gyansa-Lutterodt 2009). The average cost of drugs per claim also grew, from 1.32 Ghanaian cedis (¢) (approximately US$0.90) per claim in 2006, to ¢3.8 (approximately US$2.62) in 2007, and to ¢5.21 (approximately US$3.60) in 2008.

Some regional variation in benefit use also occurred. In 2008, enrollment in the NHIS across Ghana's 10 regions ranged from 13 percent in Central to 70 percent in Upper West. However, drug expenditure patterns did not necessarily match the enrollment figures. For example, Upper West had the highest enrollment but the lowest drug claims cost per capita. The average drug cost per claim also varied from ¢1.76 in the Upper West to ¢9.31 in the Volta Region (see figure J2 for complete data).

Current Challenges

The NHIS enjoyed two years without cash shortages, thanks to an accrual from social security taxes before its operations began. But by 2008, it owed

Figure J1   Drug Costs as a Proportion of Total National Health Insurance Claims Costs

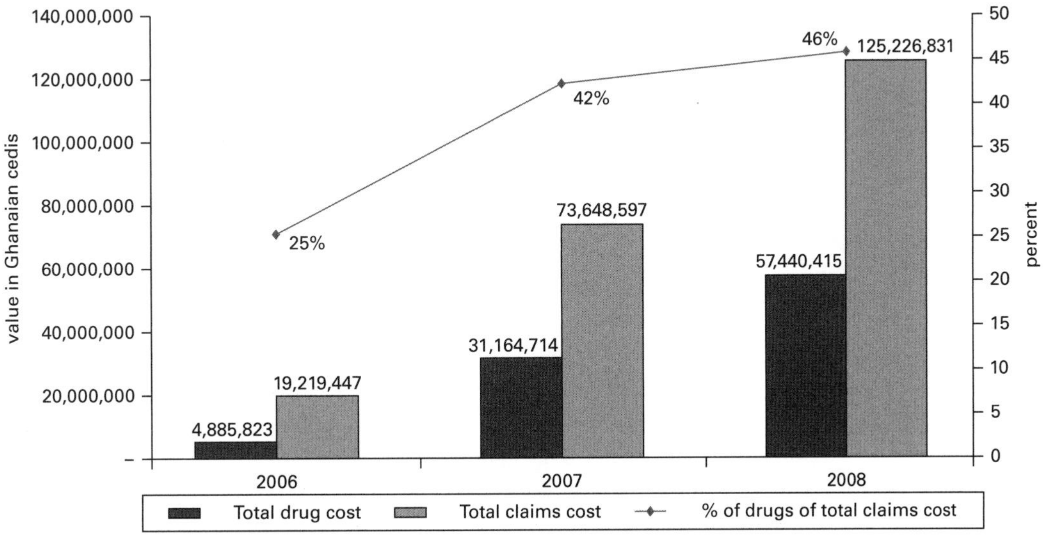

Source: Mensah and Acheampong 2009b.

Figure J2 Regional Analysis of National Health Insurance Per Capita Costs and Participation Rates

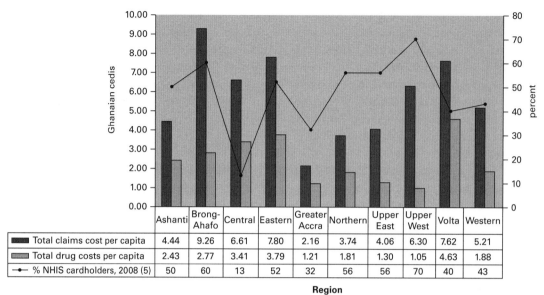

	Ashanti	Brong-Ahafo	Central	Eastern	Greater Accra	Northern	Upper East	Upper West	Volta	Western
Total claims cost per capita	4.44	9.26	6.61	7.80	2.16	3.74	4.06	6.30	7.62	5.21
Total drug costs per capita	2.43	2.77	3.41	3.79	1.21	1.81	1.30	1.05	4.63	1.88
% NHIS cardholders, 2008 (5)	50	60	13	52	32	56	56	70	40	43

Region

Source: Mensah and Acheampong 2009b.
Note: Per capita rates were calculated by dividing NHIA's total costs by the ministry of health's latest regional population estimates.

US$34 million to health facilities, mostly in the form of unpaid claims. The number of "distressed" districts also increased; the NHIA had paid 8.32 million cedis (US$5.75 million) to support them (Witter and Garshong 2009). The troubles were partly due to the low subsidy rate per exempted member that the schemes receive from the NHIS: ¢14 (or US$9.67) per year. That figure was reportedly set based on the average premium rates of pre-existing mutual health organizations. However, those organizations had offered much more limited benefits than the NHIS (Witter and Garshong 2009).

The financial shortfalls then began causing problems in the medicines supply chain. The supply system relies on revolving funds at each level. Payment delays can lead to what several authors have called "crippling levels of indebtedness" throughout the system. The mismanagement of cash at the facility level, reimbursement rates set too low for retailers to cover their costs, and the increased capital needed to meet increases in demand also led to the insufficiency of working capital (Ballou-Aares et al. 2008).

Part of the difficulty was a matter of timing. In 2008, average reimbursement time for NHIS claims was three months, which put great pressure on chronically cash-strapped health facilities (Ballou-Aares et al. 2008). As a result, in some cases, NHIS patients were denied treatment unless they paid out-of-pocket (Seiter and Gyansa-Lutterodt 2009). Also, some retailers dropped out of the scheme. About half of all district schemes had significant arrears with providers, and most schemes stopped the practice of automatically paying 40 percent of a claim immediately upon its receipt (Ballou-Aares et al. 2008; Seiter and Gyansa-Lutterodt 2009). (The 40 percent prepayment was an NHIA guideline meant to ease providers' liquidity problems. Increasing it to 80 percent or 90 percent has been suggested, but it is not clear how a higher percentage would be workable if even the 40 percent level is not adhered to.)

In addition to the general fiscal imbalance, part of the challenge the government faced in early 2009 came from the scheme's decentralized structure. Not all districts seemed to be up to the task of effective cash management and claims processing. Moreover, high spending in some districts, based on a large number of distinct medicines per claim, led to questions about the possibility of corruption in those areas. The main questions confronting the government were what changes to make, and how to make them, to maintain the viability of the scheme and yet retain its politically popular features.

References

Back, E., and D. Graymore. 2007. "Towards a Medicines Transparency Alliance (META) in Ghana: Preliminary Scoping Study Report." Unpublished draft, U.K. Department for International Development Health Resource Centre, London.

Ballou-Aares, D., A. Freitas, L. R. Kopczak, S. Kraiselburd, M. Laverty, E. Macharia, and P. Yadav. 2008. *Private Sector Role in Health Supply Chains*. New York: Rockefeller Foundation, Dalberg Global Development Advisors, and Massachusetts Institute of Technology–Zarazoga International Logistics Program.

Ghana NHIA (National Health Insurance Authority). 2009. *NHIS Medicines List*. Accra: Ghana NHIA http://www.nhis.gov.gh/_Uploads/dbsAttachedFiles/MedicinesFinal.pdf. [For the list with prices for some drugs, see http://www.chagghana.org/chag/assets/files/Medicines%20List.pdf.]

GSS (Ghana Statistical Service, Ghana Health Service, and Macro International). 2009. *Ghana Demographic and Health Survey 2008: Preliminary Report*. Accra: Ghana Statistical Service, Ghana Health Service and Macro International.

Mensah, S. A., and O. B. Acheampong. 2009a. "Analysis of Top 100 Drugs by Cost and Utilization: First Quarter 2009." National Health Insurance Authority, Accra.

——. 2009b. "National Claims Expenditures and Cost of Drugs: 2006–2008." National Health Insurance Authority, Accra.

NHIS (National Health Insurance Scheme). 2009. "NHIS Benefits Package." NHIS, Accra. http://www.nhis.gov.gh/?CategoryID=158&ArticleID=120&print=1.

Segre, J., and J. Tran. 2008. "What Works: CareShop Ghana—Improving Access to Essential Drugs through Conversion Franchising." World Resources Institute, Washington, DC. http://www.nextbillion.net/archive/files/CareShop%20 Ghana.pdf.

Seiter, A., and M. Gyansa-Lutterodt. 2009. "Policy Note: The Pharmaceutical Sector in Ghana." World Bank, Washington, DC.

Rajkotia, Y. 2007. "The Political Development of the Ghanaian National Health Insurance System: Lessons in Health Governance.", Health Systems 20/20 Project, Abt Associates Inc. Bethesda, MD.

USAID (U.S. Agency for International Development). 2009. "Tuberculosis Country Profile: Ghana." USAID, Washington, DC. http://www.usaid.gov/our_work/ global_health/id/tuberculosis/countries/africa/ghana_profile.html.

World Bank. 2009. *World Development Indicators*. Washington, DC: World Bank. http://econ.worldbank.org.

WHO (World Health Organization). 2006. "Country Cooperation Strategy: At a Glance—Ghana." WHO, Accra. http://www.who.int/countryfocus/cooperation_ strategy/ccsbrief_gha_en.pdf.

Witter, S., and B. Garshong. 2009. "Something Old or Something New? Social Health Insurance in Ghana." *BMC International Health and Human Rights* 9: 20.

Annex J1: Overview of the Pharmaceutical Market and Supply and Purchasing of Drugs

Note: Material in this annex is based on Seiter and Gyansa-Lutterodt (2009), unless otherwise noted.

First, some background on the market. The entire Ghanaian pharmaceutical market was estimated at US$250 million, at retail price level, in 2005 and probably grew to about US$300 million by 2008. Several major manufacturers have integrated distribution businesses in the country, including vans for delivering drugs to remote areas. There are 200–300 businesses involved in the import and wholesale distribution of drugs, along with 1,600 pharmacies and 10,000 licensed chemical sellers at the retail level. Some private doctors and midwives also sell drugs directly to patients.

About 70 percent of the market is prescription drugs, and 30 percent is over the counter. The private sector reportedly dominates the drug supply chain, with even public buyers in remote areas increasingly bypassing the public system of Central and Regional Medical Stores (CMS and RMS) and procuring directly from private suppliers. At the RMS and service-delivery point level, as much as 80 percent is purchased from the private sector rather than the public CMS, partly because private suppliers offer greater flexibility in purchasing and distribution.

Although the private sector dominates the supply chain, it is not clear how much drug purchasing is by public facilities and how much by private. However, some information on overall expenditures is available. The best rough estimates suggest that public sources account for about 65 percent of drug expenditures (see table J2 for the breakdown).

Table J2 Sources of Funding for Prescription Drug Purchases in 2008

Payer	Spending (US$ millions)
Ministry of health, including pooled donor funds	31
U.S. President's Malaria Initiative (PMI) ACT procurement	2
NHIS	120
Donors to Christian Health Association of Ghana for buying drugs (assumption)	1
Out-of-pocket spending	80
Total	234

Source: Seiter and Gyansa-Lutterodt 2009.
Note: ACT = artemisinin-based combination therapy. Figures are rough estimates except for ministry of health and PMI; includes nondrug items such as bed nets, syringes, etc.

Other facts relevant to the public-private balance include the following:

• Korle Bu, Ghana's premier, semiautonomous teaching hospital, represented US$2 million worth of drug procurement in 2007, with 70 percent coming from private suppliers. Korle Bu Hospital's providers write about 2,000 prescriptions per day, probably the largest volume of any facility in Ghana.

• The Christian Health Association of Ghana (CHAG) runs 144 hospitals and health centers that serve about 35 percent to 40 percent of Ghana's population, mostly in rural areas. Though private, CHAG receives between 45 percent and 60 percent of its funding from the Ghanaian government and collaborates closely with the Ghana Health Service. Because of the unique relationship between CHAG and the government, it would be difficult to categorize CHAG facilities' drug purchases as public or private.

• Up to one-fifth of the Central Medical Store's sales are to private entities, including private hospitals, mission hospitals, and nongovernmental organizations (Ballou-Aares et al. 2008).

Reflections on the Ghana Case

The Ghana case vividly illustrates the dilemma facing a low-income country that is trying to respond to citizen dissatisfaction with the costs of medicines. As discussed in chapter 2, political leaders are especially sensitive to that aspect of the pharmaceutical system. Indeed, popular dissatisfaction about Ghana's cash-and-carry system for medicines and health care was critical to the NPP's ability to defeat the ruling NDP in the elections of 2000.

But a major challenge for government is how to raise the funds to provide these benefits. The NHIS system that Ghana created is often called "social health insurance," but the Ghanaian version is far from the ideal form. In particular, contributions from those covered provide little revenue. Instead, the main funding source for Ghana's NHIS is a dedicated VAT. Because it is a dedicated tax, citizens were apparently relatively willing to accept the rate increase involved. In a country such as Ghana, with large rural and informal sectors to the economy, the burden of such a tax is likely to be slightly progressive (although there is no technical analysis to demonstrate that), unlike the generally regressive impact of a VAT in industrial economies. But for Ghana, passing the new law was the easy part; making it work over time has turned out to be more difficult.

The new system seems to have met some of its goals. Financial protection has improved, satisfaction is up, and price barriers to effective access have gone down enough so that utilization has increased. That increase, however, is both a sought-for result and a longer-run problem. In the early years the NHIS was partly financed by surpluses from the pension system; those funds have now been depleted. Moreover, as the system took hold, drug costs began to rise steeply, reaching 46 percent of total system expenditures per year. But VAT revenues will generally grow only as quickly as the economy grows. The demand for medicines is likely to grow much faster, especially when people no longer have to pay for them out-of-pocket. Thus a long-run fiscal crisis in Ghana's NHIS was more-or-less inevitable.

Decentralization has only made matters worse. It has necessitated the creation of numerous claims processing units in a country that is hard-pressed to find the technical expertise to run such activities. As discussed in chapter 10, activities like claims processing, with large economies of scale, and in which uniformity is valuable, are probably not the ones a country ought to consider for decentralization.

In Ghana, decentralization was included in the design in part because it allowed the two main political parties to control the operation of the system in the areas where they controlled the local government. But as with other examples of "decentralization of corruption," that political fact raises the question of whether the high levels of (probably partially fraudulent) claims payments to some sellers were facilitated by payoffs to local party leaders (as some informants suggested).

As fiscal pressures on Ghana's NHIS have increased, slow payment of bills has depleted the working capital in the system, making it difficult to operate. The question posed at the end of the case is what the NDP government, newly returned to power, should do about the situation.

No easy or simple answers are available. Without a clear electoral mandate, the option of disassembling the NHIS is not advisable. Recentralizing some of the claims processing to cut down on corruption and overuse is one possibility. Trying to enforce more appropriate use of medicines, through monitoring of prescribing patterns or by enforcing clinical guidelines, will be much more difficult in a country with a large rural population and where many sellers maintain only minimal records. Narrowing the list of drugs covered seems like a potentially useful step—provided the government can withstand the political opposition that would likely arise from the pharmaceutical industry and some patient groups. Meanwhile, contacts in Ghana suggest that the government is hoping that revenue from newly discovered oil reserves may solve its problem, at least for the medium term. Otherwise, it is difficult to see how the current benefit package and financing system can survive in the long run without significant modifications.

GLOSSARY

Accountability for reasonableness (A4R). The principle (proposed by Norman Daniels) that decision-making processes should be open and transparent and decisions should be reached on the basis of explicit criteria and justified by publicly available reasoning.

Allocative efficiency. A condition in an economic system in which the correct set of products is produced and distributed to the appropriate consumers, in order to maximize the performance of the system as a whole.

Barriers to entry. Conditions that limit the ability of additional sellers to compete in a given market. These could be due to government action (e.g., patent protection), the efforts of existing sellers (e.g., heavy advertising of brand-name products), or underlying technology (e.g., only very large-scale and expensive production facilities can reach the lowest costs).

Benchmarking. The process of comparing one's rate of performance to some external standard, such as the quality level of acknowledged industry leaders or the health status results reached by other similar countries.

Blockbuster drug. A medicine that while still on patent achieves global sales over $1 billion per year (typically in upper-income-country markets) and produces significant profits for the originator company.

Brand-name drug. A medicine produced by a specific manufacturer that has been sufficiently advertised and promoted so that consumers recognize the trade name (which may be a protected trademark) under which that medicine is sold.

Branded generic. A brand-name drugs that either no longer is, or never was, protected by patents but that still has name recognition in the marketplace.

Cash-and-carry. Retail or wholesale trade in which customers pay cash and carry the goods away themselves. Typical in private sector retail transactions, cash-and-carry has historically also been used in some public sector drug supply systems.

Community financing. Locally controlled small-scale social insurance schemes in low-income countries, typically based on a village or a collection of adjoining villages. In some versions the fund is supplemented by transfers from higher levels of government, especially for poorer locations.

Control knobs. Specific arenas in which governments can intervene to improve the functioning of their health systems in general and their pharmaceutical sectors in particular. The five control knobs are financing, payment, organization, regulation, and persuasion.

Counterfeit medicines. Products that falsely represent their source or contents, whether on the container, the packaging, or the labeling, or the product itself.

Decision space. The different dimensions of authority that managers have over an organization's activities, such as purchasing, budgeting, pricing, or personnel. The concept, proposed by Thomas Bossert, is particularly relevant for describing the degree of decentralization in a larger system.

Diagnostic tree. An analytical device used to systematically describe the causes, and the causes of causes, of an identified weakness in the performance of a health or pharmaceutical system.

Disability Adjusted Life Years (DALY). An index to measure the burden of disease in a population by comparing its actual quality and quantity of life with an ideal situation in which everyone lives to an advanced age, free of disease and disability.

Discriminatory pricing. The practice whereby a seller charges different prices to different buyers, with higher prices charged in markets where demand is less price-sensitive. In pharmaceutical markets, the practice of charging higher prices for on-patent medicines in higher income countries.

Effective availability. An aspect of access that takes into account whether barriers such as price, hours of operation, and culture make it difficult for patients to procure goods or services that are physically available.

Epidemiological transition. The transition from a disease burden dominated by infections to one consisting of non-communicable conditions, as is happening in some low- and most middle-income nations.

Essential medicines list. A list of medicines compiled by a national government (and by other organizations) to guide one or more arenas of decision making, such as procurement, insurance reimbursement, provider prescribing, or the regulation of the private pharmaceutical sector.

Exclusive relationships. A tactic used by a seller (often a wholesaler) in a particular market to deter new entrants and limit competition by contracting with manufacturers and retailers to only sell to, or only buy from, the company in question.

External benchmarking. The use of the rate of performance in another country or company as a basis for judging one's own performance.

Financial protection. A characteristic of a nation's system for financing and paying for health care services in general and pharmaceuticals in particular. It is the extent to which that system protects citizens from having to pay a significant fraction of their total income out of pocket for health-related goods and services.

First-in-class medicine. The first medicine of a particular kind or class that is targeted to treating a specific condition. This first entry often has many advantages in the marketplace because patients and doctors become familiar with it in the period before it has any imitators.

First mover advantage. The advantages (contacts, experience, reputation, etc.) gained by a competitor in a market who is the first to follow a specific strategy, develop a particular line of business, or introduce a new product. Such advantages typically flow to firms that introduce first-in-class medicines.

Generic drug. A medicine that has the same active ingredients and is pharmacologically equivalent to a *brand-name drug*, but which is not sold under that brand name. Instead, it is sold either under some form of the (generic) chemical name of its main active ingredient or under its own brand name as a *branded generic*.

Historic benchmarking. The use of a country's (or an organization's) own previous achievements for setting performance goals.

Ideal benchmarking. The use of an ambitious goal, or a goal based on an analysis of the best that is technologically feasible, as a standard for judging the performance of an organization or a country.

Internal benchmarking. Setting performance goals based on the achievements of the best-performing organizations or geographical subunits within a system.

Intersectoral action. The process of improving performance (in the pharmaceutical sector) through efforts outside the health arena, such as improving road access in rural areas.

Leakage. The disappearance of medicines from the public sector supply chain due to theft, either for resale or for personal or family use.

Markups. The difference between the seller's cost and the selling price, expressed as a percentage of the seller's cost. The total markup to the final customer depends on all the markups taken along the supply chain, by importers, wholesalers, retailers, and others.

Me-too drug. A medicine introduced a few years after a *first-in-class medicine*, typically while the latter is still on patent, and whose main active ingredient is chemically similar to—but not identical with—the originator compound.

Moral hazard. Situations in which individuals or institutions do not face the full consequences of their actions, and therefore have a tendency to act less carefully than they otherwise might act. For example, individuals whose health insurance subsidizes the costs of drugs have an incentive to overuse covered medicines.

Off-patent medicine. A medicine that is no longer protected by a nationally recognized patent because that patent has passed the end of its term.

On-patent medicine. A medicine that has been granted a period of exclusive access to the marketplace by a recognized national government and that is still within the time period of that protection.

Originator brand. Typically, the brand name version of a patented *first-in-class medicine* that has been extensively distributed and marketed in many countries (although that name may vary from country to country).

Parallel imports. A situation made possible by discriminatory pricing in which an on-patent medicine is bought in a market where the price is lower and then is imported into—and resold in—a higher-price market without the original manufacturer's and distributor's consent.

Patent evergreening. When the manufacturer of an on-patent medicine seeks to extend its patent protection by developing, patenting, and selling variations of the original compound, for example, by offering the compound in new dosage forms or in combination with other ingredients.

Performance monitoring. A system of recording and reporting a set of metrics and measurements that allows senior managers to determine whether different subunits in an organization are functioning effectively.

Pharmerging markets. Those national pharmaceutical markets large enough to be significant on a world-wide scale and growing in recent years at a rapid (double-digit) rate. One list (proposed by IMS Health) includes Brazil, China, India, Mexico, Russia, South Korea, and Turkey.

Physical availability. An aspect of access that considers whether a good or service is actually present (e.g., whether particular medicines are in stock) at a particular location. This does not, however, guarantee their *effective availability*.

Polypharmacy. Situations in which patients request, physicians prescribe, or retailers sell multiple medicines for treating a particular condition experienced by an individual patient.

Preferential purchasing. The policy of some national governments of maximizing their pharmaceutical purchasing from local manufacturers (as opposed to relying on imports) even if doing so adversely affects costs or quality.

Price erosion. The decrease in the price of an on-patent medicine over time as it experiences increasing competition from me-too drugs and then eventually goes off patent.

Price maker. A seller in a marketplace who has such limited competition (e.g., due to patent protection) that they can independently set the price of their own product without regard to other sellers' pricing decisions.

Price taker. A seller in a competitive market who has no choice but to sell their product at the prevailing market price.

Quality Adjusted Life Years (QALY). An index measuring the impact of policy changes on the health status of an individual or a population that combines the impact of such decisions on both the quality (morbidity) and quantity (mortality) of life.

Rational use. A situation in which patients use the least costly alternative medicine that is clinically appropriate, and do so in the correct doses and for an adequate period of time.

Reference pricing. A method for setting the prices that a social insurance system pays for medicines. Medicines are divided into therapeutic classes and the government sets a price (the reference price) for all compounds in that class based on the prices of all medicines in that class. Consumers then have to pay any difference between the reference price and the retail price out of pocket.

Rescue medicine. The practice of spending large sums of money on the treatment of acutely ill patients who face a significant risk of death.

Risk pooling. The fundamental mechanism used to create any insurance system, in which a group of individuals or organizations subject to a certain risk all make payments (called premiums) into a joint fund (the insurance pool). Those who suffer the adverse event are then allowed to draw a specified amount from the fund to cover their losses or expenses.

Risk protection. A situation in which individuals do not have to pay the costs of expensive medical treatment when they become seriously ill. This can be achieved either through an insurance mechanism or by the creation of an effective, tax-subsidized public health care system that provides treatment at low cost to patients.

Risk spreading. One way to characterize the effects of an insurance system. The costs of an adverse event are "spread" over—that is, shared among—all of the policy holders who contribute to a particular insurance fund. See also *risk pooling*.

Satisficing. A term coined by the economist Herbert Simon to describe many actual human decision processes, especially when obtaining information and making decisions are costly. In this model, individuals follow simplified plans of action (decision rules) and only readjust those rules when they yield unsatisfactory results. Once changes in these rules, and in their own behavior, yield outcomes that are "good enough" (satisfactory), people cease trying to improve the situation further.

Rule of rescue. The moral principle that justifies *rescue medicine*—namely, that human beings are obligated to do whatever they can to save another individual in imminent danger of death when it is within their capacity to do so.

Social franchising. A reform strategy that creates a set of relationships between a central organization (the brand owner) and a group of retail operators who provide certain specified goods or services in order to achieve certain social goals, such as improved access to quality medicines. The operators agree to use certain products and to follow certain business practices. In return they are granted a *franchise*—that is, the right to use the brand name and to advertise themselves as being part of the restricted distribution system.

Social marketing. The application of commercial advertising and marketing techniques to influence individuals to change their behavior in ways that advance social goals.

Stakeholder analysis. An approach to analyzing the political situation confronting policy makers that is based on identifying key individual and organizational actors, their political resources, their positions, and their degree of commitment to a particular issue.

Stock out. When a particular medicine is not physically available at a particular location.

Substandard medicines. Medicines that do not meet relevant quality standards and specifications.

Supply chain. The system of organizations, people, technology, activities, and information that is involved in moving pharmaceutical (and other) products from manufacturers to customers.

Technical efficiency. A situation in which goods and services are produced at minimum cost. In the public pharmaceutical sector, this means buying drugs at the lowest possible prices and keeping the operating costs of public supply chains as low as possible, consistent with meeting delivery objectives.

Tiered co-payment. An incentive system used by some health insurance companies in which payments by individuals toward the purchase of medicines varies according to the insurance plan's decisions about which products are most appropriate and cost-effective. Medicines whose use the insurance plan wants to discourage are assigned to higher tiers and thus require higher out-of-pocket payments from patients.

Transaction costs. The time and effort that buyers and sellers devote to reaching decisions and agreements, including the costs of identifying options, acquiring information, and engaging in negotiations.

Utility. A concept in classical economics, coined by the 19th-century British philosopher Jeremy Bentham, that refers to the subjective level of happiness, satisfaction, or well being experienced by individuals as a result of their decisions. Economists generally assume individuals act in ways designed to make their level of utility as high as possible.

Wastage rates. The proportion of the total inventory of a product (such as medicines) that is never delivered because it deteriorates in quality or becomes expired in storage.

Willingness to pay. The concept in economics that refers to the amount of money a person would hypothetically be willing to give up in order to receive a particular good or service.

INDEX

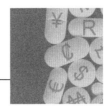

Page numbers followed by *f* or *t* refer to figures or tables, respectively.

essential medicines list compilation, 157–158

impact of pharmaceutical policy, 1

inappropriate spending on medications, 3

international comparison of originator brand and generic prices, 135–136, 135*f*

local monopolies, 134–135

in markets with limited competition, 29–30, 130, 134

mistake costs, 171

moral hazard in social insurance, 107

pharmaceutical share, 3–4

price control regulation, 178–179

price control strategies in private distribution chain, 132–133, 138

price elasticity of demand, 134

price markups, 130, 131, 132*t*, 133–134

price perceived as quality indicator, 187

in private health insurance systems, 108–109

quality regulation and, 171–172

reasons for high prices, 55–56

reference pricing, 137, 166

retailer motivation to sell higher-priced product, 133–134

significance of, for policy reform, 17–18

in social insurance systems, 107

subsidized pricing, 28–29, 137

taxation of medicines, 105

tiered co-payment system, 137, 139–140

transaction costs, 171

transport costs, 131

ultimate performance goals affected by, 57

very expensive medications and procedures, 64

see also financial aspects of pharmaceutical system; financial protection; financing, pharmaceutical system; payment system; spending

counterfeit drugs, 3, 6, 55, 112, 174, 175–176
  case study, 267–277

D

Daniels, N., 69

decentralization, 19, 32, 93, 152–154
  case study, 260–263

Department for International Development (U.K.), 13

diabetes, 2

diagnostic procedure
  assessment of local conditions in, 76, 78
  evidence-based approach, 78–79

example, 77–79

identifying supply- and demand-side problems, 82

intermediate performance goals in, 79–82, 87

need for explicit approach to, 75, 76

open-mindedness in, 87

in policy development process, 22–23, 75, 87–88, 197

transparency in, 76

tree diagram, 77–78, 77*f*, 197

value of diverse points of view in, 76

Disability Adjusted Life Years, 59–60

dispensing and sales of medications
  accreditation reform case study, 255–263, 265–266

accredited private sellers, 174–175

agency relationship in, 28

consumer ignorance and, 28

facility licensing, 176–177

gatekeeping role in, 177

government facilities for, 138–139

government regulation of, 6, 49–50

herbal and folk medicines, 97

influence on consumer health behavior, 189–190

informal sellers, 135, 188

local monopolies, 134–135

manifestations of poor clinical quality of pharmaceutical system, 80–81

motivation to sell higher-priced product, 133–134, 138

in pharmaceutical system, 5

prescribing authority combined with, 111, 190, 225–231, 232–233

private sector problems in, 55

problems with out-of-pocket financing, 111

product differentiation strategies, 30

professional licensing, 177

public health interventions at locations for, 188

quality oversight, 174–175

reform case study, 225–231, 232–233

retail markup, 133–134

social franchising operations, 155

Doha Declaration, 48

E

economic development, 66–67, 71
  epidemiological transition, 2, 108

efficiency of pharmaceutical system, 79–80, 83

egalitarian liberalism, 62–63, 68

epidemiological transition, 2, 108
equitable distribution of social goods
  classification of policy outcomes, 103
  cost-effective policy design and, 63
  distribution of problem outcomes in
      pharmaceutical system
      performance, 57–58
  egalitarian liberal philosophy, 62–63
  impact of pharmaceutical financing
      options, 103–115, 118
  international context, 67–69
  as measure of pharmaceutical system
      performance, 63
  pharmaceutical quality regulation and,
      171–172
  policy considerations, 63, 70–71
  political decision making, 91
  taxation of medicines and, 105
essential medicines list, 157–158, 201–209
ethical considerations
  case studies, 71
  cash incentives to improve health
      behavior, 192
  communitarian approach, 63–65, 66
  comparison of ethical approaches, 65t
  consequentialist view, 58
  decision making processes incorporating,
      69–70
  in economic development goals, 66–67
  essential medicines list, 157–158, 201–209
  global context of pharmaceutical systems
      and, 67–69
  in identifying and choosing reform
      priorities, 20, 21–22, 70–71
  liberal approaches in, 61–63, 66, 68
  misoprostol registration case study,
      211–220, 222–223
  in regulatory regime, 171
  in rescue medicine, 64, 201
  utilitarian approach to policy
      development, 58–61, 66
  value conflicts in reform, 12, 21
  see also equitable distribution of social
      goods

F

financial protection
  definition, 4, 15
  pharmaceutical sector problems related
      to, 57
  selection of pharmaceutical financing
      system for, 115–117
  social distribution of effects from
      lack of, 57

as target pharmaceutical policy reform,
      15–17
financing, pharmaceutical system
  case study, 119
  community financing systems, 109–110,
      117
  comparison of choices for, 115–117, 117t
  determinants of public sector financing,
      102
  distributional outcomes, 103–115
  donor assistance, 113–115
  in Flagship Framework, 24–25
  fraud and corruption in, 118
  health care system financing and,
      102–103
  market failures, 26–30
  marketization of public sector
      organizations, 149–151
  organizational revenue sources, 148
  out-of-pocket spending, 4, 55, 58–59,
      101–102, 107, 110–113, 118
  performance-based budgeting, 156
  price subsidies, 28–29
  pricing strategies, 44–46
  private health insurance systems,
      108–109
  registration process, 173
  significance of, in determining system
      performance, 101–102, 115, 118
  social insurance systems, 106–108, 117
  tax revenue for, 104–106, 117, 118
  see also cost of medications and health
      care; financial protection; spending
Flagship Framework, 16f, 32–33
  basic approach in, 7, 11–12
  control knobs, 24–26, 101, 123, 192
  diagnostic process in, 87
  economic development goals, 66–67
  ethical perspective, 60, 63, 65, 70
  keys to organizational performance
      improvement, 144–145
  problem identification in, 11–12
  purpose, 11, 196
  quality dimensions of pharmaceutical
      sector, 80–81
  ultimate goals, 13–16, 79
Flagship Program on Health Sector Reform,
      7
Food and Drug Administration (U.S), 38,
      97–98
foreign aid
  ethical perspectives, 67–69
  for medicine purchases, 103, 113–115
franchise model, 86

G

Gaal, P., 146
Gates Foundation, 174–175, 258
General Agreement on Tariffs and Trade, 47–48
generic drugs
  appeal of brand name products, 28
  availability in low-income countries, 135
  branded, 46, 168
  causes of inappropriate spending on drugs, 3
  competition with brand-name drugs, 46
  consumer perceptions of quality of, 136, 188
  consumer purchasing decisions, 182, 188
  industry trends, 46–47
  international comparison of prices, 135–136, 135*f*
  patent expiration trends, 40
  protection for first market entrant, 168
Germany, 19, 59–60
Ghana, 18, 58–59, 104, 106, 107, 117, 130, 133, 138, 153, 174, 301–313
Glaxo Wellcome, 42
Glenn, John, 127
Global Alliance for Vaccines and Immunizations, 103, 115
Global Fund to Fight AIDS, Tuberculosis and Malaria, 5, 103
Grassroot Soccer, 186
Grimes, D., 97–98
GSK, 42

H

Haiti, 191–192
Health Action International, 16
Hirschman, A., 146
HIV/AIDS, 48, 115, 125, 191–192
  case study of public health intervention, 289–299
hypertension, 2

I

implementation of policy
  consideration of, in policy development, 23–24, 198
  decentralization strategies, 154
  overcoming worker resistance to change, 160–161
  phased, 24
  pilot and demonstration projects, 24
  regulatory regime, 168, 170
  sources of government failure in, 31
India, 36, 37–38, 38*f*, 42, 50, 154, 155

Indonesia, 190, 191
infectious disease
  effectiveness of modern medicines, 1–2
  mortality, 2
  See also specific disease
injections, 3, 17, 55, 190
innovation, 43
insurance
  adverse selection, 108
  case study of Ghana's national health insurance scheme, 301–313
  pharmaceutical system in context of national policies on, 40, 41, 47, 50, 94, 101
  price sensitivity in markets with, 134
  private, 108–109
  reference pricing for medications, 137
  risk pooling in, 15–16, 106, 108
  social insurance systems, 106–108
  tiered co-payment system, 137
intellectual property rights
  international agreements, 47–49
  me-too drugs, 45
  patent expirations, 46
  patent ownership patterns, 39
  price competition and, 28–29
  protection for first market entrant with generic drug, 168
  purpose, 47
IQWiG, 59–60
Iran, 105

J

Japan, 50

K

Kenya, 115, 116*f*, 155
Korea, 92, 97, 111, 225–231, 232–233

L

labeling, 175–176
Lakin, J., 93
liberal philosophy of ethics, 61–63, 66
Liberia, 114, 114*t*, 151
libertarianism, 61–62, 66
local conditions
  community financing schemes, 109–110
  consideration of, in diagnosis process, 76, 78
  decentralization outcomes, 153, 154
  sensitivity to, in policy development, 7, 12, 23, 197
  use of local expertise in policy development, 12

logistics system reform case study, 235–246
low- and middle-income countries
  access to patent medicines in, 48
  availability of generic drugs in, 135
  capacity for medicine procurement,
    126–127, 129
  cost–performance trade-offs in
    pharmaceutical policy, 19
  drug research and development in, 38
  economic development goals, 66–67
  future of drug research and
    development, 40
  impact of pharmaceutical policy, 1
  international comparison of originator
    brand and generic prices, 135–136,
    135*f*
  mortality patterns and trends, 2, 2*t*
  pharmaceutical consumption, 3–4, 36–37,
    36*f*, 37*f*
  pharmaceutical financing options,
    115–118
  pharmaceutical industry marketing in,
    44
  pharmaceutical manufacturing in, 41
  pharmaceutical production, 36
  pharmaceutical sector workers, 145–146
  pharmaceutical trade patterns, 41–42, 41*t*
  private sector pharmaceutical spending,
    4, 55
  scope of government involvement in
    pharmaceutical system, 6, 8
  tax policies and collection, 104–105
  treatment-seeking behaviors in, 187–188

M

malaria, 3, 111–112, 137, 189, 263
Management Sciences for Health, 175,
  258–263
manufacturing and distribution
  case study of logistics reform, 235–246
  compulsory licensing of patent
    medications, 48–49
  economies of scale, 154
  evolution of global production capacity,
    41
  global market, 35–36, 37–38, 38*f*
  government role, 6
  inducements to sellers, 111, 133
  industrial policy for pharmaceutical
    system, 8
  in pharmaceutical system, 5
  pricing strategies, 44–46
  quality regulation, 173
  resistance to regulation, 166

transport costs, 131, 151–152
  see also supply chains, pharmaceutical
market failures, 26–30, 32, 56, 165, 170
marketing of drugs
  consolidation of research and
    development companies, 43
  pricing strategies, 44–46
  response to patent expiration, 46
  social marketing strategies, 184–185
marketization of public sector
  organizations, 149–151
Mectizan Donation Program, 186–187
media campaigns, 186
Medicare, 107
Medicines Transparency Alliance, 13, 23
Mexico, 92–93, 152, 155
Mill, John Stuart, 58
misoprostol, 64, 211–220, 222–223
misuse of drugs
  case study of campaign to prevent,
    279–283, 285–287
  causes, 3, 55
  challenges in preventing, 181
  drug purchases without medical
    consultation, 188
  incomplete antibiotic regimen, 191
  low prices leading to, 187
  observed compliance requirements, 177
  out-of-pocket spending and, 111, 112
  payment system incentives leading to, 122
  price subsidies and, 28, 137
  regulatory intervention to prevent, 176–177
  societal costs, 3, 29, 60
  ultimate performance goals affected by, 57
  utilitarian ethics approaches to policy
    making and, 60
monitoring and evaluation of policy reform
  effects
  evaluating regulatory outcomes, 166
  government contract oversight, 152
  intermediate process and output
    measures, 83–84
  in reform cycle, 24, 198
  selection of outcome measures, 20
monopolies, 29, 44–45, 134–135, 178
moral hazard, 107
mortality
  effect of public health interventions, 1–2
  projections, 2
  sources of, 2, 2*t*
Mozambique, 145–146
multidrug-resistance, 3, 29, 60, 191
  case study of campaign to prevent,
    279–283, 285–287

persuasion of stakeholders in reform
    process
  consumer perceptions, 136
  Flagship Framework, 24–25
Peru, 279–283, 285–287
pharmaceutical system
  evolution, 40*f*
  global market characteristics, 35–42
  government failure, 30–32
  industrial policy, 8
  performance assessment, 7–8, 11–12
  scope of government involvement, 6, 47
  scope of stakeholder interests in, 195–196
  subsystems, 5, 5*f*
  see also organizational structure of
      pharmaceutical system;
      performance of pharmaceutical
      system
pharmacies. *see* dispensing and sales of
    medications
pharmerging markets, 36, 44
Philippines, 96
pilot projects, 24
placebo effect, 189
policy development, generally
  application of ethical considerations in,
      69–70
  choice of decision making venue, 93
  consequentialist approach to ethics in, 58
  diagnostic process in, 75, 87–88
  economic development goals, 66–67
  equity considerations, 63
  forms of government failure in, 30–31
  liberal approaches to ethics in, 61–63
  managing participation in, 87
  political context, 20, 86–87, 89–91
  process, 85–87
  in reform cycle, 23
  resources for, 85–86
  self-interest in, 90–91
  utilitarian approaches to ethics in, 58–61
  see also reform of pharmaceutical policy
political functioning
  advantages of democratic process in
      policy formulation, 21, 90
  case studies of pharmaceutical reform,
      96–98
  challenges to reform, 192
  choice of decision making venue, 93
  coalition building, 93–94
  consideration of, in policy development,
      23, 197
  definition, 89–90
  electoral politics, 20, 93

forms of government failure in policy
    reform, 31–32
  governance structure and, 92–93
  in identifying and choosing reform
      priorities, 20–22, 31
  international interests, 96
  logrolling, 94
  in performance of public sector
      employees, 146–147, 148
  pharmaceutical policy reform to improve
      citizen satisfaction, 14–15
  power adjustments, 95
  in process of policy making, 20, 86–87,
      89–91, 98
  in reference pricing system for
      medications, 137
  stakeholder analysis, 91–93, 95
  strategy development to promote reform,
      93–95
  support for regulatory regime, 169
  transparency in governance, 124
  uses of scientific evidence, 97–98
population health
  equity considerations in policy goals, 63,
      70
  measurement of, 59–61
  pharmaceutical sector problems related
      to, 57
  significance of pharmaceutical policy, 1–2
  as target pharmaceutical policy reform,
      13–14
prescribing practices
  authority to prescribe and sell drugs, 111,
      190, 225–231, 232–233
  causes of inappropriate spending on
      drugs, 3
  government regulation, 50
  influence on consumer health behaviors,
      189–190
  reform case study, 225–231, 232–233
President's Emergency Plan for AIDS
    Relief, 103
price subsidies, 28–29, 105, 137
  to influence health behaviors, 186–187
  negative outcomes, 28–29, 112, 137
  trends, 105
procurement
  case study, 238–239, 247–253
  contracting out, 127, 139
  corruption risk, 123, 124–125, 125, 127–128
  decentralization, 19
  formal procedures, 124–125
  fragmentation of public sector systems
      for, 125

government function, 6
international medicine brokerage
    business, 126
in pharmaceutical system, 5
private sector systems for, 125
quality testing in, 128–129
technical demands, 126–127
transparency in, 127–128
value of trusted relationships in, 125–126
Promoting the Quality of Medicines, 128
public health efforts
    case study of anti-HIV campaign,
        289–299
    challenges in changing health behaviors,
        181
    community-based, 191–192
    determinants of financing, 102
    effectiveness, 1–2
    logistics system reform case study,
        235–246
    pharmaceutical company involvement,
        103
    pharmaceutical financing strategies,
        103–115
    in private sector drug shops, 188
    strategies for improving health
        behaviors, 181
public opinion and understanding
    access to medications, 4–5
    advantages of democratic process in
        policy formulation, 21
    citizen satisfaction as goal of
        pharmaceutical policy reform, 14–15,
        57, 58–59, 171
    reframing policy proposals to gain
        support, 95
    social franchise pharmaceutical
        operations, 155
    social marketing to influence health
        behaviors, 184–187
    support for regulatory regime, 169–170
    value of public education about
        pharmaceutical uses and choices, 71
    see also consumers

Q
Quality Adjusted Life Years, 14, 59–60
quality of products and services
    benchmarking approach to managing,
        53–54
    clinical aspects, 80
    consumer capacity to evaluate, 170
    consumer perception of generic drugs,
        136

consumer sensitivity to, 81, 170
folk and traditional remedies, 171, 172
government role, 6
intermediate performance goals, 79,
    80–81
manufacturing oversight, 173
nonclinical aspects, 80–81
packaging and, 188
price perceived as quality indicator, 187
process and output measures, 83
regulation of, 170–176
resources for monitoring, 166
retail market oversight, 174–175
social distribution of problems in, 58
strategic planning to improve, 81
systems approach to process
    improvement, 84–85
testing, 128–129, 174
ultimate performance goals affected by
    problems in, 57

R
rapid diagnostic tests, 112, 189
reference pricing, 137, 139–140, 166
reform of pharmaceutical policy
    benchmarking approach to goal setting,
        53–54
    broader policy context, 50
    broader policy context of, 66–67
    challenges in, 54–55, 196
    coalition building for, 93–94
    coherency in, 6
    cost considerations in goal setting, 17–19
    cycle of, 22–24, 22f
    drawing from experiences of similar
        countries for, 85–86
    evidence-based approach, 26, 78–79
    forms of government failure in, 30–32
    global context, 67–69
    goal setting in, 75, 196–197
    goals for, 5, 7, 13, 17, 195–196
    implementation considerations, 23–24,
        198
    implications of global market for, 35, 42,
        50
    to improve citizen satisfaction, 14–15, 57,
        58–59, 171
    to improve population health, 13–14
    interactions among tools for, 192
    intermediate performance goals, 79–82
    international interests opposed to, 96
    limitations of expert advice, 21, 23
    marketization of public sector
        organizations, 149–151

SmithKline Beacham, 42
social franchising, 154–155, 179
social insurance systems, 106–108, 107f, 117, 138
social marketing, 184–187, 189
South Africa, 92–93, 178, 289–299
spending
  drug research and development, 38–40, 39t
  ethical allocation of public resources, 70–71
  global market characteristics, 36–37, 36f, 37f
  income elasticity of demand, 105
  per capita, 4
  pharmaceutical expenditures, 3–4, 4t
  private sector, in low-income countries, 4, 55
  rescue medicine, 70
  research and development, 38–39
  willingness to pay as measure of utility, 59
  see also cost of medications and health care; financing, pharmaceutical system; out-of-pocket spending; payment system
Sri Lanka, 96, 211–220, 222–223
statin drugs, 2
Strategies for Enhancing Access to Medicines, 174–175, 258–260
subsidized prices, 28–29
sulfadoxinepyrimethamine, 3
supply chains, pharmaceutical
  case study, 235–246
  decentralization, 153
  facility licensing, 176–177
  government role, 6, 49–50
  in pharmaceutical system, 5
  price control strategies in private distribution chain, 132–133
  price markups, 130, 131, 132t, 133–134
  problems in public sector performance, 56
  weak link intervention, 159–160
  wholesale market, 129–133
  see also dispensing and sales of medications; manufacturing and distribution

T

Taiwan, China, 111, 190
Tanzania, 179, 255–263, 265–266
tax policy, 56, 102, 104–106, 117, 118
therapeutically equivalent drugs, 166
trade, international
  global markets, 37–38, 38f

international system of patent protection, 47–48
  in pharmaceutical system, 5
  safety concerns, 38
  top pharmaceutical importing countries, 41–42, 41t
trade policy, 8
  ethical perspectives, 68
  purpose of licensing regulation, 49
  tax revenue from, to finance pharmaceutical system, 104
transparency
  for corruption prevention, 124
  in diagnostic procedure, 76
  in essential medicines list compilation, 158
  in policy making processes, 69–70
  in procurement, 127–128
  in registration process, 173
transport costs, 131, 151–152
treatment-seeking behavior, 187–189
TRIPS, 48–49
tuberculosis, 3, 177

U

Uganda, 41–42, 133
Ukraine, 153
United Kingdom, 59
United States, 38–39, 97–98, 107, 128
U.S. Pharmacopeia, 128, 174
utilitarian ethics, 58–61, 66

V

vaccines and immunizations, 8
value-added tax, 104, 105, 106
value conflicts
  among health workers, 145–146
  in policy formulation, 12–13
value conflicts in policy formulation, 21

W

Wagner, A., 115
workforce, health care
  compensation, 146
  contract employees in public sector, 157
  decentralization outcomes, 154
  as determinant of pharmaceutical sector performance, 144–145, 161
  in implementation of process improvement, 159
  influence of political leadership on performance of, 146–147, 148
  managers, 145, 147–149
  in marketization of public sector organizations, 150, 151

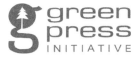